Pediatric Endocrinology

THE REQUISITES IN PEDIATRICS

SERIES EDITOR **Louis M. Bell**, M.D.
Patrick S. Pasquariello, Jr. Chair in General
    Pediatrics
Professor of Pediatrics
University of Pennsylvania School of Medicine
Chief, Division of General Pediatrics
Attending Physician, General Pediatrics and Infectious
    Diseases
The Children's Hospital of Philadelphia
Philadelphia, Pennsylvania

OTHER VOLUMES IN
**THE REQUISITES IN PEDIATRICS
SERIES**

Orthopaedics and Sports Medicine

COMING SOON IN
**THE REQUISITES IN PEDIATRICS
SERIES**

Nephrology and Urology

Toxicology

Pulmonology

Cardiology

Infectious Diseases

Hematology and Oncology

Gastroenterology

Pediatric Endocrinology

THE REQUISITES IN PEDIATRICS

Thomas Moshang, Jr., M.D.
Professor of Pediatrics, Emeritus
University of Pennsylvania School of Medicine
Senior Endocrinologist
Division of Pediatric Endocrinology
The Children's Hospital of Philadelphia
Philadelphia, Pennsylvania

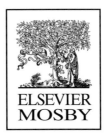

ELSEVIER
MOSBY

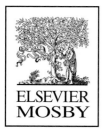

ELSEVIER
MOSBY

THE REQUISITES
THE REQUISITES
THE REQUISITES
THE REQUISITES
THE REQUISITES

THE REQUISITES is a proprietary trademark
of Mosby, Inc.

11830 Westline Industrial Drive
St. Louis, Missouri 63146

PEDIATRIC ENDOCRINOLOGY: THE REQUISITES
IN PEDIATRICS   ISBN 0-323-01825-4
Copyright © 2005 Mosby, Inc.

Notice

Pediatrics is an ever-changing field. Standard safety precautions must be followed,
but as new research and clinical experience broaden our knowledge, changes in
treatment and drug therapy may become necessary or appropriate. Readers are
advised to check the most current product information provided by the
manufacturer of each drug to be administered to verify the recommended dose,
the method and duration of administration, and contraindications. It is the
responsibility of the treating physician, relying on experience and knowledge of
the patient, to determine dosages and the best treatment for each individual
patient. Neither the Publisher nor the editor assumes any liability for any injury
and/or damage to persons or property arising from this publication.

The Publisher

First Edition 2005.

Library of Congress Cataloging-in-Publication Data

Pediatric endocrinology: the requisites in pediatrics / [edited by] Thomas Moshang.
— 1st ed.
   p.   cm. — (The requisites in pediatrics series)
      ISBN 0-323-01825-4
   1. Pediatric endocrinology. I. Moshang, Thomas. II. Series.
      [DNLM: 1. Endocrine Diseases—Child. WS 330 P3718 2004]
   RJ418.P346 2004
   618.92′4–dc22

                                                    2004040241

Acquisitions Editor: Hilarie Surrena
Developmental Editor: Kimberley Cox
Project Manager: Jeff Gunning

Printed in the United States of America.

Last digit is the print number: 9   8   7   6   5   4   3   2   1

To Mary Anne and my children, Beth, Tom, Peter, and Ali.

And also to my mentors, Al Bongiovanni and Walter Eberlein,
as well as all the Residents and Fellows who have taught me so much.

Contributors

Craig A. Alter, M.D.
Clinical Associate Professor, Department of Pediatrics, University of Pennsylvania School of Medicine; Pediatric Endocrinologist, The Children's Hospital of Philadelphia, Philadelphia, Pennsylvania

Neil Caplin, M.B.B.S., FRACP
Assistant Professor, Department of Pediatrics, University of Washington School of Medicine; Attending Physician, Division of Endocrinology, Children's Hospital and Regional Medical Center, Seattle, Washington

Diva D. De León, M.D.
Assistant Professor, Department of Pediatrics, University of Pennsylvania School of Medicine; Attending Physician, Division of Pediatric Endocrinology, The Children's Hospital of Philadelphia, Philadelphia, Pennsylvania

Robert J. Ferry, Jr., M.D.
Assistant Professor of Pediatrics and Cellular and Structural Biology, University of Texas Medical School at San Antonio; Research and Training Director, Division of Pediatric Endocrinology and Diabetes, Department of Pediatrics, University of Texas Health Science Center at San Antonio; Attending Physician, Department of Pediatrics, Christus-Santa Rosa Children's Hospital, and Department of Medicine, South Texas Veterans Administration Health Care System; Texas Medical Ranger, Alamo Medical Response Group, Medical Reserve Corps, Texas State Army Guard, San Antonio, Texas

Adda Grimberg, M.D.
Assistant Professor, Department of Pediatrics, University of Pennsylvania School of Medicine; Attending Physician, Division of Pediatric Endocrinology, The Children's Hospital of Philadelphia, Philadelphia, Pennsylvania

Daniel E. Hale, M.D.
Professor of Medicine, University of Texas Medical School at San Antonio; Chief, Division of Endocrinology and Diabetes, Department of Pediatrics, University of Texas Health Science Center at San Antonio; Senior Attending Physician, Department of Pediatrics, Christus-Santa Rosa Children's Hospital, and Senior Physician, Department of Pediatrics, University Health System; Director, The Children's Center, Texas Diabetes Institute, San Antonio, Texas

Maria J. Henwood, D.O.
Assistant Professor, Department of Pediatrics, The Ohio State University College of Medicine and Public Health; Attending Physician, Division of Endocrinology and Diabetes, Columbus Children's Hospital, Columbus, Ohio

Saraswati Kache, M.D.
Clinical Instructor, Department of Pediatrics, Stanford University School of Medicine; Attending Pediatric Intensivist, Lucille Packard Children's Hospital, Stanford, California

Lorraine E. Levitt Katz, M.D.
Assistant Professor, Department of Pediatrics, University of Pennsylvania School of Medicine; Attending Physician, Division of Endocrinology, and Diabetes, The Children's Hospital of Philadelphia, Philadelphia, Pennsylvania

Howard E. Kulin, M.D.
Professor of Pediatrics, Emeritus, Department of Pediatrics, Pennsylvania State College of Medicine, Hershey, Pennsylvania

Mary M. Lee, M.D.
Associate Professor, Department of Pediatrics, University of Massachusetts School of Medicine; Director, Division of Pediatric Endocrinology and Diabetes, UMass Memorial Health Care, Worcester, Massachusetts

Peter A. Lee, M.D., Ph.D.
Professor, Department of Pediatrics, Pennsylvania State College of Medicine; Attending Physicians and Chief, Division of Pediatric Endocrinology and Metabolism, Milton S. Hershey Medical Center, Hershey, Pennsylvania

Sheela Magge, M.D.
Fellow, Instructor in Pediatrics, University of Pennsylvania School of Medicine; Instructor, Division of Pediatric Endocrinology, Department of Pediatrics, The Children's Hospital of Philadelphia, Philadelphia, Pennsylvania

Madhusmita Misra, M.D.
Instructor in Pediatrics, Harvard Medical School; Assistant in Pediatrics and Assistant in Biology, Massachusetts General Hospital, Boston, Massachusetts

Thomas Moshang, Jr., M.D.
Professor of Pediatrics, Emeritus, University of Pennsylvania School of Medicine; Senior Endocrinologist, The Children's Hospital of Philadelphia, Philadelphia, Pennsylvania

Wilma C. Rossi, M.D.
Clinical Associate Professor, Department of Pediatrics, University of Pennsylvania School of Medicine; Pediatric Endocrinologist, The Children's Hospital of Philadelphia, Philadelphia, Pennsylvania

Paul S. Thornton, M.B., B.Ch., MRCPI
Medical Director, Department of Endocrinology and Diabetes, Cook Children's Medical Center, Fort Worth, Texas

Stuart A. Weinzimer, M.D.
Assistant Professor, Department of Pediatrics, Yale University School of Medicine; Attending Physician, Yale-New Haven Medical Center, New Haven, Connecticut

Weizhen Xu, M.D.
Assistant Professor, University of Medicine & Dentistry of New Jersey Robert Wood Johnson Medical School; Physician, The Cooper Health System, Camden, New Jersey

Foreword

What are the essential elements of pediatric endocrinology? How can this fascinating (and challenging) specialty, which involves recognizing and treating disorders of carbohydrate metabolism, growth, and thyroid function vital to health and life, be presented in an accessible manner? Will this book help those of us who are not endocrinologists in diagnosis, early treatment, and the decision to refer to our subspecialty colleagues if necessary?

Fortunately, Thomas Moshang, in *Pediatric Endocrinology: The Requisites in Pediatrics*, has met the challenge posed in these questions with a clear, concise, and well-organized work.

The book is divided into seven sections: Carbohydrate Disorders, Sexual Development, Growth, Thyroid, Adrenal Gland, Calcium, Phosphorus, and Bone and Vasopressin and Disorders of Fluids and Electrolytes. The most important aspects of each of these topics are the subjects of the chapters in that section. For example, Section 6 includes chapters on calcium regulation and hypocalcemic disorders, hypercalcemic disorders, and osteoporosis. Embryology, anatomy, and normal physiology are discussed in each of the sections where appropriate. Normal values and interpretation of abnormal values are outlined as well.

As an example of the consistent relevance of the book's content, Section 1, on carbohydrate disorders, includes an outstanding chapter on type 2 diabetes mellitus in children and adolescents, by Daniel E. Hale and Stuart A. Weinzimer. These authors point out that the

increasing incidence of type 2 diabetes mellitus is now considered a pediatric problem. The rising incidence is a "harbinger of an epidemic" of childhood obesity. I fear that it will be extremely important for primary care providers to understand the pathophysiology and feel comfortable with the treatment options for this disease for years to come.

This second installment of **The Requisites in Pediatrics** fulfills the expectation for this series, which is to present information on the most common (and emerging) diseases in pediatrics and the required medical knowledge for students, nurse practitioners, resident physicians, and primary care physicians.

I would like to thank Dr. Moshang and the contributors to this book for offering a useful, updated discussion of the most important topics in pediatric endocrinology. We hope you enjoy this second volume in the **Requisites in Pediatrics** series.

Louis M. Bell, M.D.
Patrick S. Pasquariello, Jr. Chair in General Pediatrics
Professor of Pediatrics
University of Pennsylvania School of Medicine
Chief, Division of General Pediatrics
Attending Physician, General Pediatrics and Infectious Diseases
The Children's Hospital of Philadelphia
Philadelphia, Pennsylvania

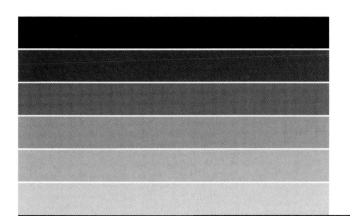

Preface

Information and new knowledge pertaining to pediatric endocrinology, as in all of medical science, are expanding at an exponential rate. In fact, new hormones are being discovered to the degree where it is not yet clear how these hormones (such as leptin, resistin, adiponectin, and gherelin) are related to clinical disease. We know that many clinical disorders can be confirmed by analyzing specific genes, yet many of these gene studies are not available except in research laboratories. Specific hormones can be measured precisely in microunits, especially important in evaluating developmental changes in children. Yet despite all of the new technology, the genetic advances, and relevant discoveries, there is still a need for understanding the basic paradigms of clinical medicine.

In medicine, the term *requisites* is interpreted as the basic knowledge that is necessary for practice or board review. This book was designed to be consistent with the premise of the other volumes in the Requisites in Pediatrics series—that there should be a series of books that provide required basic information important for pediatric residents, pediatricians, primary care physicians and nurse practitioners caring for children. In that context, this volume of the Requisites series provides a basic tutorial by each of the various authors in areas of pediatric endocrinology that are important for the care of children. Each chapter is to be read as if a trainee wishes to obtain basic information in a certain area in a tutorial fashion, not as a reference text or source book. Although many of the authors are involved in research, all are clinicians with a strong focus on pediatric endocrine care, and they wrote their chapters with clinicians in mind.

It is important to include discussion of disorders not previously thought to be within the purview of pediatric endocrinology, such as type 2 diabetes mellitus and osteoporosis. Type 2 diabetes mellitus, previously identified as "adult-onset diabetes mellitus," is increasing in our adolescent patients in epidemic proportions. The chapter written by Daniel Hale and Stuart Weinzimer addresses not only the diagnosis and management of type 2 diabetes mellitus in adolescents but also some of the issues of increasing obesity in children. The technology and information for assessing bone density and osteoporosis are focused on the elderly, thereby making assessment and therapy in children difficult, as well as limiting management options, because of the lack of data in the pediatric population. In fact, even normative data for bone density based on age (because onset of puberty is variable in the normal adolescent population) may be inaccurate. These issues are still to be resolved, but clinicians caring for children with potential problems of bone formation should be aware of the many different issues as addressed in the section on osteoporosis.

I appreciate the difficulty faced by academic clinicians writing chapters focused on requisite information: It is always easier to be exhaustively inclusive for fear of omissions. As the editor, I have the same concern that in selecting the requisite clinical issues important in pediatric endocrinology for clinicians, medical students, and residents, I have omitted important topics. Nevertheless, having made my choices, I wish to thank the various contributors for their efforts. Any important omissions are my responsibility, not that of the authors.

Thomas Moshang, Jr., M.D.

Contents

Color Plate section starts on page xv.

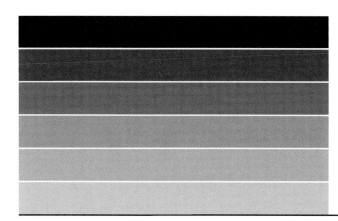

Color Plates

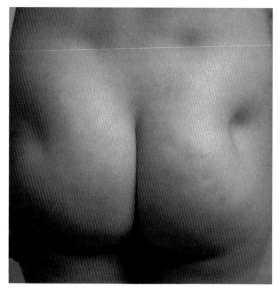

Plate 1-1 Lipoatrophy of the buttocks secondary to insulin injections. This sequela is less common today with the use of human insulin. (From Wales JKH, Wit JM, Rogol AD: Pediatric Endocrinology and Growth, 2nd ed, Philadelphia, 2003, Saunders.)

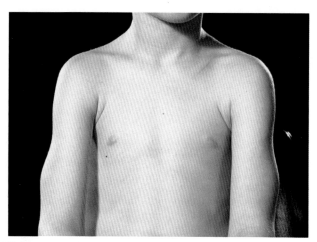

Plate 1-2 Lipohypertrophy in the upper arms due to repeated injections of insulin in the same area. (From Wales JKH, Wit JM, Rogol AD: Pediatric Endocrinology and Growth, 2nd ed, Philadelphia, 2003, Saunders.)

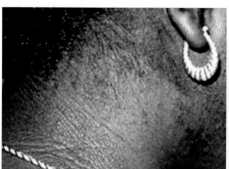 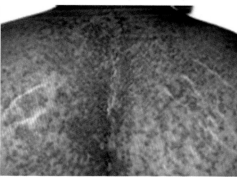

Plate 2-1 Severe acanthosis nigricans associated with insulin resistance. The patient was a 15-year-old African-American girl with type 2 diabetes mellitus and obesity. Note the thickened, vellous black areas on back and neck.

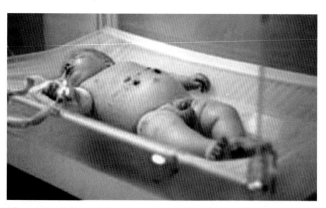

Plate 3-1 Infants with severe hyperinsulinemic hypoglycemia are born very large for date, appearing extremely large generally.

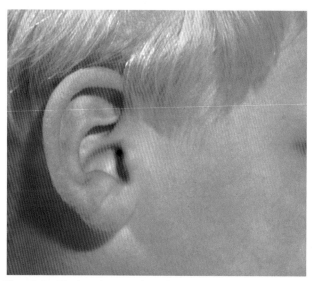

Plate 3-2 The large hyperinsulemic hypoglycemic infant must be distinguished from the infant with Beckwith-Wiedemann syndrome, who will have gigantism as well as other features including a large tongue and ear creases, as seen here. (From Wales JKH, Wit JM, Rogol AD: Pediatric Endocrinology and Growth, 2nd ed, Philadelphia, 2003, Saunders.)

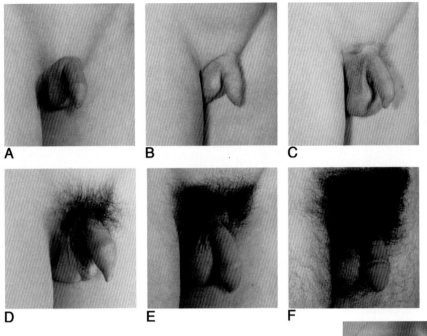

Plate 4-1 Normal male penile and pubic hair development. **A**, Tanner 1 pubic hair and testicular and penile development. **B**, Early testicular development—Tanner 2 genital development but still Tanner 1 pubic hair. **C**, Tanner 2 pubic hair and Tanner 3 genital development. **D**, Tanner 3 pubic hair and genital development. **E**, Tanner 4 for both pubic hair and genital development. **F**, Tanner 5. (From Wales JKH, Wit JM, Rogol AD: Pediatric Endocrinology and Growth, 2nd ed, Philadelphia, 2003, Saunders.)

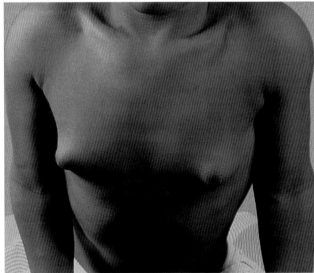

Plate 4-3 Adolescent male gynecomastia. From 25% to 50% of adolescent males, especially heavy boys, will develop a mild degree of gynecomastia. Occasionally, as in this patient, the degree of gynecomastia may be severe enough to cause psychological problems, and surgical mammoplasty will be necessary. (From Wales JKH, Wit JM, Rogol AD: Pediatric Endocrinology and Growth, 2nd ed, Philadelphia, 2003, Saunders.)

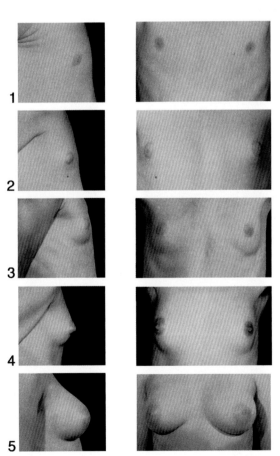

Plate 4-2 Normal female breast development, from Tanner stage 1 (prepubertal) to Tanner stage 5 (adult breast). (From Wales JKH, Wit JM, Rogol AD: Pediatric Endocrinology and Growth, 2nd ed, Philadelphia, 2003, Saunders.)

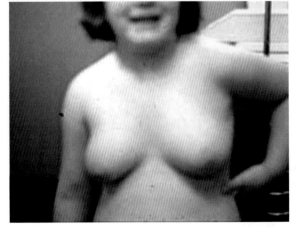

Plate 5-1 Precocious puberty. As seen in this 5-year-old patient with central precocious puberty, excessive weight is a not uncommon problem in girls with early puberty.

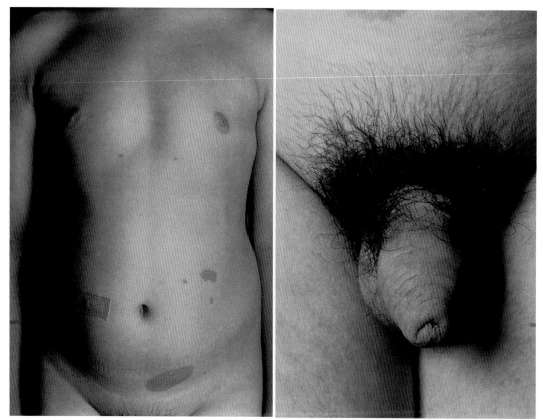

Plate 5-2   Male precocious puberty. Precocious puberty is more likely in males than in females to be secondary to a central nervous system lesion. These two photographs demonstrate multiple café-au-lait spots with regular smooth borders (the adhesive bandage covers an injection site) and the changes characteristic of central precocious puberty in a boy with neurofibromatosis, who was found to have an optic glioma. (From Wales JKH, Wit JM, Rogol AD: Pediatric Endocrinology and Growth, 2nd ed, Philadelphia, 2003, Saunders.)

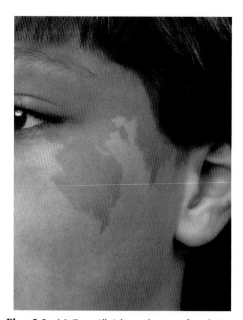

Plate 5-3   McCune-Albright syndrome: café-au-lait macule. The triad in McCune-Albright syndrome consists of precocious puberty, polyostotic fibrous dysplasia, and café-au-lait macules. The macules are large, with irregular borders, and often are asymmetrical in location, as in this patient. This syndrome is due to an abnormally activated G protein mutation in the cyclic adenosine monophosphate (cAMP) system. (From Wales JKH, Wit JM, Rogol AD: Pediatric Endocrinology and Growth, 2nd ed, Philadelphia, 2003, Saunders.)

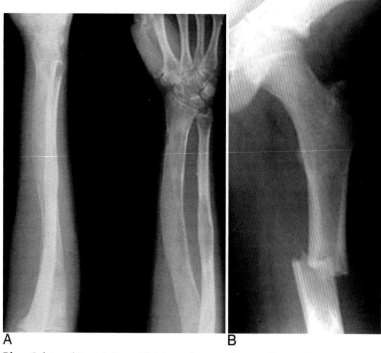

Plate 5-4 A and **B**   McCune-Albright syndrome: polyostotic fibrous dysplasia. These radiographs demonstrate the large cystic lesions in bone (especially in the radius) seen in this syndrome. In **B,** a spontaneous fracture through one of the cystic lesions in the femur can be seen.

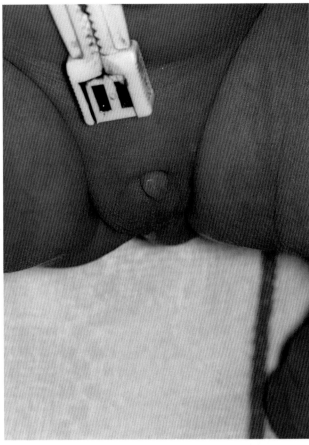

Plate 6-1 Microphallus. In this newborn boy, microphallus and cryptorchidism were secondary to panhypopituitarism. Microphallus is most frequently associated with gonadotropin deficiency. (From Wales JKH, Wit JM, Rogol AD: Pediatric Endocrinology and Growth, 2nd ed, Philadelphia, 2003, Saunders.)

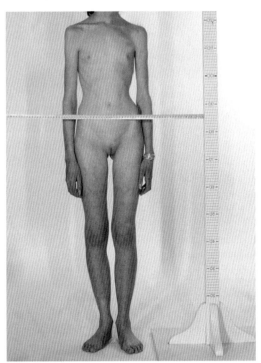

Plate 6-2 Delayed sexual development may be due to anorexia nervosa, as in this female patient. (From Wales JKH, Wit JM, Rogol AD: Pediatric Endocrinology and Growth, 2nd ed, Philadelphia, 2003, Saunders.)

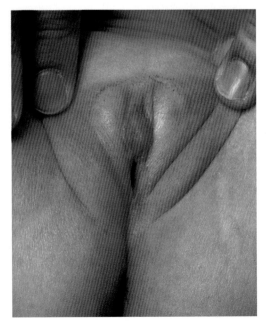

Plate 7-1 Ambiguous genitalia in a female infant. Virilization of the genitals, with an enlarged clitoris and fusion of the labia, can be seen. The underlying disorder was the 21-hydroxylase deficiency form of congenital adrenal hyperplasia. (From Wales JKH, Wit JM, Rogol AD: Pediatric Endocrinology and Growth, 2nd ed, Philadelphia, 2003, Saunders.)

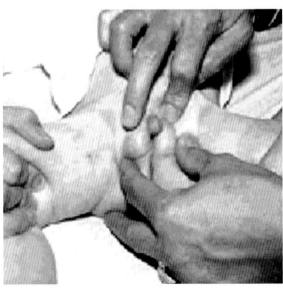

Plate 7-2 Ambiguous genitalia in a male infant. A small phallus, (with hypospadias) and incomplete fusion of scrotum, with both testes descended, can be seen. The underlying disorder was 3β-hydroxysteroid dehydrogenase deficiency.

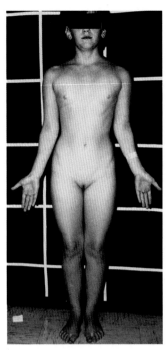

Plate 8-1 Turner syndrome: body habitus and other features. This 15-year-old patient demonstrates some of the classic features of Turner syndrome, including short stature, sexual infantilism, triangular facies, cubitus valgus (increased carrying angle of upper extremities), broad chest, and hypoplastic nipples. Many children with Turner syndrome will have only short stature, however, and need not have the phenotypic features pictured here. (From Wales JKH, Wit JM, Rogol AD: Pediatric Endocrinology and Growth, 2nd ed, Philadelphia, 2003, Saunders.)

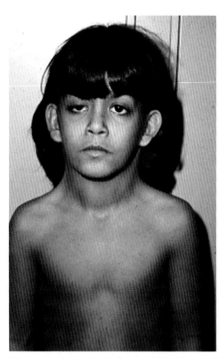

Plate 8-2 Turner syndrome: facial features. This 13-year-old patient demonstrates the classic triangular facies with ptosis of the eyelids. She has sexual infantilism and short stature.

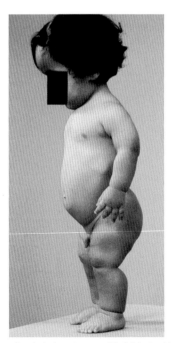

Plate 8-3 Achondroplasia in a 2-year-old child. At this age, the achondroplasia is represented by the short limbs, especially the proximal limbs. There is already a suggestion of lordosis; note also the disproportionately large head. (From Wales JKH, Wit JM, Rogol AD: Pediatric Endocrinology and Growth, 2nd ed, Philadelphia, 2003, Saunders.)

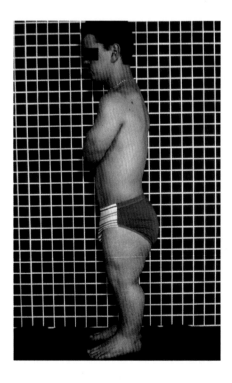

Plate 8-4 Severe hypochondroplasia in a young adult (note the short limbs, especially the proximal limbs). Hypochondroplasia may be very mild and demonstrated only by careful measurements of extremities. The shortened limbs distinguish these patients from those with growth hormone deficiency, who are normally proportioned. As well, patients with hypochondroplasia have a normal bone age, whereas growth hormone–deficient patients have delayed skeletal maturation. (From Wales JKH, Wit JM, Rogol AD: Pediatric Endocrinology and Growth, 2nd ed, Philadelphia, 2003, Saunders.)

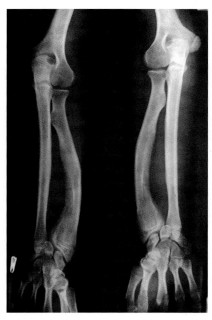

Plate 8-5 Leri-Weil syndrome. This short stature syndrome is due to a mutation or deletion of the *SHOX* gene and is characterized by short limbs, especially the distal limbs. There is often a dyschondrosteosis of the radius, with a Madelung deformity, as illustrated in this radiograph. (From Wales JKH, Wit JM, Rogol AD: Pediatric Endocrinology and Growth, 2nd ed, Philadelphia, 2003, Saunders.)

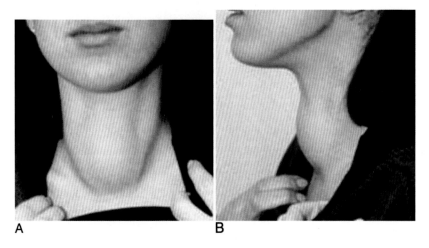

Plate 9-1 A and **B** Goiter. The patient was a 15-year-old girl with a large cystic goiter.

A   B

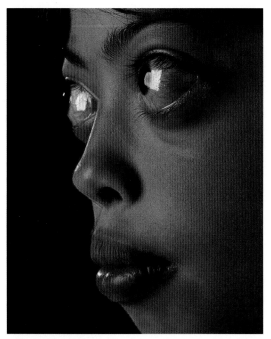

Plate 9-2 Exophthalmos in a young woman with Graves disease. (From Wales JKH, Wit JM, Rogol AD: Pediatric Endocrinology and Growth, 2nd ed, Philadelphia, 2003, Saunders.)

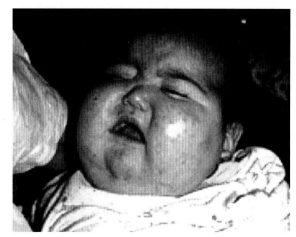

Plate 10-1 Cushing syndrome in an infant due to an adrenal carcinoma. At 3 months of age, the child shows the typical "moon facies" with acne and plethoric cheeks.

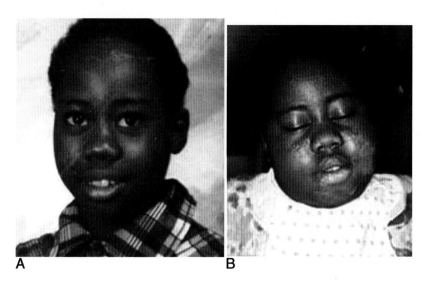

A   B

Plate 10-2 A and **B** Cushing syndrome in childhood secondary to an adrenal carcinoma. **A,** The patient's appearance in a school photograph 1 year before onset of Cushing syndrome. **B,** The dramatic changes are clearly different from obesity.

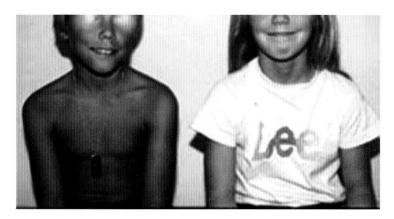

Plate 10-3 A boy with Addison's disease, pictured with his sister, showing the diffuse hyperpigmentation typical of the disorder.

7

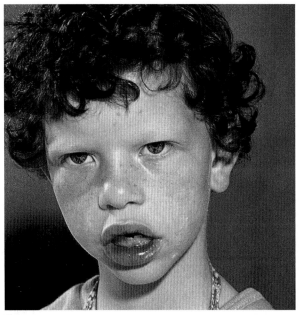

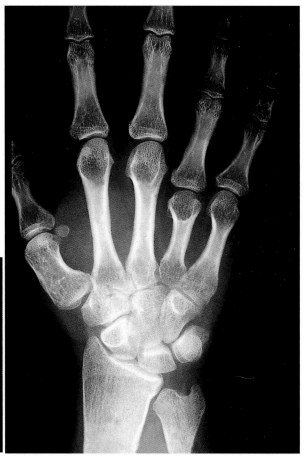

Plate 11-1 The short fourth and fifth metatarsals characteristic of pseudohypoparathyroidism may be less obvious in the hands of a child, as seen in the photograph. The abnormality is more readily appreciated on the radiograph. (From Wales JKH, Wit JM, Rogol AD: Pediatric Endocrinology and Growth, 2nd ed, Philadelphia, 2003, Saunders.)

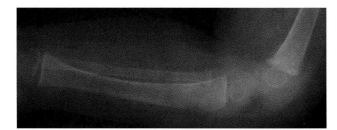

Plate 12-1 Williams syndrome. This patient has some of the phenotypic features of Williams syndrome; note the "elfin facies" with an upturned philtrum of the upper lip. (From Wales JKH, Wit JM, Rogol AD: Pediatric Endocrinology and Growth, 2nd ed, Philadelphia, 2003, Saunders.)

Plate 13-1 Osteoporosis. This radiograph shows the decreased bone density seen in many conditions of osteoporosis, such as osteogenesis imperfecta. The patient was a child with juvenile idiopathic osteoporosis. Decreased bone density is better quantified by either DEXA or quantitative CT. (From Wales JKH, Wit JM, Rogol AD: Pediatric Endocrinology and Growth, 2nd ed, Philadelphia, 2003, Saunders.)

CARBOHYDRATE DISORDERS

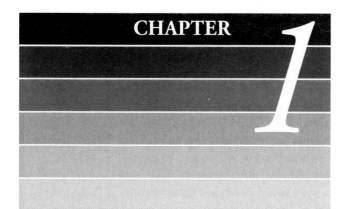

Type 1 Diabetes Mellitus in Children

STUART A. WEINZIMER

SHEELA MAGGE

TABLE OF CONTENTS>
Introduction
Epidemiology
Genetics
Pathogenesis
Pathophysiology
Diagnosis and Differentiation of Type 1 Diabetes Mellitus
Management of and Treatment Options for New-Onset Type 1
Diabetes Mellitus
Diabetic Ketoacidosis
Complications
Medical Therapy of the Child with Type 1 Diabetes Mellitus
   General Principles
   Insulin Regimens
   Self-Monitoring and Problem-Solving
   Nutritional Management
   Exercise and Physical Fitness
   Psychological Aspects
   Medical Follow-up
Conclusions
Major Points

INTRODUCTION

Although the ancient Egyptian physicians first described polyuria, it was Aretaeus, a Greek physician and disciple of Hippocrates who lived in the second century C.E., who first coined the term *diabetes*, from the Greek word for "siphon." He described the ailment as "a melting down of the flesh and limbs into urine," as accurate a description of the disease as any in use today. Currently, *diabetes* may be defined as chronic hyperglycemia due to an absolute or relative deficiency of insulin. The criteria for the diagnosis of diabetes, as established by the National Diabetes Data Group and World Health Organization, are (1) a casual (at any time of day, regardless of timing of food intake) plasma glucose greater than 200 mg/dL in the presence of symptoms of

diabetes, (2) fasting (>8 hours) plasma glucose greater than 126 mg/dL, or (3) a 2-hour post–75-gram glucose load glucose level greater than 200 mg/dL via oral glucose tolerance test. The oral glucose tolerance test is rarely useful in children. In the absence of obvious symptoms of diabetes (see Diagnosis section) or medications known to elevate the blood glucose (such as glucocorticoids), a casual or 2-hour postprandial blood glucose level greater than 200 mg/dL on two occasions is sufficient for the diagnosis.

Diabetes encompasses several diseases with distinct genetic, pathophysiological, and therapeutic aspects. The predominant form of diabetes in children is type 1 (previously named insulin-dependent or juvenile) diabetes mellitus (T1DM), a state of absolute insulin deficiency caused by immunologically based destruction of the islets of Langerhans. Type 2 (non–insulin-dependent or adult-onset) diabetes, a state of relative insulin deficiency usually accompanied by insulin resistance, is becoming increasingly more common in the pediatric population and, hand-in-hand with obesity, represents an emerging public health problem. Less common varieties of diabetes include the MODY (maturity-onset diabetes of youth) phenomenon, a family of single-gene dominantly inherited disorders of regulation of insulin secretion, cystic fibrosis–related diabetes and other varieties related to pancreatic agenesis or damage, mitochondrial disorders, and pharmacologically induced forms of the disease. This section focuses on the genetics, epidemiology, pathophysiology, clinical presentation, and aspects of the treatment of T1DM only. Type 2 diabetes mellitus is discussed in a separate chapter.

EPIDEMIOLOGY

Diabetes is the second most common chronic disease in childhood, after asthma, and occurs in 1 of every 1500 children by the age of 5 and in 1 of every 350 children by age 18. There are two peaks in age of presentation: the first occurs at ages 5 to 7 and the second occurs in early puberty. One third of people with T1DM do not present until adulthood, although T1DM rarely occurs after age 45. Diabetes affects boys and girls equally.

T1DM is primarily a disease of whites of northern European, especially Scandinavian, background. The highest incidence rates of T1DM worldwide are found in Finland, Sweden, and Denmark, about 30 new cases annually per 100,000 population. For comparison, the annual incidence rate in the United States is about 12 to 15 per 100,000 population, whereas that in Africa is about 5 per 100,000 per year and that in east Asia is less than 2 per 100,000 per year. There are striking geographical differences related to diabetes incidence: countries located at a greater distance from the equator and with lower mean annual temperatures have greater incidence rates for diabetes, although whether this finding is related to genetic differences in populations or to exposure to certain infectious agents is unclear. Migrant studies show increased rates of diabetes in populations moving from areas of lower diabetes incidence to those with higher diabetes incidence. However, because general trends of migration are from poor, tropical, developing countries to more affluent, temperate countries in the Western world, confounding influences such as diet and lifestyle make the implication of certain geographical areas problematic.

GENETICS

It has long been recognized that diabetes occurs more frequently in families with a previously affected member. First-degree relatives of an affected proband have an approximately 3% to 5% risk of developing diabetes, a 10-fold increase over that of the general population, and concordance rates for diabetes in identical twins are about 30% to 50%. It is clear that diabetes, as well as other autoimmune disorders such as Addison disease and thyroiditis, are associated with an increased frequency of certain human leukocyte antigens (HLAs) of the major histocompatibility complex (MHC). This system, located on chromosome 6, regulates the immune response and recognition of self from nonself through the expression of certain antigens on the cell surface. The inheritance of HLA antigen DR3 or DR4 increases the risk of development of diabetes approximately 3-fold, whereas the inheritance of both DR3 and DR4 confers about a 10- to 15-fold increase in risk. More than 90% of all whites with diabetes carry HLA antigen DR3 or DR4, although these alleles are present in more than 50% of the general white population. T1DM in African Americans is associated with the same HLA genes as in whites.

The homozygous absence of an aspartic acid residue at position 57 (Asp57) within the DQβ chain is associated with an approximate 100-fold risk of diabetes susceptibility, whereas individuals heterozygous for non-Asp57 also have an increased risk relative to Asp57/Asp57 homozygotes. The frequency of non-Asp57 is directly proportional to the incidence of T1DM within a given population. Similarly, the absence of arginine at position 52 of the DQα chain is also associated with increased susceptibility to T1DM. It is thought that the changes at positions 52 and 57 alter the tertiary structure of the HLA molecule, so that a normally closed "groove" is opened up, allowing greater access of the HLA antigen to T-cell receptors and triggering an immune response.

PATHOGENESIS

The current model for the development of diabetes is that the susceptibility to the disease, rather than the disease itself, is inherited through specific genetic sequences with the MHC. This is followed by a triggering event, or "second hit," that initiates the misdirected inflammatory process against the pancreatic islets. Recognition of β-cell stimulates T-lymphocyte activation, leading to the release of inflammatory cytokines, production of toxic free radicals, and β-cell killing, which in turn results in further β-cell antigen release and escalation of the immune process. T-cell infiltration of the islets is noted in pancreatic specimens of diabetics, akin to the infiltrates seen in other autoimmune disorders such as Hashimoto thyroiditis. There also is evidence that at disease onset, there is an alteration in the ratio between killer and helper T cells.

The inflammatory process against the islets is accompanied by the development of serum antibodies that contribute to the inflammatory process. These islet cell antibodies (ICAs) are present in the serum of more than 80% of diabetic persons at diagnosis. The predominant autoantibody is GAD65, directed against the enzyme glutamic acid decarboxylase, which catalyzes the conversion of glutamate to γ-aminobutyric acid (GABA), but antibodies to insulin and other β-cell antigens (ICA512 or IA-2) are also seen. These autoantibodies may be detected in the blood years before the development of clinical diabetes, suggesting a smoldering, indolent, silent inflammatory destruction of β-cell mass that manifests clinically with carbohydrate intolerance when 90% of the β-cell mass is destroyed.

The triggering event that leads to the destructive autoimmune process is thought to be a viral infection, either by molecular mimicry of a specific virus toward a β-cell antigen or through a nonspecific viremia. Certain viruses, such as rubella, mumps, coxsackievirus, and cytomegalovirus, may be directly toxic to pancreatic β-cells, whereas other viral infections may trigger the disease by producing a widespread, generalized immune response. The observations that breast-fed infants have lower incidences of diabetes and that many new-onset diabetic persons have antibodies to bovine serum albumin have led to concerns that early introduction of cow's milk–based formulas may trigger diabetes, especially in susceptible individuals. Large-scale prospective studies have been initiated to answer this question. Similarly, whether environmental toxins, such as nitrosamine compounds produced in the smoking of meat, are associated with increased diabetes risk, remains an unanswered question, although it is intriguing that populations with a typical Western diets, which are relatively antioxidant deficient, are associated with higher diabetes incidence than populations ingesting the higher antioxidant-containing diets of the developing world. Antioxidant therapy for the prevention of diabetes, however, remains entirely speculative.

PATHOPHYSIOLOGY

Insulin is an anabolic hormone that regulates the body's balance of storage versus mobilization of body stores. It is stimulated by a rise in glucose levels in the peripheral bloodstream and, via a receptor-mediated mechanism, allows the uptake of glucose (through specific glucose transporters) into the cells of the peripheral tissues. In the liver, insulin stimulates glycogen synthesis and inhibits gluconeogenesis and glycogenolysis. Insulin also increases hepatic lipid synthesis from triglycerides and glycerol. In adipose tissues, insulin serves to favor lipid storage *(lipogenesis)*. In skeletal muscle, insulin stimulates increased amino acid uptake, as well as protein and glycogen synthesis. Insulin action is inhibited by catecholamines, such as epinephrine, and by the other counterregulatory hormones, growth hormone and cortisol.

In the absence of insulin, the body acts as if in the fasting state, despite being fed. Existing serum glucose cannot be used by peripheral tissues, because of the dependence of the peripheral tissue glucose transporters on insulin. Hepatic glycogenolysis and gluconeogenesis are stimulated, resulting in further hyperglycemia. As serum glucose levels exceed the renal threshold (180 mg/dL), an osmotic diuresis occurs, leading to significant urinary losses of fluids and electrolytes such as potassium, sodium, calcium, phosphorus, and magnesium. Continued glucose production along with decreased peripheral glucose uptake, combined with urinary water losses, leads to a slowly progressive dehydration and hyperosmolarity.

The disruption in protein and fat metabolism also contributes to the metabolic destabilization. Insulin deficiency triggers lipolysis in adipose tissue, fatty acid oxidation in the liver, and proteolysis in muscle, leading to an accumulation of the ketones β-hydroxybutyrate and acetoacetate and subsequent metabolic acidosis. Progressive dehydration and acidosis stimulate production of the counterregulatory hormones epinephrine, growth hormone, and cortisol. These hormones further antagonize insulin action and thereby exacerbate hyperglycemia, catabolism, and metabolic acidosis through the stimulation of glycogenolysis, gluconeogenesis, lipolysis, and ketone production, perpetuating the vicious cycle.

DIAGNOSIS AND DIFFERENTIATION OF TYPE 1 DIABETES MELLITUS

Classically, children with T1DM present with a triad of polyuria, polydipsia, and polyphagia. However, there is great variation within the spectrum and severity of presentation, and a wide differential diagnosis can exist. Furthermore, the fact that the initial presentation of T1DM is often triggered by an intercurrent illness can also confound the diagnosis. In children with T1DM, polyuria and compensatory polydipsia result once the renal threshold for glucose has been exceeded (at serum glucose concentrations of about 180 mg/dL), and glucosuria occurs. Hyperglycemia and the hyperosmolar state cause an osmotic diuresis, leading to the polyuria, polydipsia, and often enuresis. On presentation, these symptoms have often been present for several weeks. This is all the more true in infants and active adolescents, in whom it is difficult for parents to note the symptoms of excessive urination. Progressive insulin deficiency leads to weight loss, fatigue, and general malaise, as protein and fat stores are lost. As counterregulatory hormones increase and ketosis worsens, symptoms of acute illness develop, including nausea, anorexia, abdominal pain, and vomiting. At this point, the acute worsening of dehydration and acidosis may produce symptoms of lethargy, confusion, stupor, even coma, and the respiratory compensation for the metabolic acidosis produces hyperpnea, the deep-sighing *Kussmaul respirations*. Box 1-1 summarizes the typical symptoms present at diagnosis. Other important historical points that should be elicited at presentation include family history of diabetes or other autoimmune conditions (thyroiditis, Addison disease) and recent use of medications known to raise the blood sugar.

The physical examination should focus on the state of hydration and include careful evaluation of heart rate and blood pressure and a description of mucous membranes, capillary refill, pulses, and warmth of extremities. A rough

Box 1-1   Symptoms of Type 1 Diabetes Mellitus
Polyuria Polydipsia Polyphagia Weight loss Recurrence of enuresis in previously trained child Candidal vaginitis Lethargy Blurred vision Abdominal pain* Vomiting* Difficulty breathing* Obtundation*

*Indicative of diabetic ketoacidosis.

Box 1-2   Physical Findings in Type 1 Diabetes Mellitus

Dehydration
    Dry mucous membranes
    Decreased skin turgor*
    Delayed capillary refill*
    Tachycardia*
    Hypotension*
Vulvovaginitis
Fruity odor to breath*
Kussmaul respirations*
Ileus, guarding*
Depressed level of consciousness*

*Indicative of diabetic ketoacidosis.

estimation of dehydration status ($\approx$5%, 10%, or 20%) should be made to calculate the fluid deficit and facilitate rehydration therapy. A careful examination and written documentation of the neurological status are also critical, to serve as a baseline in case of deterioration in neurological status later in therapy. General physical examination should include respiratory and abdominal examinations, as well as a search for an intercurrent illness that may have served as the "trigger." Evaluation of the thyroid for goiter and skin for hyperpigmentation allows for the diagnosis of potential comorbidities such as thyroiditis or Addison disease. Girls should be evaluated for the presence of candidal vulvovaginitis, and both boys and girls should have documentation of height, weight, and sexual maturity rating. The discovery of a "fruity" odor to the breath is characteristic of diabetic ketoacidosis (DKA), but significant ketosis may be present even in the absence of this finding. Box 1-2 summarizes common findings at diagnosis of T1DM.

Appropriate laboratory studies begin with the measurement of serum blood glucose. As mentioned earlier, random "casual" blood glucose levels are indicated in the setting of a child with symptoms suggestive of diabetes. In the symptomatic child, blood glucose should be checked promptly; children should *not* be instructed to have a fasting blood glucose level measured the next day. In the obviously well-appearing child, minimal laboratory testing is required: electrolytes, blood urea nitrogen, and creatinine, along with a formal urinalysis for glucose and ketones, may suffice. In children with clinical evidence of more severe dehydration and/or other organ system signs, the evaluation should be expanded to include complete metabolic panel, blood count with differential, venous or arterial blood gas, and, in the setting of fever or shock, blood culture. Other studies depend on the clinical scenario and should be individualized.

A careful history, physical examination, and laboratory investigation should allow the diagnosis of diabetes mellitus to be deduced in a rapid, efficient manner. The presence of polyuria, polydipsia, and weight loss in a child should be considered T1DM until proved otherwise. The primary differential diagnosis for T1DM in children is urinary tract infection, due to the symptoms of excessive or frequent urination. If the symptoms of polydipsia and polyuria predominate, diabetes insipidus should be considered. However, formal urinalysis can easily differentiate the two conditions, as the urine of diabetes mellitus contains glucose, ketones, and osmotically active electrolytes, whereas the urine of diabetes insipidus is bland and dilute. If the presentation includes dehydration and vomiting, gastroenteritis should be considered, as should streptococcal pharyngitis and pneumonia. Pneumonia or asthmatic exacerbation may also be suggested in the setting of metabolic acidosis and Kussmaul respirations. In children presenting with fever, vomiting, and abdominal pain, appendicitis or other acute abdominal events may also be possibilities, a situation made more confusing by the fact that children in DKA often have leukocytosis. Other conditions in the differential diagnosis of T1DM include toxic ingestion, pelvic inflammatory disease in a sexually active adolescent, and, in any age, sepsis. Patients with persistent hyperglycemia may also present with various forms of fungal infections. Infants and toddlers may have thrush and/or diaper candidiasis, and adolescents may present with genital yeast infections. Patients and parents are often unaware that these symptoms are in any way related to diabetes. Thus, a careful genitourinary examination is necessary on admission. In a prepubertal child, the presence of candidiasis should always trigger blood glucose testing by the primary care physician. It should also be stressed that the diagnosis of diabetes requires measurement of blood glucose; the finding of glucosuria alone is not sufficient. Renal glycosuria, a benign condition in which the threshold for urinary excretion of glucose occurs even at normal blood glucose concentrations, may occasionally masquerade as diabetes in the child in whom routine urinalysis is performed in the absence of true symptoms of diabetes. Table 1-1 summarizes the differential diagnostic considerations in T1DM.

MANAGEMENT OF AND TREATMENT OPTIONS FOR NEW-ONSET TYPE 1 DIABETES MELLITUS

The goals of management of the child with new-onset T1DM are metabolic stabilization of the child and education of the family to care for the child after the stabilization has been completed. Treatment of the newly diagnosed child with T1DM depends on the acuity of the illness at presentation: the ambulatory, well-appearing child without severe dehydration may be handled quite differently than the acutely ill, dehydrated patient with vomiting. It is still generally accepted that the newly diagnosed diabetic child requires acute hospitalization, in that

the frequent monitoring that is required cannot yet be accomplished in the ambulatory setting by an untrained family still recovering from the shock of the diagnosis. Small pilot projects by Chase and colleagues have, however, demonstrated that outpatient management of the new-onset diabetic patient may be accomplished in some situations. The development of diabetes in the sibling of a known patient may easily be managed in an ambulatory setting if the child is not acutely ill and the family is well trained in diabetes management.

In the newly diagnosed patient without vomiting or ketoacidosis, initiation of subcutaneous insulin by injection is appropriate. In the case of a child with hyperglycemia alone, a dosage of approximately 0.3 to 0.5 unit/kg/day may suffice, whereas if ketosis is also present, a dosage of 0.7 unit/kg/day or more may be required. A child presenting in DKA and transitioning to subcutaneous insulin often requires 1 unit/kg/day or more. The management of a child presenting in DKA is discussed in a separate section.

The total daily dose is divided into rapid- and intermediate-/long-acting insulin, typically Humalog (Lispro, Eli Lilly and Company, Indianapolis, IN) or Novolog (Aspart, Novo Nordisk, Bagsvaerd, Denmark) along with NPH, given in a three shot-per-day regimen. After calculating the

Table 1-1   Differential Diagnoses in Type 1 Diabetes Mellitus and Tests to Consider

Clinical Findings	Differential Diagnosis	Tests/Interpretation
Polyuria, nocturia, enuresis	Urinary tract infection (UTI), benign nocturnal enuresis	Urinalysis demonstrates glycosuria with/without ketonuria characteristic of diabetes, instead of pyuria and other markers of UTI
Polydipsia	Psychogenic polydipsia, diabetes insipidus	Urinalysis demonstrates glycosuria with/without ketonuria in diabetes, instead of low specific gravity (alone)
Weight loss	Anorexia nervosa, gastrointestinal or chronic disease	Careful history should reveal behaviors and ideations characteristic of anorexia nervosa; plasma glucose diagnostic of diabetes
Vomiting	Gastroenteritis, toxic ingestion, other metabolic disorders	Serum glucose and electrolytes in vomiting child reveal diabetes; electrolyte disturbances and acidosis without hyperglycemia suggest other metabolic disorders, requiring more directed testing
Abdominal pain	Gastroenteritis, appendicitis, other intra-abdominal process	Careful history and physical should elicit typical symptoms of diabetes and exclude surgical abdomen; measurement of serum glucose and urinalysis differentiates diabetes
Hyperpnea	Pneumonia, asthma, anxiety	Kussmaul respirations (deep sighing breaths) suggest metabolic acidosis, whereas tachypnea suggests a primary respiratory disorder; no rales or wheezes; serum glucose and electrolytes characteristic of diabetes and metabolic acidosis
Hyperglycemia	Medication- or stress-induced hyperglycemia	May be mistaken for diabetes, although careful history does not demonstrate characteristic prodromal weight loss or urinary symptoms
Glycosuria	Benign renal glycosuria	May be mistaken for diabetes; measurement of serum glucose differentiates diabetes from renal glycosuria

total daily dose, approximately 50% is given as NPH and 15% is given as rapid-acting insulin before breakfast, approximately 10% is given as NPH and 15% as rapid-acting insulin before dinner, and approximately 10% is given as NPH at bedtime. In toddlers, in whom meal intake is unpredictable, insulin may be administered after meals, by giving a set amount of long-acting insulin and dosing the rapid-acting insulin according to the prior carbohydrate intake (see description of carbohydrate counting later). In infants, generally only a long-acting insulin is given in a two or three shot-per-day regimen. Blood sugars are checked before meals, at bedtime, and at 2 to 3 AM (or before feedings in infants), and all urine output is checked for glucose and ketones by dipstick.

For the child admitted to the hospital with only hyperglycemia and no ketosis, "touch-ups" of rapid-acting insulin can be given before meals in addition to the scheduled dose. Infants and toddlers may require only 0.5 unit of rapid-acting insulin to decrease the serum blood sugar by 100 mg/dL. In young school-age children, 1 unit may decrease the blood sugar by about 100 mg/dL, and in older school-age children, 75 mg/dL. In teenagers, in whom insulin resistance is typical, 1 unit may bring the blood sugar down by only about 30 to 50 mg/dL. These insulin "touch-ups" should generally be administered after the premeal or presnack blood glucose checks (to avoid hypoglycemia) and should be done with the goal to correct the blood sugar to approximately 120 mg/dL. In addition, it should be remembered that these rough guidelines should be individualized based on patient response.

If a child also presents with ketosis, another treatment regimen, known as "sick day rules," may be implemented. Blood glucose levels and urine ketones are checked every 2 hours. An additional 10% of the total daily dose of insulin is given as rapid-acting insulin every 2 hours until the urine ketones clear. This is continued even if the blood sugars are not elevated, as the presence of ketones indicates the need for supplemental insulin. Supplemental fluids should be given to restore intravascular fluid volume and hasten the excretion of ketones. In the child tolerating oral rehydration, a fluid "dose" of 1 ounce per year of age per hour serves as a rough guideline, of which the sugar content depends on the serum glucose. For blood sugar levels greater than 200 mg/dL, sugar-free fluids should be given; between 120 and 200 mg/dL, a mixture of sugar-free and sugar-containing fluids; and for less than 120 mg/dL, all sugar-containing fluids. "Sick day rules" are useful not only in the hospital setting but also to families at home trying to manage a diabetic child with an intercurrent illness. If emesis precludes normal oral intake, the intermediate- or long-acting insulin should be discontinued, and small, frequent doses of short- or rapid-acting insulin only should be given.

Once the ketones have cleared and the child is tolerating an oral diet, the family may resume the normal routine.

Newly diagnosed patients and their families should be taught carbohydrate counting. This allows dietary flexibility, as the child can adjust the rapid-acting insulin dose according to the mealtime or snack-time carbohydrate intake. A typical approximate starting ratio would be 0.5 unit of insulin for 15 to 30 grams of carbohydrate in the infant or toddler, 1 unit per 15 grams in the younger school-age child, and 1 unit per 10 grams in an adolescent. These ratios should be individually titrated based on the 2-hour postprandial blood glucose measurement.

Before discharge, an assessment of the family's overall level of coping and functioning should be made. Special situations, such as blended families or alternate/additional caretakers in the home, should be worked out before hospital discharge. Families typically experience shock and grief at the child's diagnosis, but consideration should be made for referrals for psychosocial counseling if grief, anxiety, or depression appears to be excessive or interferes with diabetes education.

On hospital discharge, the total daily insulin dose is typically decreased by 20% to 30%, as children are generally much more active at home and therefore require less insulin. Families are instructed to check for urine ketones if the blood sugar is greater than 240 mg/dL or if the child is sick. Close contact with the newly discharged patient is critical to monitor the safety and efficacy of the prescribed insulin regimen and the coping skills of the family.

DIABETIC KETOACIDOSIS

DKA is a life-threatening, preventable complication of diabetes mellitus characterized by inadequate insulin action, hyperglycemia, dehydration, electrolyte loss, metabolic acidosis, and ketosis. It is associated with a significant mortality rate and is the most frequent cause of death in children with T1DM. Children whose diabetes has not yet been diagnosed may present with DKA, so the diagnosis must be considered in any child with confusion or coma of undetermined etiology. In children whose diabetes has already been diagnosed, DKA can usually be prevented by patient and family education, frequent monitoring of blood glucose and urinary ketones during intercurrent illness, adequate oral hydration, and supplemental insulin ("sick day rules").

Diabetic ketoacidosis is defined as a blood sugar level of greater than 240 mg/dL, ketonemia/ketonuria, and pH less than 7.3. The primary abnormality is insulin deficiency, which leads to hyperglycemia because of both decreased glucose utilization and increased gluconeogenesis. As glucose levels exceed the renal threshold of 180 mg/dL, an osmotic diuresis occurs, resulting in the loss of extracellular water and electrolytes and worsening of the hyperglycemia. Insulin deficiency also leads to accelerated lipolysis, with subsequent conversion of free fatty acids to β-hydroxybutyric and acetoacetic acids. This results in a metabolic acidosis. (Acetone is also formed and gives a fruity odor to the patient's breath, but it does not contribute to the acidosis.) Potassium, primarily an intracellular ion, is transported out of the cell into the plasma in exchange for hydrogen and is lost in the urine. Thus, virtually all patients with DKA develop a "total body" deficiency of potassium, regardless of their serum potassium level. Phosphate, another predominantly intracellular ion, is handled similarly. Deficiency of 2,3-diphosphoglycerate, a phosphate-containing glycolytic intermediate in red blood cells that facilitates release of oxygen from hemoglobin, may contribute to the development of lactic acidosis complicating the ketoacidosis. Although insulin deficiency is the principal abnormality, elevated counterregulatory hormones (glucagon, cortisol, catecholamines, and growth hormone) contribute to both the accelerated gluconeogenesis and lipolysis.

DKA is not difficult to recognize in a child with known diabetes who is dehydrated, hyperventilating, and obtunded. In the child whose diabetes has not yet been diagnosed, however, it may be confused with Reye syndrome, toxic ingestion (especially salicylate or alcohol), and central nervous system infection or trauma. Persistent vomiting may suggest gastroenteritis or, with abdominal pain, acute appendicitis or another intra-abdominal process. The diagnosis of diabetes (if not already established) is suggested by a history of polyuria, polydipsia, polyphagia, nocturia, or enuresis in a previously toilet-trained child. Weakness and unexplained weight loss may also be presenting features. When the diagnosis of DKA is suspected, an attempt should be made to identify precipitating causes (e.g., infection, stress, or noncompliance). In a child with known diabetes, it is important to review briefly the recent blood sugar history and to ascertain not only the usual insulin dosage but also the quantity and timing of the most recent injection.

The physical examination should focus initially on the adequacy of the airway, breathing, and an assessment of the circulatory status (pulse, blood pressure, peripheral perfusion), degree of dehydration (including weight if possible), and mental status. Deep, rapid respirations (Kussmaul breathing) and a fruity odor to the breath are classic signs but are not present in every patient. A careful search should be made for a source of infection that may have precipitated the episode of DKA. Bedside determination of the blood glucose with a glucose monitoring device and evaluation of the urine for glucose and ketones should be performed as quickly as possible, and treatment should be initiated without waiting for the results of the laboratory assessment to become available.

The laboratory evaluation of patients suspected to have DKA includes determination of the blood glucose, plasma or urinary ketones, serum electrolyte concentration, blood urea nitrogen (BUN), creatinine, osmolarity, and a baseline calcium and phosphorus. A baseline blood gas measurement should also be made to determine the pH and P_{CO_2}. Although venous blood gas measurements may suffice in milder episodes of DKA, an arterial blood gas measurement should be obtained in patients suspected to have incomplete respiratory compensation and/or those expected to require bicarbonate therapy (see later). If hyperlipidemia is present, the serum sodium concentration may be artifactually lowered. Similarly, the serum sodium is reduced approximately 1.6 mEq/L for each 100-mg/dL rise in glucose because of the reequilibration of the intracellular and extracellular compartments at a higher osmolarity. In the presence of ketones (and lactate), a large anion gap acidosis is present. The degree of elevation of the BUN and creatinine, as well as the hematocrit, may indicate the extent of dehydration (and the possibility of renal damage). The initial serum potassium may be low, normal, or high, depending on the degree of acidosis and the quantitative urinary losses.

The acute management of DKA is directed at correction of the dehydration, electrolyte loss, hyperglycemia, and acidosis (Box 1-3). Initial fluid therapy is aimed at rapid stabilization of the circulation to correct impending shock but, as in other forms of hypertonic dehydration, too rapid fluid administration must be avoided. Fluid replacement in excess of 4 $L/m^2/24$ hr has been associated with the development of potentially fatal cerebral edema in DKA. For this reason, an initial fluid bolus is usually advised to expand the vascular compartment and improve peripheral circulation, but once the patient has been stabilized, subsequent rehydration is accomplished with caution. Typically, one aims to correct the fluid defect gradually, over 36 to 48 hours. Gradual correction is particularly important in children at an increased risk of developing cerebral edema. This includes children with altered mental status, history of symptoms for longer than 48 hours, pH of less than 7.0, glucose of greater than 1000 mg/dL, corrected sodium of greater than 155 mEq/L, extreme hyperosmolality (>375 mOsm/L), or age younger than 3 years. A corrected sodium level that fails to rise with treatment may signify excessive free water accumulation and an increased risk of cerebral edema. Therefore, rehydration fluids should contain at least 115 to 135 mEq sodium chloride/L to ensure a gradual decline in serum osmolality and minimize the risk of cerebral edema. Early potassium replacement is also important, to correct the potassium depletion that occurs because of both the severe initial intracellular losses and the

Box 1-3	**Guidelines for Management of Diabetic Ketoacidosis**
Insulin	A continuous intravenous infusion of 0.1 unit/kg/hr is typical. For very young or severely acidotic, hyperosmolar patients, 0.05 unit/kg/hr may be initiated to prevent rapid changes during metabolic stabilization. In hyperglycemic, hyperosmolar, nonketotic coma (which is rarely seen in children except in some adolescents with type 2 diabetes), insulin may be withheld during the first several hours.
Fluids	A 10 to 20 mL of 0.9% saline/kg bolus to restore intravascular volume. Repeat as needed to treat shock. Base subsequent fluid administration on estimated degree of dehydration, and plan to replace deficit evenly over 48 hours.
Sodium	Na^+ deficit at presentation generally resolves with administration of isotonic fluids during resuscitation phase. Measured $[Na^+]$ typically underestimates true Na^+ levels due to effects of hyperglycemia. Calculation and assessment of true $[Na^+]$ over time may decrease risk of cerebral edema.
Potassium	K^+ deficit at presentation requires aggressive therapy. Replacement depends on serum $[K^+]$ at presentation; 20-60 mEq (½ as KCl and ½ as K^+ phosphate) added to each liter of rehydration fluid is typical.
Glucose	Added to rehydration fluids once the blood glucose level falls <300 mg/dL. Goal generally to reduce blood glucose 50 to 100 mg/dL/hr, although recent evidence suggests that rapid fall in blood glucose may not increase risk of cerebral edema.
Bicarbonate	Considered in extreme acidosis only; bicarbonate use may increase risk of cerebral edema.
Clinical monitoring	Assess vital signs, neurological status, state of hydration, and fluid intake and output at least hourly.
Laboratory monitoring	Measure blood glucose hourly and electrolytes and pH at least every 2 hours until stable. Follow blood urea nitrogen, creatinine, calcium, and phosphate if abnormal at presentation.

subsequent potassium shift from the extracellular to the intracellular compartment (this occurs when treatment with insulin is initiated and the acidosis is corrected). Potassium is administered only after urine output is ensured to prevent hyperkalemia in the setting of unrecognized renal impairment. Potassium is usually given at a dose of 20 to 60 mEq/L of fluid, half as the chloride salt and half as the phosphate salt, to replace the phosphate losses simultaneously. Electrocardiographic monitoring facilitates early recognition of either hyperkalemia (peaked T waves) or hypokalemia (flat or inverted T waves) and the development of potentially dangerous cardiac arrhythmias. Serum calcium should be monitored if phosphate is given, because phosphate administration may precipitate hypocalcemia.

Insulin therapy is typically initiated after the patient has been stabilized with an initial fluid bolus. As with fluid replacement, the aim of therapy is gradual correction: reduction of the blood glucose by 50 to 100 mg/dL/hr. Usually, the glucose falls significantly with initial rehydration alone. Continuous "low-dose" insulin infusion is the preferred route in most patients because of the predictability of the rate of fall in blood glucose, the ability to closely titrate the insulin dose to the metabolic needs, and the avoidance of erratic absorption from subcutaneous sites during dehydration. The usual dosage is 0.5 to 1.0 U/kg/hr, which may be titrated up or down according to the clinical response. Dextrose is added to the intravenous solution when the serum glucose level falls below 300 mg/dL and is

titrated to provide a continued gradual decline in blood glucose to target levels. This is easily accomplished with the simultaneous use of two intravenous solutions, which differ only in the dextrose concentration. Usually the lowering of the blood glucose concentration precedes the decrease in ketones. Thus, in the situation of continued acidosis with a glucose level of less than 300 mg/dL, it is important not to decrease the insulin dosage but rather to add glucose. Determination of serum ketones, although helpful diagnostically, is not an accurate guide to clinical improvement, as only acetoacetate is measured by the usual method and not β-hydroxybutyrate, which predominates early (but not later) in the course of untreated DKA.

Specific therapy for the acidosis of DKA remains controversial. Frequently, dramatic clinical improvement results simply from initial expansion of extracellular fluid volume, reestablishment of adequate peripheral perfusion, and insulin administration. An elevation in blood pH after bicarbonate administration may be attended by worsening acidosis in the central nervous system, because carbon dioxide (but not bicarbonate) diffuses across the blood-brain barrier. Furthermore, the organic acids in DKA, in contrast to metabolic acidosis from other causes, are metabolized to bicarbonate. Thus, administration of "additional" bicarbonate may result in a late alkalosis. Bicarbonate may have a place in the treatment of DKA but only in the more severe degrees of acidosis (pH < 7.0, which may be associated with myocardial depression) and in the setting of inadequate respiratory compensation. According to Glaser and associates, the use of bicarbonate in otherwise uncomplicated DKA has been demonstrated to prolong therapy and may in fact be associated with an increased risk of cerebral edema. If bicarbonate is given, the dosage is calculated to bring the pH only to around 7.2, paying attention to the sodium administered concomitantly; slow infusion is preferable to bolus injection.

Acute cerebral edema is a rare, potentially fatal complication of DKA that occurs without warning within the first 24 hours of treatment. This is to be distinguished from the asymptomatic brain swelling detectable on computed tomography scanning that may occur in some children with DKA. Although a number of causes of acute cerebral edema have been suggested from uncontrolled, retrospective studies, the etiology is not known. Increased risk of cerebral edema has been associated in many cases with rates of fluid administration greater than 4 L/m^2/24 hr and corrected sodium levels and effective plasma osmolality that decline over the course of treatment. Therefore, careful monitoring of neurological status, input/output log (I's and O's), and corrected sodium and effective osmolality is essential for early recognition of cerebral edema. Treatment of cerebral edema is aimed at lowering intracranial pressure: intravenous mannitol (an osmotic diuretic), intubation/hyperventilation, and, if needed, ventriculostomy.

It is clear that therapy requires frequent modifications based on an individual patient's response. This can only be accomplished with a carefully maintained flow sheet that includes such items as vital signs, neurological status (Glasgow Coma Scale score), intake and output volumes ("I's and O's"), weight, insulin dosage administered, and measurement of blood glucose, urinary ketones, serum electrolytes (with calculation of corrected serum sodium and effective serum osmolality), calcium, phosphorus, BUN, and creatinine (plus blood gases as necessary). Measurements are performed hourly at first and less frequently as the patient's condition stabilizes.

In contrast to those in DKA, patients with new-onset diabetes who are not significantly dehydrated and whose serum electrolytes are normal may usually be treated with subcutaneous insulin and oral fluids. In these patients, an intravenous fluid bolus may not be indicated and, in fact, may be harmful.

Rarely, a patient presents with an extremely high blood glucose level and an absent or inappropriately low urinary ketone level. This syndrome, known as hyperglycemic, hyperosmolar, nonketotic coma, usually occurs at the extremes of age and is due to a combination of severe dehydration (due to inadequate access to fluids) and insulin deficiency. It is associated with an extremely high mortality rate and must be treated with caution.

COMPLICATIONS

The complications of diabetes may be divided into early, which are frequently encountered in children, and late, which are uncommonly seen in the pediatric age group. The most common early complications of diabetes are directly attributable to insulin deficiency or excess. DKA, which may occur either as an initial presentation of diabetes or in the setting of intercurrent illness or poor glycemic control, is discussed earlier.

The most common early complication of diabetes, related to insulin treatment, is hypoglycemia. Mild hypoglycemic reactions, consisting of headache, tremors, abdominal pain, or mood changes, are considered a part of tight control. More severe hypoglycemia, however, may lead to severe alterations in consciousness, coma, seizures, and even death. Particularly in children, the chronic effects of repeated episodes of hypoglycemia on cognitive development are worrisome, thus limiting the extent to which the goals of intensive control can be applied to children. Electroencephalographic abnormalities may be documented in the majority of diabetic children with a history of severe hypoglycemia, and also in a significant percentage of diabetic children with only mild hypoglycemia. School performance and tests of neuropsychological functioning are lower in diabetic children compared with controls, particularly in children with diabetes onset before 5 years of age. Additionally, episodes of hypoglycemia may predispose to more hypoglycemia, by blunting the counterregulatory hormones glucagon and epinephrine. This hypoglycemia unawareness syndrome is extremely common in adults with diabetes but may also be seen in older children and adolescents with longer duration of diabetes. Younger children may be considered to have "functional" hypoglycemia unawareness because of limited ability to recognize and/or communicate their symptoms.

Another early complication of diabetes is lipohypertrophy, which results from the repeated subcutaneous injections of insulin into the same area, rather than rotating the sites of injections. Lipohypertrophy appears as a firm, rubbery mass in the subcutaneous space, but the problem is more than cosmetic: absorption of insulin from areas of lipohypertrophy is poor and erratic, resulting in decreasing effectiveness of insulin doses and unpredictable hypoglycemia.

Early complications of diabetes specific to childhood are delayed growth and puberty, secondary to chronic insulin deficiency and poor metabolic control. The Mauriac syndrome, or diabetic dwarfism, consisting of short stature, delayed growth and pubertal development, pallor, hepatomegaly, and thickened skin, is rarely seen in children today and is readily treatable with improved diabetes control.

Late complications of diabetes, related mainly to chronic microvascular and macrovascular disease, are the major causes of diabetes-related mortality and morbidity. The etiology and pathogenesis of microvascular disease are still under investigation but certainly involve a combination of factors, including thickening and weakening of capillary basement membranes by nonenzymatic protein glycosylation, accumulation of sorbitol and other sugar alcohols in tissues, and alterations in the paracrine/autocrine expression and action of growth factors such as insulin-like growth factor-I and transforming growth factor-β in target tissues. Risk of microvascular complications, however, is not solely related to metabolic control; the risk of development of microvascular disease is almost certainly also related to differential genetic susceptibility to the metabolic effects of diabetes, although specific susceptibility genes have yet to be identified. Hypercholesterolemia, hypertriglyceridemia, alterations in lipoproteins, and hypertension all contribute to the development of macrovascular disease.

Retinopathy is the most common microvascular complication of diabetes, and diabetic retinopathy is the leading cause of blindness in the United States. The earliest lesion is nonproliferative retinopathy, which consists of microaneurysms. More severe forms of this background retinopathy include the development of exudates and venous beading. Background retinopathy eventually develops in almost all diabetics but is not sight threatening. Proliferative retinopathy, characterized by fibrous proliferation, new blood vessel formation, and macular edema, is associated with progressive loss of vision. Proliferative retinopathy occurs in about 50% of diabetics after a disease duration of 20 years but is almost never seen in children before the age of 15. The development of retinopathy in children appears to be related not only to the duration of diabetes but also the pubertal stage; less retinopathy is seen in prepubertal children than in pubertal children with the same disease duration.

Kidney failure is one of the most common causes of death in patients with diabetes, and diabetic nephropathy is the most common cause of renal failure in the United States. Diabetic nephropathy may be divided into five stages. Glomerular hyperfiltration and renal enlargement are the earliest changes, associated with an increase in glomerular filtration rate. Hyperfiltration is correlated with hyperglycemia but is present even in patients with good metabolic control. In the second stage, which occurs 18 to 24 months after the onset of T1DM, thickening of the glomerular basement membrane and expansion of the mesangial matrix occur. Microalbuminuria (urinary albumin excretion rate of 30-300 mg/24 hr or 20-200 μg/min) may be seen but is not persistent. Persistent microalbuminuria is the hallmark of the third stage, which develops in about 25% of patients within 10 years of diagnosis. The progression to frank proteinuria, stage four, (urinary albumin excretion >300 mg/24 hr or 200 μg/min), nephrotic syndrome, and end-stage renal disease (stage 5) occurs in about 30% to 40% of patients with diabetes of 30 years' duration. Overt nephropathy is uncommon in children, but earlier stages of the disease may be seen in the pediatric diabetes population. The prevalence of microalbuminuria in children and adolescents is about 20% to 30% and, as in retinopathy, appears to depend on not only the duration of diabetes but also the number of years postpuberty.

Diabetic neuropathy develops in about 50% of diabetics within 10 years of disease diagnosis, although clinically evident diabetic neuropathy is extremely rare in children. However, decreased vibration and light touch sensation as well as decreased nerve conduction velocity, indicative of peripheral neuropathy, may be detected in children using sensitive techniques. Autonomic neuropathy is also extremely rare in children with diabetes, although abnormal cardiac autonomic testing may be demonstrated. Autonomic dysfunction in diabetics has been implicated in increased risk of hypoglycemia unawareness and sudden death ("dead-in-bed" syndrome).

Macrovascular disease and atherosclerosis are the major causes of death in adults with T1DM. Hypercholesterolemia and hyperlipidemia are frequently seen even in pediatric patients with T1DM, the extent of which is inversely proportional to the degree of metabolic control.

MEDICAL THERAPY OF THE CHILD WITH TYPE 1 DIABETES MELLITUS

General Principles

Optimal management of the child with diabetes requires an integrated approach, taking into account the overall level of functioning of the child and family, the nutritional and lifestyle patterns specific to that child, and attention to the overall developmental stages of childhood and adolescence. There is not just one appropriate insulin regimen or meal plan. The overriding principles are that the diabetes care plan should fit wherever possible into the surrounding home and school environments and that the primary childhood tasks of education, socialization, growth, and maturity should continue unhindered by the extra responsibilities that diabetes care entails. This potentially daunting task requires a multidisciplinary team, consisting of physicians, nurses, dietitians, and mental health professionals who are all trained and experienced in the nuances of diabetes care. Children with diabetes should be seen by the team at frequent intervals for assessment of glycemic control, growth, and development; evaluation for related disorders and complications; education, troubleshooting, and problem-solving; and screening for adjustment problems that may affect diabetes and/or the overall health of the child.

The rationale for this intensive approach to diabetes care comes from the Diabetes Control and Complications Trial (DCCT), a national multicenter study designed to test the hypothesis that "intensive" diabetes management would be associated with fewer long-term complications of diabetes than "standard" therapy. At the time of the DCCT, standard diabetes therapy consisted of two injections of insulin daily, infrequent home testing of the blood glucose level, and basic nutritional and exercise counseling. Intensive management entailed at least three or four injections of insulin daily or use of continuous subcutaneous insulin infusion (CSII) via programmable portable pumps ("pump therapy"), frequent self-monitoring of the blood glucose level through home glucose meter use, and frequent contact with the diabetes care team to adjust insulin dosages and the nutritional and exercise programs. In the DCCT study, intensive treatment in adults was associated with improvement in glycemic control (hemoglobin A1c [Hb$_{A1c}$] of 7.1% versus 9.0% in the standard group) and dramatically reduced incidence and progression of microvascular complications. The development and progression of retinopathy were reduced by 70%, whereas nephropathy was reduced by 35% and neuropathy was reduced by 30% to 70%. Significantly, there was an almost linear relationship between the Hb$_{A1c}$ and the risk of complications. There was no real threshold effect: the risk decreased with each improvement in the Hb$_{A1c}$ but remained elevated for any Hb$_{A1c}$ value greater than normal. However, intensive control was also associated with a 3-fold increase in severe hypoglycemia and a 2-fold increase in obesity.

The DCCT also demonstrated that intensive control was possible in adolescents. Intensively treated adolescents achieved a mean Hb$_{A1c}$ of 8.1% (versus 9.8% in the standard group). Intensive control in adolescents was associated with a 60% reduction in the risk of retinopathy and a 35% reduction in the risk of nephropathy. As in adults, adolescents undergoing intensification of therapy were at a 3-fold risk of severe hypoglycemia and a 2-fold risk of obesity. It is worthwhile to note, however, that the benefits of intensive control persisted even after the conclusion of the trial. In a 4-year follow-up study of adolescents participating in the DCCT, despite equivalent Hb$_{A1c}$ levels, subjects who had been intensively controlled during the DCCT period continued to have a 74% to 78% reduction in risk of worsening retinopathy and a 48% to 85% reduction in risk of nephropathy.

Insulin Regimens

The goal of insulin therapy is to most closely approximate the requirements of the body for basal metabolism and meals with the use of exogenous subcutaneous injection. In essence, the normally "closed loop" of the β cell, which senses the body's minute-to-minute insulin requirements and matches it with insulin production and secretion, is replaced by the "open-loop" system of the home glucose meter and insulin syringe.

Insulin has continued to evolve from an impure animal-derived pancreatic extract with poorly predictable pharmacokinetics and pyrogenic tendency to a pure, recombinantly derived human protein with reliable activity profile and low antigenicity. Many types of insulin preparations are commercially available, with different onset, peak, and duration effects, to custom design an insulin regimen to suit the particular child or clinical need. Recently, very rapid-acting insulin analogues (Lispro, Eli Lilly and Company, Indianapolis, IN; and Aspart, Novo Nordisk, Bagsvaerd, Denmark) and one very long-acting, peakless insulin analogue (Glargine, Aventis Pharmaceuticals, Bridgewater, NJ) were developed. A list of available insulin preparations is given in Table 1-2.

Before the DCCT, most children with diabetes were treated with two shots of insulin daily: a combination of short- and intermediate-acting insulin given approximately 30 minutes before both breakfast and dinner. The rationale for this approach is that the short-acting insulin (Regular) would "cover" the glycemic surge of breakfast and dinner meals and the intermediate-acting insulin (NPH, Lente) would "cover" the lunch meal and basal overnight requirements. Typically, the insulin dose would be split so that two thirds of the daily dose was given in the morning (one third of that as Regular and two thirds as NPH or Lente) and one third of the daily dose was given before dinner (half of that as Regular and half as NPH or Lente). Most children would require 0.7 to 1.0 unit/kg/day, less in younger children or those with recent onset, and frequently more in adolescents. Late-morning and late-evening hypoglycemia is a frequent complication of this regimen, as the peaks of NPH or Lente are highly variable. Additional snacks in the morning and late at night ameliorate the hypoglycemia but may predispose to weight gain.

The desire for intensive insulin therapy, the justification for which was provided by the results of the DCCT, has been aided by the development of rapid-acting insulin analogues. The rapid-acting analogues more closely match the glycemic surges after meals and are associated with less frequent postprandial hypoglycemia. An additional benefit of the rapid-acting analogues is that meals may be eaten immediately after the injection. Most children are now treated with a mixed dose of rapid- and intermediate-acting insulin at breakfast and dinner and an additional injection of intermediate- or long-acting insulin at bedtime. However, many other combinations are possible, including one or two injections of very-long acting insulin (Ultralente, Eli Lilly and Company, Indianapolis, IN; or

Table 1-2   Pharmacodynamic Properties of Common Insulin Formulations

Category	Onset (hr)	Peak (hr)	Duration (hr)
Rapid-acting			
Insulin Lispro	0.25-0.5	0.5-1	3-4
Insulin Aspart	0.25-0.5	0.5-1	3-5
Short-acting			
Regular	0.5-1	2-4	4-8
Intermediate-acting			
NPH	2-4	4-10	12-24
Lente	3-4	6-12	12-24
Long-acting			
Ultralente	4-6	6-12	18-24
Insulin Glargine	2-4	NA	24+
Premixed			
70/30 (70% NPH/30% Regular)	0.5-1	2-8	12-24
50/50 (50% NPH/50% Regular)	0.5-1	2-6	12-24
Mix 25 (75% NPH/25% Lispro)	0.25-0.5	1-2	12-24
Novolog Mix (70% NPH/30% Aspart)	0.25-0.5	1-2	12-24

Glargine, Aventis Pharmaceuticals, Bridgewater, NJ) daily plus rapid-acting analogue with each meal or snack. Clearly, the most appropriate regimen depends on the schedule and desire of the child and family.

CSII, or insulin pump therapy, has grown in popularity. Although programmable insulin pumps have been available for more than 20 years, technological advancements have made practical use feasible. Pump therapy more closely mimics the true physiological state, in that rapid-acting insulin is continuously infused at very low basal levels, with additional boluses for mealtime demands. Both the basal rates and bolus amounts are programmable. Multiple basal rates may be programmed, so that the normal early morning surge in blood glucose may be matched by an incremental increase in the insulin dose. Multiple studies in both adults and adolescents have demonstrated that CSII is associated with improvements in glycemic control, less weight gain, and less frequent hypoglycemia, and newer pump models assist in dose calculation for meals or hyperglycemia correction.

Self-Monitoring and Problem-Solving

It should be readily apparent from the discussion of intensive insulin therapy that the safety and success of any insulin regimen are dependent on frequent monitoring of blood glucose levels. Intensive diabetes control would have been impossible without the development of inexpensive, accurate, easy-to-use home glucose meters. There are many brands of glucose meters that are commercially available,

most of which have similar reliability and accuracy to within about 10% of laboratory measurements. Older models used a glucose oxidase–impregnated reagent strip that, when exposed to a drop of blood, underwent a color change that could be assayed spectrophotometrically by the meter and converted to a numerical value based on known calibration standards. Newer models instead rely on a peroxidase system that generates a small electric current, which is then converted to a numerical value based on calibration standards. The newer meters are faster (results in 5 versus 45 seconds) and require less blood (0.1 versus 1.0 µL). The smaller blood volume requirement has allowed alternate site lancing (forearm, thigh, calf), which may minimize discomfort and improve adherence to self-monitoring regimens.

Children with diabetes should routinely test the blood glucose 4 times daily (before meals and before bedtime) and record the results in a log for later review by the family and diabetes care team. A target range is established, typically 80 to 120 mg/dL at breakfast and 80 to 150 mg/dL at other times of day but may be altered based on the age of the child and the ability of the family. Ideally, 80% of the blood glucose values should fall within the target range. Information gained from frequent testing is used to titrate insulin dosages according to need. For example, a regular pattern of prebreakfast hyperglycemia should prompt the family to increase the bedtime long-acting insulin dose incrementally over several days until the majority of prebreakfast readings fall within the target range, whereas frequent hypoglycemia during school may suggest reducing the morning rapid- or intermediate-acting insulin. Additionally, supplemental insulin doses may be given when blood glucose values outside the target range are discovered, according to a predetermined formula. For example, a younger child with a pre-dinner blood glucose of 240 mg/dL may be given 1 extra unit of rapid-acting insulin analogue to reduce the blood glucose by 100 mg/dL in addition to the usual insulin dose at that mealtime. Supplemental blood glucose testing should be performed before exercise, during intercurrent illness, or after correction doses are given.

In addition to monitoring blood glucose concentrations, testing of the urine for ketones should be performed in the setting of chronic hyperglycemia or intercurrent illness. Families are instructed that the presence of urinary ketones indicates insulin deficiency, and supplemental doses of short- or rapid-acting insulin should be given frequently, along with fluids, until the ketones have "cleared." In this way, the progression to more severe ketoacidosis may be prevented in most situations.

Nutritional Management

Proper nutritional management is critical to the short- and long-term health of children with diabetes. Generally, terms such as "diet" should be avoided in favor of "meal plan," both for the negative connotation associated with the former and for the simple fact that nutritional requirements for normal growth and development are the same in diabetic and non-diabetic children. However, adherence to meal plans and accurate assessment of carbohydrate intake are important for optimal glycemic control.

The American Diabetes Association has adopted formal recommendations regarding general nutritional principles in diabetes, taking into account the short-term goals of blood glucose stabilization and the long-term goals of prevention/amelioration of macrovascular and microvascular complications of diabetes. The currently favored model of nutritional therapy is carbohydrate counting, based on the conceptual model of matching carbohydrate "doses" to insulin doses. As the carbohydrate content of foods has the greatest impact on blood glucose, the amount of carbohydrates ingested per meal or snack should be accurately assessed. Protein and fat intake, while important in the larger context of a healthy meal plan, are not counted to simplify the procedure. Recent changes in food labeling requirements have simplified the process, as most foods are clearly labeled with both the amount of carbohydrate grams per serving and the serving size. Foods less easily quantified may be weighed or estimated.

Two popular approaches to regulating carbohydrate intake are (1) consistent carbohydrate servings per meal/snack and (2) insulin-to-carbohydrate ratios. In the former, a standard amount of carbohydrates are eaten per meal or snack (e.g., 45 grams for breakfast, lunch, and dinner, and 30 grams each for midafternoon and bedtime snack). In this way, the insulin dose may be kept reasonably constant. In the latter, more flexible approach, there is no set intake. Rather, the child or parents decides upon the meal content, the carbohydrates are counted, and an insulin dose is calculated on the spot, based on a ratio of the number of insulin units per grams of carbohydrate. In younger children typical insulin to carbohydrate ratio is 1 unit: 15 gm, while an older child may require 1:10 and an insulin-resistant adolescent 1:5-7. Actual ratios of insulin to carbohydrates vary from child to child and may even vary in the same child from meal to meal or during periods of exercise.

Long-term goals of nutritional management of diabetes include maintenance of nutrient intake balance of about 50% carbohydrate, 20% protein, and 30% fat (of which no more than 10% should be saturated). Most important, growth and weight gain should be monitored, and regular follow-up with a dietitian trained in diabetes management should be encouraged to individualize a meal plan for each child based on his or her needs and food preferences.

Exercise and Physical Fitness

Establishment and maintenance of an active lifestyle should be a goal for all children, but they are especially important for children with diabetes. Exercise and increased physical fitness are associated with improved insulin sensitivity and glucose utilization, the clinical correlates of which are lower insulin requirements in general and, frequently, less pronounced blood glucose excursions after meals. Improvements in physical fitness are also frequently associated with greater self-esteem and motivation to participate in diabetes care.

The effects of exercise must be carefully considered in the context of the entire diabetes care plan, because episodic exercise may predispose to acute hypoglycemia if the insulin dose is not reduced or extra carbohydrates are added proactively. Furthermore, intense physical activity in the setting of insulin deficiency (chronically poor diabetes control or recent omission of insulin) may provoke metabolic decompensation and DKA. Children participating in school sports or other programs should be counseled to monitor blood glucose before, during, and after exercise, because the hypoglycemic effects of exercise may be delayed and/or prolonged over the next 12 to 18 hours. We frequently recommend the reduction of dinner/bedtime NPH and, for pump users, decreases in basal rates to account for these exercise effects.

Psychological Aspects

There are few disorders in childhood that affect as many aspects of life as does diabetes. A previously healthy child must rely on multiple injections of insulin daily as well as lance the skin of the fingertips, draw blood, and test for glucose levels as many as 6 to 8 times a day. Flexibility and spontaneity in meal timing and content are frequently sacrificed. School and recreational activities are interrupted by the necessity of attending to testing or injecting. The practical problem of carrying insulin bottles, syringes, lancets, and glucose records to school, on dates, and on vacations is a constant reminder of the disease and that the child with diabetes is different in nearly every way. At any time, embarrassing or dangerous hypoglycemic reactions may occur, and there is the gnawing, ever-present knowledge of the chronic complications and morbidity that may develop even with good metabolic control.

It is therefore imperative that the psychosocial functioning of the child and family is evaluated at diagnosis and periodically thereafter by the health care team, ideally a mental health professional. The diabetic child may be depressed, angry, or in denial of the severity of the disease. The parents may be feeling grief or guilt, especially if one of them has diabetes. Other siblings may be fearful of developing diabetes or jealous of the newfound attention that must be paid to the affected child. The additional stress of the diagnosis may sunder an already weakened family system to the point of divorce, violence, or neglect. Warning signs that require further psychosocial evaluation and intervention include declining school performance, isolation from friends and activities, new behavioral problems, and recurrent episodes of DKA. Frank depression and anorexia nervosa require referral to appropriate psychiatric services.

Medical Follow-up

The importance of frequent follow-up by the diabetes health care team cannot be overemphasized. At each visit, the blood glucose logbooks should be reviewed and appropriate dosage or schedule changes should be instituted as needed. A detailed interim history should include questions relating to general health, energy, fatigue, polyuria or nocturia, intercurrent illnesses, hypoglycemic episodes, and the presence of abdominal symptoms such as pain, bloating, or diarrhea. It is important to remember the comorbidities of other autoimmune disorders that occur with an increased frequency in children with T1DM: thyroiditis, adrenal insufficiency, and celiac disease. The child should be weighed and measured at each visit, and pulse and blood pressure also documented. Physical examination of the child should focus not only on the general organ systems

but also on examination of the skin and insulin injection/pump insertion sites (for signs of lipohypertrophy or pigmentary changes), palpation of the thyroid, and determination of the sexual development stage. In older children or those with longer diabetes duration, examination should include the feet. A deceleration in growth, delay in sexual development, or finding of goiter may herald hypothyroidism, which occurs in approximately 5% of children with T1DM. The astute clinician should also consider that frequent, unexplained hypoglycemia or reduction in insulin requirements in the absence of exercise or activity may be a subtle indicator of hypothyroidism or adrenal insufficiency. Similarly, although the history of frequent, foul-smelling, greasy diarrhea are more obvious indicators of celiac disease, which occurs in about 2% of children with T1DM, the presence of abdominal pain, poor weight gain, and unexplained hypoglycemia may be the first and only signs.

Measurement of Hb_{A1c} should be performed at each clinic visit. The Hb_{A1c} is an indirect indicator of the overall glycemic control based on the phenomenon that glucose binds in an irreversible, nonenzymatic manner to serum proteins at a rate proportional to the mean serum glucose concentration. The level of glycosylation of a given protein, therefore, depends on its exposure to glucose and its own rate of breakdown. For example, because the life span of the human red blood cell is about 90 to 120 days, measurement of glycosylated hemoglobin gives a measure of the mean glucose concentrations of the preceding 3 months. The most common measure of glycosylated hemoglobin is the Hb_{A1c}, and the conversion of the Hb_{A1c} to the mean blood glucose level may be estimated by the formula:

$$Glucose_{mean} \ (mg/dL) = [Hb_{A1c} \ (\%) \times 30] - 60$$

In children with decreased red cell survival time, however, such as occurs in sickle cell disease or spherocytosis, the Hb_{A1c} may be artificially low, because the time available for glycosylation is decreased. In these children, Hb_{A1c} measurements are not useful, and measurement of other glycosylated proteins, such as albumin, should be considered for analysis of long-term control.

The availability of small, portable laboratory equipment that measures the Hb_{A1c} with a small sample of capillary blood in the clinic setting and offers results within minutes has greatly benefited the diabetes clinician. In this way, the Hb_{A1c} may be reviewed with the family at the clinic visit and compared with the logs. Discrepancies between the logs and the Hb_{A1c} may suggest improper testing technique or, more seriously, falsification of the data. In the case of the latter, deeper questioning into the family dynamics and psychosocial functioning of the child is warranted.

Monitoring of the diabetic child for complications is an important function of the clinic visit, because many early complications do respond to prompt intervention. Urinary albumin excretion may be measured in a spot sample by comparison with urinary creatinine; the urinary albumin/creatinine ratio should be less than 30 mg albumin/1 g creatinine. Elevated spot samples should be confirmed by collections of first morning void or a timed overnight period to eliminate the confounding variable of benign orthostatic proteinuria. If the first morning void or timed overnight collection demonstrates microalbuminuria (>30 mg albumin/1 g creatinine, or >30 mg albumin excretion/24 hr), treatment with angiotensin-converting enzyme inhibitor or referral to pediatric nephrologist may be indicated. All diabetic children with hypertension, regardless of albumin excretion status, should be referred to a pediatric nephrologist for consideration of angiotensin-converting enzyme inhibitor therapy.

Other screening studies for complications of diabetes includes measurement of serum lipid concentrations and referral for dilated retinal examination, both of which should be performed on a yearly basis in all pubertal children with diabetes or even in prepubertal children with diabetes duration of at least 5 years. Current guidelines suggest maintaining serum low-density lipoprotein concentrations below 100 mg/dL and serum triglycerides below 150 mg/dL in adults with diabetes, but there are no published recommendations specifically for children. Treatment for hypercholesterolemia and hyperlipidemia should include intensification of diabetes control and dietary interventions. There are little data on the efficacy and safety of specific lipid-lowering therapeutic agents in the pediatric population.

Recent developments have brought some new promise in the areas of diabetes prevention and islet cell replacement. Preliminary studies involving newer immunomodulatory agents have demonstrated improved survival of transplanted islet cells and reversal of clinical diabetes in experimental animals. The well-publicized Edmonton protocol demonstrated that a nonsurgical transplantation of donor islet cells into the liver followed by a glucocorticoid-free immunosuppressive regimen allowed seven people with T1DM to remain insulin free and in good metabolic control for more than 1 year. These studies are now being replicated in multiple centers in the United States.

A simultaneous development in diabetes treatment has been the use of novel insulin delivery systems and glucose monitoring technologies. Clinical trials have shown inhaled insulin to be a potentially viable alternative to injection of rapid-acting insulin, and intraportal insulin delivery systems may hold some promise over current continuous subcutaneous insulin pumps. Minimally invasive blood glucose monitoring, using subcutaneous or transcutaneous sensors, at the present time function as adjuncts to routine finger-stick blood glucose monitoring and prototype systems in which these sensors communicate with insulin pumps in a "closed-loop system" are under development. Whether the next revolution in diabetes management will be such "artificial β-cell" systems or true islet cell replacement, the goal of all diabetes clinicians at this time should be to optimize the metabolic control in their patients to maintain their health and their hope until such treatments become routine.

CONCLUSIONS

The treatment of T1DM has evolved greatly since Leonard Thompson was given the first injection of insulin in 1921. In more than 80 years, T1DM has changed from a universally fatal disorder to an eminently manageable chronic condition, albeit one that requires a great deal of effort and expense to treat effectively. It is frequently said that insulin is not a cure for diabetes; the risk of long-term complications still looms large in the minds of diabetic patients and their loved ones.

Efforts to prevent or reverse T1DM have historically been disappointing. Clinical trials of glucocorticoids, cyclosporin, nicotinamide, insulin, and other immunomodulatory agents have not been shown to significantly reduce the risk of diabetes in high-risk subjects. Pancreatic transplants are complicated surgical procedures, and the small number of viable donor specimens and the necessity of long-term immunosuppressive therapy have limited their general applicability.

MAJOR POINTS

Diabetes is defined by the finding of an elevated blood glucose (BG); random BG greater than 200 mg/dL, fasting BG greater than 126 mg/dL, or, with an oral glucose tolerance test, 2-hour BG greater than 200 mg/dL.

T1DM occurs in approximately 1 in 350 children under age 18 in the United States; about 15 new cases occur per 100,000 children per year.

The gene or genes for T1DM are associated with the human leukocyte antigens of the major histocompatibility complex, located on chromosome 6.

T1DM is caused by an autoimmune-mediated destruction of pancreatic β-cells in genetically susceptible individuals after a triggering event, usually a viral infection.

At the present time, there is no available treatment to halt this autoimmune process and prevent the onset of T1DM.

The classic symptoms of polyuria, polydipsia, and weight loss occur in the majority of children with T1DM.

Continued

> ### ◄ MAJOR POINTS—Cont'd ►
>
> *Diabetic ketoacidosis* is defined as the presence of hyperglycemia (glucose >240 mg/dL), ketosis (positive serum or urinary ketones), and acidosis (pH < 7.30 and/or serum bicarbonate <15 mEq/L).
>
> The Diabetes Control and Complications Trial demonstrated that lowering mean BG levels dramatically reduced the incidence and progression of microvascular complications such as retinopathy, nephropathy, and neuropathy.
>
> Optimal management of children with T1DM includes insulin therapy, self-monitoring of blood glucose, medical nutrition therapy, exercise, and attention to the developmental and psychosocial needs of children dealing with chronic illness.
>
> Technological advances such as insulin pump therapy and continuous glucose monitoring offer the promise of artificial β-cell replacement therapy.

SUGGESTED READINGS

American Diabetes Association Task Force for Writing Nutrition Principles and Recommendations for the Management of Diabetes and Related Complications: American Diabetes Association position statement: evidence-based nutrition principles and recommendations for the treatment and prevention of diabetes and related complications, J Am Diet Assoc 2002;102:109.

American Diabetes Association: Standards of medical care for patients with diabetes mellitus, Diabetes Care 2002;25 (suppl 1):S33.

Becker DJ, Coonrod BA, Ellis D, et al: Influence of age, sex, blood pressure, and glycemic control on microalbuminuria in children and adolescents with IDDM. In Weber B, Berger W, Danner T, editors: Structural and Functional Abnormalities in Subclinical Diabetic Angiopathy, Basel, 1992, Karger.

Boland E, Grey M, Oesterle A, et al: Continuous subcutaneous insulin infusion: a new way to lower risk of severe hypoglycemia, improve metabolic control, and enhance coping in adolescents with type 1 diabetes mellitus, Diabetes Care 1999;22:1779.

Chase HP, Crews KR, Garg S, et al: Outpatient management vs. in-hospital management of children with new-onset diabetes, Clin Pediatr 1992;31:450.

Cryer PE: Hypoglycemia is the limiting factor in the management of diabetes, Diabetes Metab Res Rev 1999;15:42.

Diabetes Control and Complications Trial Research Group: Effect of intensive diabetes treatment on the development and progression of long-term complications in adolescents with insulin-dependent diabetes mellitus: Diabetes Control and Complications Trial, J Pediatr 1994;125:177.

Diabetes Control and Complications Trial Research Group: The effect of intensive treatment of diabetes on the development and progression of long-term complications in insulin-dependent diabetes mellitus, N Engl J Med 1993;329:977.

Diabetes Control and Complications Trial (DCCT)/Epidemiology of Diabetes Interventions and Complications (EDIC) Research Group: Beneficial effects of intensive therapy of diabetes during adolescence: outcomes after the conclusion of the Diabetes Control and Complications Trial (DCCT), J Pediatr 2001;139:804.

Duck SC, Wyatt DT: Factors associated with brain herniation in the treatment of diabetic ketoacidosis, J Pediatr 1988;113:10.

Glaser N, Barnett P, McCaslin I, et al: Risk factors for cerebral edema in children with diabetic ketoacidosis, N Engl J Med 2001;344:264.

Gregory RP, Davis DL: Use of carbohydrate counting for meal planning in type 1 diabetes, Diabetes Educator 1994;20:406.

Harris GD, Fiordalisi I, Harris WL, et al: Minimizing the risk of brain herniation during treatment of diabetic ketoacidemia: a retrospective and prospective study. J Pediatr 1990;117:22.

Harris GD, Fiordalisi I: Physiologic management of diabetic ketoacidemia: a 5-year prospective pediatric experience in 231 episodes, Arch Pediatr Adolesc Med 1994;148:1046.

Rovet JF: Diabetes. In Yeates KO, Ris MD, Taylor HG, editors: Pediatric Neuropsychology: Research, Theory, and Practice, New York, 2000, Guilford Press.

Sanders LJ: A Philatelic History of Diabetes, Alexandria, VA, 2001, American Diabetes Association.

Shapiro AM, Lakey JR, Ryan EA, et al: Islet transplantation in seven patients with type 1 diabetes mellitus using a glucocorticoid-free immunosuppressive regimen, N Engl J Med 2000;343:230.

Sochett E, Daneman D: Early diabetes-related complications in children and adolescents with type 1 diabetes: implications for screening and intervention, Endocrinol Metab Clin North Am 1999;28:865.

Tamborlane WV, Bonfig W, Boland E: Recent advances in treatment of youth with type 1 diabetes: better care through technology, Diabet Med 2001;18:864.

CHAPTER 2

Type 2 Diabetes Mellitus in Children and Adolescents

DANIEL E. HALE

STUART A. WEINZIMER

INTRODUCTION

Although there have been case reports of type 2 diabetes mellitus (T2DM) in individuals less than 18 years of age as early as 1979, until recently these cases were viewed as interesting phenomena rather than as the harbingers of an epidemic. However, by 1998, it was apparent that T2DM was increasingly seen in all pediatric endocrine centers with substantial minority populations. In response to concerns raised by pediatric endocrinologists in the United States and Canada, meetings took place at the Texas Department of Health (Austin, Texas), the Centers for Disease Control and Prevention (CDC) (Atlanta, Georgia), and the

National Institutes of Health (Washington, D.C.). Subsequently, an expert committee sponsored by the American Diabetes Association (ADA) and the American Academy of Pediatrics (AAP) formulated a statement acknowledging that T2DM was now a pediatric problem, and specific guidelines for screening for this condition were published. In response, the CDC, the NIH, and other public and private institutions announced plans for funding research projects to establish the prevalence of T2DM in the pediatric population, to develop strategies for prevention, and to initiate pediatric-specific pharmaceutical and behavioral treatment trials. Most of these initiatives and projects are now in their first or second year; others are still in the planning phases.

As a consequence of the relatively recent widespread acknowledgment that T2DM is also a pediatric disease, there are few peer-reviewed publications on the treatment of T2DM in children and adolescents. Therefore, until clinical trials demonstrate clear efficacy of a specific approach, the approach to the management of pediatric T2DM is drawn from four primary sources: experience with type 1 diabetes (T1DM) in children, understanding of T2DM in adults, knowledge about obesity in children, and clinical experience of pediatric endocrinologists with children with T2DM.

With reference to pediatric T1DM and adult T2DM, scholarly papers, erudite books, and innovative continuing medical education programs are widely available and cover every aspect of treatment from glycemic control to birth control, from hypertension to hypothyroidism, and insulin resistance to insulin pump therapy. There is more than 70 years' worth of knowledge and experience with T1DM in children as they progress from home care to school care, from dependence to independence, and from childhood to parenthood. Strategies for dealing with these transitions, as well as with day-to-day management, and the integration of

T1DM into family life are generally accepted and used by the pediatric diabetes community. Although T1DM management is evolving at a rapid pace, there is strong consensus on the major goals and ideal outcomes of T1DM treatment. Similarly, there is a vast experience with the effective management of T2DM in adults, a sizable array of medications for achieving glycemic control, and broad agreement on the aims and optimal outcomes of T2DM management. There is an increasing literature on the effective treatment of pediatric obesity. This is of particular relevance to pediatric T2DM, given the central role of obesity in the pathogenesis of this condition. Finally, there are pediatric endocrinologists in North America who have substantial clinical experience in the treatment of pediatric T2DM and have been willing to share their expertise. In the following sections, the basic pathophysiology of T2DM is briefly summarized, the diagnostic issues are reviewed, and the concepts and experiences from diverse sources are united into a coherent plan for the management of pediatric T2DM.

PATHOPHYSIOLOGY OF TYPE 2 DIABETES MELLITUS

It is increasingly clear that both insulin resistance and β-cell dysfunction, and the resultant relative or absolute insulin deficiency, play a role in the etiology of T2DM. Assessment of the relative contribution of each to the pathogenesis of T2DM is confounded by methodological problems in examining β-cell function; insulin secretion and action are physiologically interconnected, so that an initial defect in either is likely to lead to a deficit in the other function over time. Both insulin resistance and impaired insulin release precede and predict T2DM in prospective studies in adults. Genetic analysis has not yet provided definitive answers as to the basic molecular defect in T2DM that would elucidate true etiological factors.

Several important factors support the role of insulin resistance in the etiology of T2DM. Insulin resistance is found in the majority of patients, even in the earlier stages of impaired glucose tolerance, and predicts subsequent development of the T2DM in prediabetic and normoglycemic states. Insulin resistance is only partially reversible by any form of treatment. A key cellular mechanism of skeletal muscle insulin resistance (defective stimulation of glucose transport, phosphorylation, and glycogen storage) is detectable not only in individuals with T2DM but also in normoglycemic offspring of affected individuals.

Given the tight homeostatic control of glucose, relative or complete β-cell dysfunction is a sine qua non for the development of diabetes. Although the defect in insulin secretion in T2DM is functionally severe, β-cell mass is reduced by only 20% to 40% in patients with long-standing T2DM. Moreover, the insulin secretory deficit is worsened with hyperglycemia and recovers, at least partially, on improving glycemic control. This suggests that part of the β-cell dysfunction is acquired (via glucose toxicity, lipotoxicity, or both). Further, although insulin insufficiency is necessary for diabetes, it may not be sufficient to cause T2DM. Subtle defects in β-cell response to glucose may be widespread in the population and cause hyperglycemia only when obesity and insulin resistance stress the secretory capacity of the β-cell.

DIAGNOSIS AND DIFFERENTIATION OF TYPE 2 DIABETES MELLITUS

Diagnosis of Diabetes

The diagnosis of diabetes is based solely on the blood glucose level. These guidelines are clearly delineated in publications from the ADA and are summarized in Box 2-1.

Diagnosis of Type 2 Diabetes Mellitus and Differentiation From Type 1 Diabetes Mellitus

A basic tenet of pediatric diabetes has been that there was no need to screen for diabetes because all children with diabetes would eventually develop severe symptoms and seek medical care. Although this is true for T1DM, it may not be the case for T2DM. In adults, about 40% of those

---

Box 2-1 Criteria for the Diagnosis of Diabetes Mellitus

The diagnosis of diabetes may be made using **any one*** of the following criteria:
1. Symptoms and a casual plasma glucose of ≥200 mg/dL (11.1 mmol/L). Symptoms include polyuria, polydipsia, and unexplained weight loss. *Casual* is defined as any time of day, without regard to the time of last meal.
2. Fasting plasma glucose of ≥126 mg/dL (7.0 mmol/L). *Fasting* is defined as no caloric intake for 8 hours.
3. Two-hour postprandial glucose of ≥200 mg/dL (11.1 mmol/L) on an oral glucose tolerance test. An oral glucose tolerance test requires the equivalent of 1.75 g/kg (to a maximum of 75 grams) of anhydrous glucose dissolved in water.

*In the absence of overt hyperglycemia with acute metabolic decompensation, these criteria should be confirmed by repeat testing on a different day.

affected by T2DM are unaware of their condition. Because there have been no widespread screening studies for diabetes in the pediatric population, it is impossible to estimate the number of children with T2DM, whether diagnosed or undiagnosed before the screening.

Of those children known to have T2DM, the great majority have been members of high-risk ethnic or minority groups, including Native Americans (First Nations Peoples in Canada), African Americans, Hispanics (Mexican Americans, Puerto Ricans), and Pacific Islanders (Guamese and Samoans). However, a number of pediatric diabetes centers are now reporting non-Hispanic white children with T2DM, so T2DM should be considered as a possible diagnosis in children of all ethnic and racial groups.

Family history may be helpful in distinguishing T1DM from T2DM. Only about 3% of first-degree relatives of children with T1DM have T1DM. In contrast, T2DM is much more prevalent in the families of children with T2DM, ranging from 48% to 99%. Thus, a strong family history of diabetes is more suggestive of T2DM or maturity-onset diabetes of youth than of T1DM. At the time of diagnosis, the majority of children with T2DM are 10 years old or older. However, younger children with T2DM have been reported: the youngest Pima child reported was age 4; Mexican American, age 6; and African American, age 8. Most youth with T2DM present in midpuberty or postpubertally. The onset of puberty is associated with increased production of growth hormone that in turn increases insulin resistance. It is possible that the onset of puberty plays a role in transforming covert insulin resistance into overt-type T2DM in the overweight, genetically susceptible child.

The medical history is often helpful in the differentiation of T2DM from T1DM. In contrast to the relatively rapid onset of T1DM, youth with T2DM may have symptoms or signs for months or even years before the diagnosis. The classic triad of polyuria, polydipsia, and polyphagia, especially when accompanied by weight loss, usually leads to the correct diagnosis in T1DM. In contrast, the signs and symptoms of T2DM may be missed in the adolescent. Polyphagia may be interpreted as a normal adolescent eating pattern, polyuria may not be observed because the bathroom habits of teenagers are generally not topics of family discussion, and high-volume fluid intake is viewed as normal, particularly in warmer climates. Furthermore, weight loss in an obese adolescent may be viewed a positive event or attributed to other factors (e.g., loss of "baby fat," normal response to adolescent growth spurt) and therefore may not prompt a visit to the physician. Although large prospective descriptive studies have not been undertaken, symptoms such as nocturia, recurrent vaginal or urinary tract infections, and unintentional weight loss in a youth who

has been overweight for a prolonged period of time may be indicative of new-onset T2DM.

On physical examination, there are some findings that may lead the clinician to suspect the diagnosis, although these abnormalities are also common in obese children without T2DM. Almost all children with T2DM are overweight or obese at the time of diagnosis. In San Antonio, Texas, 97% of children with T2DM had a body mass index (BMI) of greater than 20 kg/m^2 and 83% of children had BMI of greater than 25 kg/m^2. Most children with T2DM are at, or above, the expected height for age and demonstrate advanced sexual development for age, likely related to hyperinsulinemia. Some affected youth appear cushingoid, with round faces, prominent cheeks, and facial redness. An occasional adolescent may appear acromegalic with prominent jaws and large hands and feet. Acanthosis nigricans (AN) is present in the majority of children with T2DM, although it is also a very common finding in obese children without T2DM. Generally, AN is thought to reflect insulin resistance rather than diabetes per se. Clinical experience suggests that the appearance and disappearance of AN may lag substantially behind changes in body weight. AN is also easier to detect in some groups of children (e.g., Mexican American) than in other groups of children (e.g., non-Hispanic white). In some series, AN has been shown to be the most reliable differentiating factor between T1DM and T2DM.

The physical findings may be affected by the duration of obesity, rapidity of onset, and alterations in lifestyle that have occurred before the medical evaluation. For example, children who have experienced recent rapid weight gain may have significant striae over the lower abdomen and hips, whereas the child who has been steadily gaining weight since infancy may have few or no striae. The adolescent who has intentionally lost 20 pounds in the 6 to 8 weeks before the office visit may have substantial fading of AN.

Screening for Diabetes in Asymptomatic Children

The expert panel convened by the ADA in 2000 to address T2DM in youth published recommendations for screening, as given in Box 2-2.

Initial Laboratory Evaluation of Children with T2DM

The majority of children with T2DM are not ill enough to require hospitalization at the time of diagnosis. Table 2-1 summarizes the laboratory tests that should be considered in the child presenting with signs or symptoms suggestive of diabetes or in the child who has been found to be hyperglycemic on screening.

Box 2-2 Criteria for Screening for Diabetes in Asymptomatic Children

IF	AND ANY 2 OF THE FOLLOWING ARE PRESENT	AND	THEN
Body mass index is >85% for age and gender	High-risk ethnic group Family history of diabetes mellitus Sign or symptom associated with type 2 diabetes mellitus, including hyperlipidemia, hypertension, polycystic ovarian syndrome	Physical signs of puberty *Or* Age ≥10 years	Screen*

*Screening should be done every 2 years in the absence of symptoms. The preferred method of screening is a fasting plasma glucose test.

Table 2-1 Laboratory Tests at the Time of Initial Presentation

	Laboratory Test	Rationale and Commentary
Glucose related	Fasting glucose Oral glucose tolerance test Fasting plasma insulin C-peptide Hb_{A1c}	An elevated glucose is required for diagnosis (see Box 2-1). The insulin and C-peptide levels are often elevated in type 2 diabetes mellitus (T2DM) and may be useful in the diagnosis of T2DM. For youth who are acidotic or who have experienced significant weight loss, these may be low secondary to "glucose toxicity." An Hb_{A1c} that is normal does not rule out T2DM; however, an elevated Hb_{A1c} suggests persistent hyperglycemia and guides the choice of initial therapy.
Lipids	Triglycerides Total cholesterol High-density lipoprotein cholesterol	Hyperlipidemia is a common finding in individuals with T2DM and the leading cause of mortality. If the child is acutely ill, it is recommended that these studies be deferred until glycemic control is well established.
Thyroid	T_4 (or free T_4) Thyroid-stimulating hormone	Hypothyroidism at the time of diagnosis is uncommon; however, this establishes a baseline.
Liver	ALT, AST Total and direct bilirubin	In adults, 5% to 10% with T2DM have nonalcoholic fatty liver disease (NAFLD). If the liver enzymes are elevated >3 times normal, this may affect the choice of medication. If persistently elevated, a liver biopsy or a search for other etiologies is recommended.
Gonadal (pubertal females)	Luteinizing hormone, follicle-stimulating hormone, androstenedione, dehydroepiandrosterone sulfate	Hyperandrogenism, hirsutism, dysmenorrhea, and polycystic ovarian syndrome are common in obese girls. Correction of these may occur with weight loss or reduction of hyperinsulinemia.
Islet cell	Anti–islet cell antibodies Anti-GAD65 antibodies	If negative, these rule out type 1 diabetes mellitus (T1DM); however, 10% to 20% of adults with clinical picture of T2DM have positive antibodies. Positivity increases the likelihood that the patient requires insulin treatment. Lack of positivity is supportive of the diagnosis of T2DM (or other non-T1DM types of diabetes, such as maturity-onset diabetes of youth [MODY]).
Kidney	Protein (microalbumin), blood urea nitrogen, creatinine	The true duration of diabetes in generally unknown in T2DM. These tests ensure that there is no evidence of overt dysfunction at diagnosis and establish a baseline. If protein is not found on urinalysis, then urine should be tested for microalbuminuria.
Specialty testing	24-Hour urinary free cortisol	Cushing syndrome should be considered in some cases (e.g., the child is short for age).
	Insulin-like growth factor-I	Acromegaly must be considered if the youth has consistent clinical findings (prominent jaw, large hands and feet, etc.).
	MODY genes	These studies are not all commercially available. They may be of use in the evaluation of the atypical patient (e.g., the nonobese male who does not require insulin). The identification of a MODY variant has implications for treatment. Presently, the diagnosis of MODY is often made on clinical grounds.

MANAGEMENT OF TYPE 2 DIABETES MELLITUS

General Principles

Given the primary role of obesity and insulin resistance in the pathophysiology of T2DM, the major focus of management must be placed on those strategies that address these problems (e.g., reducing caloric intake, decreasing fat mass). Implementation of effective dietary and exercise strategies is of utmost priority, which as necessary should be supported by self-monitoring of blood glucose and medication.

Before addressing treatment per se, it is essential to consider the treatment environment and how it differs between T1DM and T2DM. This environment includes the health care system, the social milieu, cultural attitudes, family dynamics, economic trends, and political climate. Most currently practicing pediatricians had some exposure to T1DM in children during their training; can access general pediatric textbooks detailing the pathophysiology, diagnosis, and treatment of T1DM; and can consult competent pediatric endocrinologists in their communities. In contrast, few active pediatricians had any exposure to T2DM in children during their training, there is minimal information on T2DM in general pediatrics, and only a limited number of pediatric endocrinologists have experience with T2DM. Many of the medications used to treat T2DM and its comorbidities are not yet tested or approved for use in the pediatric population, so there is minimal literature on any unique benefits or problems related to their use in children. Some studies that address these issues are under way or in the planning phase.

As in many chronic disease models, family structure, culture, and belief systems have a significant impact on how the family perceives and manages T2DM in youth. In contrast to T1DM, almost all children with T2DM are adolescents: most are in middle school or high school. Although the implications specific to T2DM have not been explored, there are well-documented developmental and social differences that occur with the onset of adolescence. Children newly diagnosed with T1DM are often significantly symptomatic at diagnosis, 40% to 80% may be hospitalized, and as many as half of those require intensive care. On the other hand, few children with T2DM have severe symptoms at diagnosis, and even fewer require hospitalization or intensive care. Most families of children with T1DM have little or no experience with diabetes, whereas most families of children with T2DM have one or more family members already affected by the disease. In the former case, diabetes is unfamiliar and frightening, whereas in the latter case, diabetes is familiar and the only threat is perceived to be in the far future, if at all. Furthermore, in the case of T2DM, not only is diabetes familiar but also the affected family members often have been unsuccessful in adequately managing their diabetes. Access to health care may be more limited for children with T2DM: it is well documented that minority communities have less access to care due to both geographic (e.g., fewer neighborhood health care providers) and economic (e.g., fewer children with health insurance) issues.

Eating behaviors, food preferences, and food choices are largely established in early childhood and are often limited by parental experience, background, and income. Families in which multiple caretakers work to support the family may have limited time to prepare healthful, lower-calorie meals, opting instead for less-nutritious, higher-fat "fast" foods. Even if efforts are made to prepare food at home, supermarkets may be less accessible to economically challenged families, who then purchase their groceries at corner convenience stores, where fresh fruits and vegetables may be more expensive, of lower quality, and less available.

There is a common perception that obesity is a significant source of social distress or discomfort to adolescents. This may be true is some communities but is by no means true in all communities. In schools where 45% of the children are overweight or obese, there may be no adverse social consequences (e.g., teasing) related to being overweight. In fact, there may be some advantages to being overweight, because the youth with T2DM often is taller than average and more sexually mature.

Even for motivated, educated, middle-class adults, weight control or weight loss is difficult. As a consequence, weekly meetings or weekly visits are a routine part of most of popular weight loss programs. In the successful pediatric obesity programs, the initial intervention requires weekly interactions for several weeks, followed by biweekly or monthly reinforcement for an additional time period. It is unrealistic to think that effective strategies for weight loss, or related behaviors, that are crucial to T2DM management can be instituted and sustained with the quarterly visit to the diabetes clinic that has been standard for T1DM care. Therefore, a key element of T2DM care is frequent contact. Other components of management include family involvement, school participation, and health care team familiarity with the individual child, as well as the child's family, neighborhood, and school.

Clarity and simplicity are the key concepts in managing adolescents and children with T2DM. Youth, like adults, have competing priorities that often interfere with diabetes management. Furthermore, the capacity of youth for long-term planning is limited. Within this context, it is crucial that the diabetes care team understands the individual youth's priorities and attempts to match those priorities with those of diabetes care—a task that is made more difficult by the reticence of many teenagers to talk openly to any adult. It is imperative to sharply limit the goals of any particular interaction and to provide education consistent with the adolescent's life experience and education.

Medical Nutrition Therapy

The goals of medical nutrition therapy are to normalize serum glucose and lipid levels, achieve weight loss or stabilization, and develop healthy and sustainable eating habits. There are no dietary guidelines specific to children and adolescents with T2DM. Until such guidelines are developed, the ADA guidelines for adults with T2DM should be adequate and appropriate, as summarized in Box 2-3. The safety and efficacy of alternative approaches to dietary restrictions and modifications (high fat, low fat, high protein, low carbohydrate) in children with obesity, insulin resistance, or T2DM have not been established. Although carbohydrate counting is now widely used for children with T1DM, it is not always a wise choice for the adolescent with T2DM because there is a greater need to be attentive to the total caloric content as well as to the amount and composition of the fats. From a practical point of view, some of the more complex concepts such as "calorie" and "ratio and proportion" are beyond the educational level of many children and parents. Greater benefit may be achieved by focusing on eating behaviors rather than on food choice and caloric content per se. Finally, concern has been expressed regarding encouraging weight loss in children and possible dire consequences on adult height and psyche. However, weight stabilization or modest supervised weight loss in overweight children is safe; therefore, it is reasonable to assume that the same is true with regard to weight loss in children with T2DM.

Educational efforts must be targeted at all individuals who make choices about the child's meals: the adolescent, parents, grandparents, school cafeteria personnel, and after-school program personnel. In general, the initial focus is on the person who is most responsible for the youth's intake. For the younger adolescent with T2DM, this is often the

parent or grandparent. The older adolescent may in large part be responsible for his or her own intake and have an independent source of money from a job or access to food through a job or school. Dietary education is guided by the education and sophistication of the family and by their willingness and ability to make requisite dietary changes. Some core principles that can be taught to most families and children with T2DM concern eating regular meals, eliminating unnecessary calories, limiting portion size, reading labels, having low-calorie foods and beverages accessible, avoiding eating in front of the television, and making the process a "team effort."

Physical Activity

Some background on contemporary levels of physical activity may serve to reinforce both the critical importance of getting all children to be more physically active and the stark sociocultural environment that works contrary to this recommendation. Regular participation in physical activity during childhood and adolescence has been demonstrated to help develop and maintain healthy bones, muscles, and joints; control weight, increase lean muscle, and reduce fat; prevent, delay, or reverse the development of hypertension in some adolescents; and reduce feelings of depression and anxiety. There is also evidence that regular physical activity may improve academic performance and social well-being. With respect to children with T2DM, additional benefits such as improved glycemic control, insulin sensitivity, and hyperlipidemia would also be expected.

Despite these proven benefits, a 1999 survey of physical activity from a nationally representative sample of students in grades 9 to 12 showed that among U.S. high school students, 35% did not participate regularly in vigorous physical activity, 44% did not play on any sports teams, 44% were not enrolled in a physical education (PE) class, and only 29% attended daily PE classes. Activity also decreased with age: regular participation in vigorous physical activity dropped from 73% of 9th graders to 61% of 12th graders, and enrollment in PE dropped from 79% in 9th grade to 37% in 12th grade.

There are no specific recommendations related to exercise for children with T2DM. Until the time that such recommendations are available, general guidelines for children, established by the AAP, should be the benchmark. Many children with T2DM are overweight and poorly conditioned, so appropriate modifications may need to be made. Reasonable activity guidelines are 60 minutes of age-appropriate and developmentally appropriate physical activity from a variety of activities every day of the week, of which at least 30 minutes should be aerobic. Physical activity other than formal exercise should be incorporated into

Box 2-3 Nutrient Intake and Distribution	
NUTRIENT	**DISTRIBUTION**
Protein	10-20% of total calories
Total fat	<20% of total calories
Saturated fat	<10% of total calories
Polyunsaturated fat	<10% of total calories
Carbohydrate	>60% of total calories
Fiber	25-35 g/day
Sodium	<3000 mg/day

all aspects of daily life, such as walking to and from school, biking to friends' homes, walking the dog, climbing stairs in public buildings, and parking in the parking lot at the maximum distance from the store or shopping mall. Youth with T2DM should not be excused from the requirements for PE at school. Instead, PE teachers should assist the youth in steadily increasing activity throughout the school year. Participation in organized physical activity should be actively encouraged, facilitated, and promoted by the family, school, after-school program, and neighborhood organizations.

As a general rule, the major problems seen in adulthood that might preclude or limit physical activity are rarely seen in youth, and therefore the investigation for these problems as a prelude to the development of an exercise program is not usually indicated. Hypertension does not prevent participation in physical activity, but there are specific guidelines approved by the AAP for evaluation and monitoring of hypertensive youth participating in various physical activities. Orthopedic evaluation of the joints of lower body (hips, knees, ankles) may be required if the child already has complaints about pain or discomfort in these areas. Pulmonary problems such as asthma should not be allowed to interfere with physical activity.

Critical to the success of an exercise program, like a diet program, is individualization. Whatever program is initiated should be fun for the child, use available facilities, and, when possible, incorporate other family members or friends as "exercise partners."

Attention should be paid not only to active behaviors but also to sedentary behaviors, the majority of which revolve around television, video, and video games. The average child currently watches more that 3 hours of television and/or video each day. A recent study found that 32% of 2- to 7-year-olds and 65% of 8- to 18-year-olds have television sets in their bedrooms. Time spent with various media may displace other more active pursuits, such as exercising or playing with friends.

The goal of the AAP is to reduce utilization of television to less than 2 hours per day. This goal is equally applicable to children and adolescents with T2DM. The putative benefits include increasing caloric expenditure as a result of increased movement and decreasing caloric intake due to "unconscious eating" (snacking while watching television with little attention to portion control).

Most families and physicians are completely unaware of the AAP recommendations regarding television use. Few families have ever actually considered the amount of time that the child watches television or the impact of advertising on their child. Increasing awareness of the consequences of sedentary behaviors and limiting television or video time are important steps to meeting activity goals.

Diabetes Medications

The primary goal of treatment with medication is normalization of the glycosylated hemoglobin. Secondary goals include weight stabilization or weight loss, and normalization of blood pressure and hyperlipidemia. This should be addressed in such a way as to minimize frequency of medication administration, side effects, and interference with daily routines and schedules.

Because T2DM is a relatively new entity for pediatric endocrinologists and diabetologists, published reports of therapy are in large part anecdotal and based on personal experience and bias rather than controlled clinical trials. The ADA consensus panel consisting of eight experts in diabetes in children, complemented by representatives from National Institute of Diabetes and Digestive and Kidney Diseases (NIDDK), the CDC, and the AAP, developed a position paper on the treatment of children with T2DM. The recommendations are that for asymptomatic or mildly symptomatic children, initial management should consist of medical nutrition therapy with behavior modification strategies for lifestyle changes. If treatment goals are not met (hemoglobin A1c [Hb_{A1c}] <7% and fasting blood glucose [FBG] <126 mg/dL), pharmacological therapy is indicated. The first oral agent recommended is metformin, which is now approved by the Food and Drug Administration (FDA) for use in children with T2DM. In a 16-week double-blind placebo-controlled trial of metformin in new-onset T2DM in children, metformin resulted in significantly lower Hb_{A1c} (7.5% versus 8.6%, $P < 0.001$) and lower FBG (−43 mg/dL versus +21 mg/dL, $P < 0.001$) compared with placebo. Metformin was well tolerated, with adverse event rates similar to those observed in the adult population. Intensification of therapy is recommended when monotherapy with metformin is not successful over a 3- to 6-month period. Intensification may include oral insulin secretagogues, alternative or additional insulin sensitizers (e.g., thiazolidinediones [TZDs]), or exogenous insulin therapy.

For the patient who is symptomatic at presentation with evidence of severe insulin deficiency and greatly elevated blood glucose and Hb_{A1c}, with or without ketonuria, the recommendation is to initiate insulin therapy. When glucose control is established, metformin could be added with tapering of insulin, if feasible. A survey of 130 clinical practices of members of the Lawson Wilkins Pediatric Endocrine Society in North America revealed that approximately 48% of youth with T2DM were treated with insulin (typically twice a day) and 44% were treated with oral hypoglycemic agents. Among the latter, 71% received metformin, 46% received sulfonylureas, 9% received TZDs, and 4% received a meglitinide (non-sulfonylurea secretagogue). Some would argue in favor of using insulin on all children who are newly diagnosed with T2DM. It is our opinion that insulin usage in T2DM places an overemphasis on medication, when this should be the third priority of treatment. Obviously insulin is important and required for the minority of children presenting with ketoacidosis or hyperosmolar nonketotic dehydration, or when optimal control cannot be achieved with oral therapy.

As is the case with T1DM, the type of insulin to be used is dependent on the child's pattern of eating and activity. Therefore, insulin treatment alone, or in combination with insulin-sensitizing agents, must be individualized. Even if the child is to be managed with diet and exercise alone or with oral agents, all families and adolescents should be taught how to inject insulin and instructed on the circumstances under which to use it, such as intercurrent illness with vomiting, high blood glucose, and large urinary ketones. These special circumstances and procedures should be reviewed at least on an annual basis. For acute illness in T2DM, we prefer to use regular insulin, primarily because it has a longer half-life than the analogue insulins Humalog

(Lispro, Eli Lilly and Company, Indianapolis, IN) and Novolog (Aspart, Novo Nordisk, Bagsvaerd, Denmark). For chronic use, the major problem associated with insulin use is increased weight gain. This must be balanced against the risks of poor glycemic control.

Premixed insulins (70/30, 50/50, Mix 25 [Eli Lilly and Company, Indianapolis, IN], Novolog Mix [Novo Nordisk, Bagsvaerd, Denmark]) are often a mainstay of therapy for children with T2DM near the time of diagnosis. Their use obviates the need for insulin mixing and minimizes the number of medications and procedures that the family must learn. In our experience, it has been well tolerated and well accepted. There have been rare problems with hypoglycemia, which has almost always been associated with vigorous physical activity in the preceding 12 hours or after a prolonged period of decreased or absent intake. If the child requires insulin as initial therapy, we prefer to use 70/30, Mix 25, or Novolog Mix BID almost exclusively, with initial doses of 0.5 to 1 unit/kg/day. It is not unusual to use substantially more (2 units/kg/day), especially in the first

Table 2-2   Insulin Use in Type 2 Diabetes Mellitus

Insulin Type	Comments
Rapid (analogue) Humalog Novolog	Analog insulin is typically used preprandially to reduce postprandial hyperglycemia. It improves the postprandial glycemic profile compared with regular insulin and is associated with less late postprandial hypoglycemia.
Short-acting Humulin R Novolin R	Short-acting insulin is used preprandially to reduce postprandial hyperglycemia. It may result in more hypoglycemia in the postprandial period than the analogue insulins. It is used acutely during significant illness and surgery when oral intake of medications is precluded.
Intermediate-acting Humulin N Novolin N Humulin L Novolin L	In adults, intermediate-acting insulin has a lower risk of hypoglycemia than Ultralente, at least when used on a single-dose-a-day regimen given at bedtime. A single bedtime dose of $\cong 0.25$ unit/kg is widely used to reduce fasting glucose. Some adolescents respond favorably to 2 injections per day of an intermediate-acting alone or, in combination with an analogue or short-acting insulin, as a supplement to insulin sensitizers.
Long-acting Ultralente	Humulin Ultralente is used as a basal insulin supplement to oral medications. In adult clinical trials, this has a higher risk of hypoglycemia than insulin Glargine or NPH. We have minimal experience using Ultralente in children and adolescents with T2DM.
Sustained action Insulin Glargine Lantus	Insulin Glargine is used as a supplement to oral medications. In adults, it results in improved glycemic control and lower Hb_{A1c} compared with NPH or Ultralente, with a lower risk of hypoglycemia. A regimen of evening (either presupper or bedtime) insulin Glargine ($\cong 0.4$ unit/kg) has been well tolerated in adolescents and anecdotally improved glycemic control.
Premixed	Premixed insulins are used as a supplement to insulin sensitizers. Head-to-head comparison with patient-mixed insulin has not been reported. The theoretical advantage is simplicity (see text). These have been used in adolescents on both an HS and a BID schedule.

few days or weeks after diagnosis or when the youth has an intercurrent infection. The dosage is generally divided with about 65% given in the morning and 35% given in the evening, but the distribution varies significantly, depending on the child's eating and physical activity patterns (e.g., many adolescents have the great majority of their calories between 4 PM and 10 PM and therefore need relatively more insulin in the evening dose than in the morning dose). We have some experience in using insulin Glargine (Aventis Pharmaceuticals, Bridgewater, NJ) in combination with repaglinide (Prandin, Novo Nordisk, Bagsvaerd, Denmark) in place of Humalog or Novolog in several teenagers with T2DM with a variable eating pattern: this has been successful in improving Hb$_{A1c}$ and glycemic control without leading to weight gain. Table 2-2 reviews the types of insulin preparations currently available and their use in T2DM.

Insulin-Sensitizing Agents

Metformin is an insulin sensitizer that improves glycemic control by enhancing liver insulin sensitivity, reducing hepatic gluconeogenesis, and possibly by improving muscle insulin sensitivity. It has been in clinical use for more than 40 years and is proved to be efficacious and safe in adults. It is the only oral antidiabetic agent that is approved by the FDA for use in children with T2DM. The majority of youth with T2DM are obese with significant insulin resistance. A weight-stabilizing effect has been reported in adult studies, and this may be an added benefit of metformin. In the United Kingdom Prospective Diabetes Study (UKPDS), metformin was the only medication that reduced diabetes-related death, heart attack, and stroke. Metformin has beneficial effects on cardiovascular risk factors, including dyslipidemia, elevated plasminogen activator inhibitor I levels, and other fibrinolytic abnormalities. The major serious potential complication of metformin is lactic acidosis, which should not occur if prescribing guidelines for metformin are followed. In the clinical trial of metformin in pediatric patients, the medication was well tolerated: similar side effects to those reported in adult studies, such as flatulence and diarrhea, were reported by subjects with a similar frequency (20% to 30%). The side effects tended to resolve within 2 weeks and were less likely to occur if the initial dose was low ($\leq$500 mg BID). In most cases, adult doses and dosing schedules are indicated, because almost all youth with T2DM have body weights approaching or exceeding those of the average adult. Extended action forms of metformin (Glucophage XR, Bristol-Myers Squibb, New York, NY) and combinations of metformin and glyburide (Glucovance, Briston-Myers Squibb) have become available for adults. A pediatric clinical trial is under way for Glucovance. Anecdotally, both the extended-release form of metformin

(Glucophage XR) and the metformin/glyburide combination (Glucovance) have been well tolerated in pediatric patients and effective in improving compliance and glycemic control.

There is very little pediatric experience with the TZDs rosiglitazone (Avandia, GlaxoSmithKline, Philadelphia, PA) and pioglitazone (Actos, Takeda Pharmaceuticals, Lincolnshire, IL), although pediatric clinical trials are under way. TZDs are potent insulin-sensitizing agents that can reverse insulin resistance and profoundly improve many of the features of the dysmetabolic syndrome. These compounds appear to enhance insulin action by modulating the activity of the nuclear receptor peroxisome proliferator-activated receptor-γ. In adult clinical trials, TZDs were effective, safe, and well tolerated, not only when used as monotherapy but also when used in combination with sulfonylureas or metformin. A potential advantage of the TZDs is that they may preserve β-cell function by ameliorating lipotoxicity and lowering free fatty acid levels. However, adult trials with TZDs have demonstrated weight gain and fluid retention and, in some elderly patients, heart failure.

Insulin Secretagogues

Glipizide (Glucotrol, Pfizer, New York, NY) or other insulin secretagogues were the first line of therapy for T2DM used in adults throughout most of the past two decades. When the initial adolescents with T2DM were seen in the early and mid 1990s, this was also the first drug that was chosen and used in most locales. With the approval of metformin for adults in the United States, increasing familiarity and experience with metformin in the pediatric age range, and the recent FDA approval of this medication for the pediatric population, metformin is now considered first-line therapy for pediatric T2DM. Insulin secretagogues are more frequently used as adjunctive therapy. The starting dosage of glipizide is 5 mg BID and can be increased to 10 mg BID or TID. It is well tolerated. Insulin secretagogues are associated with symptomatic hypoglycemia, especially in youth who have successfully lost weight, recently instituted a vigorous exercise program, or gone for prolonged periods without eating while continuing to take medication.

A primary goal of treatment of T2DM is β-cell preservation. The UKPDS showed that β-cell function in adults with T2DM on long-term sulfonylurea declines as a function of time. Sulfonylurea therapy does not spare β-cell function and is associated with worsening of insulin resistance. Furthermore, the use of exogenous insulin does not seem to preserve β-cell function. Both the prolonged secretagogues, like glipizide, and insulin have the disadvantage of weight gain, an undesirable outcome in youth with T2DM. The theoretical advantages of short-acting secretagogues, such as repaglinide, are that there is less chronic hyperinsulinemia and that the dose can be adjusted to intake; the disadvantage is that family must be taught carbohydrate counting. The concepts intrinsic to carbohydrate counting may encourage increased intake or suboptimal food habits. The pediatric experience with newer secretagogues is limited. In our clinical practice, it has been well tolerated with few side effects. There have been some problems with adherence at school because the child must go to the nursing station to get a pill before lunch. Furthermore, to optimize dosing postprandial glucose monitoring must be done on a regular basis.

Acarbose (Precose)

There is minimal experience with this medication in children with T2DM. It may prove to be a useful adjunct, as it has in some adults. However, there is clearly a need for carefully controlled pediatric clinical trials. Widespread use of acarbose (Precose, Bayer Pharmaceuticals, West Haven, CT) in youth may be limited due to the common intestinal side effects of diarrhea and flatulence.

For any medication choice, it is essential to evaluate whether it is safe for the affected adolescent, the requirements for taking the medication and monitoring the effects at home are understandable to the child and family, and the monitoring and other steps are acceptable to the adolescent and parents. General education regarding the various types of medication that are available and their mechanism of action should be included as part of the initial education of the patients and family. These concepts are intrinsic to the pathophysiology of diabetes (e.g., if one of the major problems of T2DM is insulin resistance, then it makes sense to treat the insulin resistance). When a child is started on any medication, the benefits and risks should be described and discussed with the family. Written instructions should be given to the family that include the dose, the approximate time(s) that the dose(s) should be given, the expected outcome, possible side effects, and special circumstances that warrant contact with the health care professional. The parent and child should be asked to review this information while in the physician's office. Extra copies of this information should be made, kept in the patient chart, and reviewed with the family and child at least annually, and more often if the dose is changed or the desired outcome is not achieved.

The choice of medication should be responsive to such factors as past experience of the parent with a particular medication and economic/insurance issues. Many parents (or related family members) of children with T2DM have experience with both diabetes and with diabetes medications. If a family member has had a particularly bad experience with a medication, it is unlikely that the parent will become an enthusiastic supporter of the use of that medication in the child. The choice of medication may also be limited by the insurer or other third-party payer. For example, many insurers reimburse

for metformin and glipizide individually but not for the combination form of these drugs. It is worthwhile to get to know which items are covered by the major insurers in a particular geographic area. It has taken a major effort in many states to educate third-party payers that medications other than insulin may be used to treat diabetes in children and adolescents. In some areas, failure to reimburse for non-insulin medications was simply a result of computer software that was set up to automatically reject certain medications for individuals who fell outside of a particular age range. For example, metformin was automatically excluded as a reimbursable medication for individuals younger than 21 years of age. Insurers have refused to reimburse for medications that are not approved by the FDA for a particular age group or medical condition. For example, the FDA has not yet approved the use of TZDs for the treatment of T2DM in pediatrics.

There are no specific protocols that have been rigorously tested and reported for therapy of T2DM in the pediatric population. We generally have adopted a scheme in which therapeutic decisions are based on an Hb_{A1c} obtained on a quarterly basis, with the benchmark Hb_{A1c} value being 7% for all except the 3-month visit after diagnosis. This strategy is summarized in Table 2-3. At the 3-month visit after diagnosis, patients are on one of four regimens: lifestyle only, metformin, metformin plus insulin, or insulin only. In general, if there has been substantial improvement or achievement of Hb_{A1c} of less than 7%, the youth is permitted to remain on his or her present regimen. If there has been deterioration, or the target has not been achieved, then the medication dosage is maximized or the regimen is augmented. Augmentation can involve the addition of another medication or increasing the dosage or frequency of insulin. Some flexibility is permitted if there is an obvious reason that a goal has not been achieved; for example, the child has not taken his or her metformin for a month preceding the visit because the family lost their insurance coverage. In this case, the focus is on ensuring a constant supply of medication, rather than on the addition of another medication.

For those children who are on insulin, we typically taper by reducing the dose by 25% every 2 weeks. Blood glucose testing is continued at least 4 times a day while on insulin and the parents are asked to call if there are two or more glucose values of greater than 250 mg/dL, or the recurrence of polyuria, nocturia, or rapid weight loss is noted. Frequent glucose testing is continued until the child has been off of all insulin for at least 2 weeks.

A variety of strategies has been used for initiating metformin. We have typically started at 500 mg BID and cautioned the child and family that gastrointestinal side effects are common in the first 2 weeks. Once initiated, we do not routinely stop metformin, regardless of the Hb_{A1c}. Occasionally, a particular child and family are successful not

Table 2-3   Therapeutic Strategy for Type 2 Diabetes Mellitus in Youth

Initial Treatment	3-Month Visit	6-Month Visit	9-Month Visit
Lifestyle	Hb_{A1c} <7, continue Hb_{A1c} >7, add M	Hb_{A1c} <7, continue Hb_{A1c} >7, maximize M	Hb_{A1c} <7, continue Hb_{A1c} <7, continue M Hb_{A1c} >7, augment
Metformin (M)	Hb_{A1c} <8, continue M	Hb_{A1c} <7, continue M Hb_{A1c} >7, maximize M	Hb_{A1c} <7, continue M Hb_{A1c} <7, continue M Hb_{A1c} >7, augment
	Hb_{A1c} >8, maximize M	Hb_{A1c} <7, continue M	Hb_{A1c} <7, continue Hb_{A1c} <7, continue M Hb_{A1c} >7, augment
		Hb_{A1c} >7, augment	Hb_{A1c} <7, continue Hb_{A1c} >7, augment
Metformin + insulin (I)	Hb_{A1c} <8, taper I, continue M	Hb_{A1c} <7, continue M	Hb_{A1c} <7, continue M Hb_{A1c} >7, augment
		Hb_{A1c} >7, maximize M	Hb_{A1c} <7, continue M Hb_{A1c} >7, augment
	Hb_{A1c} >8, maximize M	Hb_{A1c} <7, taper I	Hb_{A1c} <7, continue M Hb_{A1c} >7, augment
		Hb_{A1c} >7, intensify I	Hb_{A1c} <7, continue Hb_{A1c} >7, augment
Insulin only	Hb_{A1c} <7, taper I, add M	Hb_{A1c} <7, continue M	Hb_{A1c} <7, continue M Hb_{A1c} >7, maximize M
	Hb_{A1c} >7, continue I, add M	Hb_{A1c} <7, taper I	Hb_{A1c} <7, continue M Hb_{A1c} >7, maximize M
		Hb_{A1c} >7, maximize M	Hb_{A1c} <7, continue Hb_{A1c} >7, augment

only in achieving an Hb_{A1c} < 6%, but also in attaining and maintaining normal or near normal BMI, normal fasting and postprandial glucose levels, and a normal lipid profile. In this circumstance, we permit a trial of "lifestyle only" treatment, with continued monitoring of all parameters.

Once the metformin dose is maximized, the choices for augmentation are insulin, insulin sensitizer (TZD), and/or insulin secretagogue (glipizide, repaglinide). There is no consensus on the optimal approach: therefore, we have generally been guided by insurance reimbursement policies, family preference, medication tolerability, and simplicity of use. Once controlled clinical trials demonstrate clear efficacy of one augmentation over the other, then the choice of medication is considerably simpler (see Table 2-3).

Home Glucose Monitoring

Self-monitoring of blood glucose (SMBG) is an important tool to achieve target glycemic goal in T2DM youth treated with diet and/or oral agents and is essential for safety in insulin-treated patients. Prebreakfast fasting and 2-hour postprandial dinner SMBG may be sufficient in most cases, although children on insulin therapy or those with recently deteriorating glycemic control may require the 4-times-daily premeal, prebedtime schedule more typical of T1DM patients. The goals for glycemic control are a FBG of less than 110 mg/dL 85% of the time (six of seven mornings), 2-hour postprandial glucose less than 140 mg/dL 85% of the time (six of seven evenings after supper), and Hb_{A1c} less than 7%, consistent with ADA guidelines.

The choice of using the supper meal reflects the fact that for most people the supper meal is the largest meal of the day in terms of caloric content. Furthermore, by 2 hours after supper, most youth are at home and have access to their blood glucose monitor. In contrast, attempting to determine a 2-hour postprandial glucose after breakfast or lunch would disrupt the child's classroom activities. A "2-hour postprandial glucose" must be defined for children and families, because many families do not necessarily eat a meal; instead, they continuously snack. We strongly encourage children to have a discrete meal that is consumed in 30 minutes and to check the blood glucose level between 1¾ and 2¼ hours after the meal is finished.

The mechanical skills of proper glucose meter technique and maintenance and the interpretation of SMBG data should be taught and frequently reviewed. Patients should be taught the circumstances where additional testing may be indicated (such as during acute illness or when high Hb_{A1c} levels suggest periods of undetected hyperglycemia). As with medication choice, third-party payers may dictate the choice of meter and the frequency of testing. Parents and youth should be strongly encouraged to bring SMBG records and the meter(s) to each clinic visit, permitting the data to be downloaded and evaluated by the diabetes team. The glucose records, from either the diary or monitor memory, are useful teaching tools for instilling new ideas or refreshing old ones. For example, a pattern of consistently high glucose values 2 hours after supper is an opportunity for reviewing goals (blood glucose <140 mg/dL on six of seven nights), discussing the various possible responses to a consistently high glucose (alter intake, change medication, alter activity), identifying the actions that the youth is willing or able to make, and conversing about the potential barriers to taking these actions. In addition, the meter can be checked to be certain that the time and date are accurate, that the machine is accurate, and whether there is a need to clean or replace the monitor. Each of these activities is also an opportunity for further education for the child and family.

MEDICAL MONITORING

The goals of medical monitoring are to promote or ensure normalization of Hb_{A1c}, lipids, blood pressure, and body weight; screen for diabetes complications, including retinopathy and nephropathy, or complications related to medical therapies; and identify potential barriers to the management plan.

Although most published minimum standards suggest Hb_{A1c} be measured twice each year, more frequent monitoring (at least quarterly) is warranted in children and youth, given the probable duration of diabetes and the benefits of having multiple objective assessment parameters. Ideally, the Hb_{A1c} should be within the normal range for nondiabetic individuals. However, steady improvement with each visit is a reasonable intermediate goal. In general, at the end of each visit, a realistic target Hb_{A1c} is set for the next visit, along with possible actions that will be taken if that goal is not met.

The ADA practice guidelines recommend lipid monitoring (total cholesterol, high-density lipoprotein cholesterol, triglycerides) at least annually if the lipid profile is normal on initial evaluation and more frequently if abnormal or when pharmacological therapy is used. Additional recommendations by the ADA for individuals diagnosed with T2DM are (1) dilated eye examination at or near the time of diagnosis and repeated on an annual basis and (2) a urine test for microalbuminuria at or near the time of diagnosis, repeated on an annual basis. The 24-hour urine collections for microalbuminuria are difficult to obtain and have in large part been replaced by spot urine samples for albumin/creatinine ratios.

Protocols should be placed in each patient chart indicating which analyses are to be done on which visit, and either

Box 2-4 Recommended Frequency of Evaluation for Youth With Type 2 Diabetes Mellitus

PARAMETER	FREQUENCY
Weight/height/body mass index	At least quarterly
Blood pressure	At least quarterly
Hb_{A1c}	At least quarterly
ALT, AST	Initially and then frequency dependent on type of medication
Lipid profile	Initially and then at least annually; more frequently if on medication or if a value is abnormal
Microalbumin	Initially and then at least annually; more frequently if on medication or if a value is abnormal; if proteinuria or microalbuminuria, then additional renal studies are indicated
Other	Thyroid-stimulating hormone initially and then annually
Ophthalmologic examination	Initially and then at least annually; more frequently if abnormal
Influenza vaccine	Annually in the fall of each year
Dietitian	Initially as required for education, then at least yearly
Diabetes educator	Initially as required for education, then at least yearly

the results should be entered onto the protocol or a notation should be made by office staff when testing is done, allowing the quick assessment of longitudinal changes over time and providing quality assurance assessment. Patients should be given the rationale for the performance of various tests and procedures and written material regarding the expected frequency of testing (Box 2-4).

Hypertension

Hypertension is a common comorbidity of diabetes, affecting 20% to 60% of adults with T2DM. The Third National Health and Nutrition Evaluation Survey (NHANES III, 1988–1994) revealed that 71% of individuals with diabetes had hypertension, that 29% of those with hypertension were unaware of the diagnosis, that 43% with hypertension were untreated, and that 55% on treatment were not effectively treated. Hypertension is about twice as common in individuals with diabetes as it is in a comparable population without diabetes. Not surprisingly, there is also approximately a 2-fold higher risk of cardiovascular disease in individuals with diabetes compared with those without diabetes. In addition to its role in macrovascular disease, hypertension increases the risk for renal insufficiency, retinopathy, and possible neuropathy in diabetic individuals. In the UKPDS, each 10-mm Hg reduction in systolic blood pressure was associated with a reduction in risk of 12% for any complication related to diabetes.

Current recommendations from the ADA are to begin intervention for blood pressure when diastolic pressure is greater than 80 mm Hg and/or systolic pressure is greater than 130 mm Hg, with an initial focus on behavioral (lifestyle) treatment. If there is no benefit after 3 months, pharmacological therapy is recommended. For initial diastolic blood pressure of greater than 90 mm Hg or systolic pressure of greater than 140 mm Hg, pharmacological therapy at the outset and behavioral interventions are recommended.

Although there are no comparable data on the long-term macrovascular and microvascular risks of T2DM in children and youth, there is no reason to believe that childhood or adolescence provides any protection from these consequences. The recommendations from the Task Force on High Blood Pressure in Children and Adolescents (subsequently referred to as the "Task Force") are that blood pressures above the 90th percentile for age warrant lifestyle intervention and those about the 95th percentile merit the addition of pharmacological agents. The most recent data for children and adolescents have recognized that height is an important determinant of blood pressure in childhood and therefore that data have been normalized for age, gender, and height. For practical clinical purposes, we have used the following standards, reflecting the fact that most children with T2DM are not only overweight but also taller than expected (average about 1 SD above the mean). Therefore, for the sake of simplicity we have used normative data for children who are at the 75th percentile for height and further simplified the tables to prepubertal children (ages 6 to 10 years), pubertal (ages 11 to 15 years), and postpubertal (ages >15 years). Although lacking the precision of the Task Force, these values are a rough approximation of the published pediatric standards and segue nicely with the adult recommendations (Box 2-5).

There are potential methodological issues in blood pressure assessment, because many children with T2DM are obese; therefore, it is critical that a cuff of the appropriate size is used. The recommendations of the Task Force are that children with blood pressure at or above the 95th percentile are defined as hypertensive, whereas children with blood pressure between the 90th and 95th percentiles are high-normal and merit ongoing monitoring. No unique recommendations were given for children with T2DM who are hypertensive.

Hypertension treatment includes both nonpharmacological and pharmacological interventions. The most obvious intervention, and perhaps the most difficult to achieve in this population, is weight loss. In obese children, both systolic and diastolic blood pressures decrease with weight loss. Blood pressure also tends to decline with increasing physical fitness; therefore, a program to increase the amount of physical activity may have significant benefit. Hypertension per se is not a contraindication to exercise or participation in sporting activities. Pharmacological therapy is recommended for those individuals with blood pressure in excess of the 95th percentile. Task Force recommendations were last made in 1996, and therefore some of the newer medications were not yet available. The drugs that were recommended are listed in Table 2-4, along with specific comments related to their use in individuals with diabetes.

Hyperlipidemia

Cardiovascular disease is a major cause of morbidity and mortality in adults with T2DM. Given the assumed long duration of T2DM after the diagnosis in individuals with T2DM of childhood onset, it is advisable to both monitor and manage this problem relatively aggressively. The standards put forth by the ADA for adults are less rigorous than those put forth by the AAP for children and youth.

Box 2-5 Blood Pressure Standards (Modified)				
	DIASTOLIC (mm Hg)		SYSTOLIC (mm Hg)	
	90TH PERCENTILE	95TH PERCENTILE	90TH PERCENTILE	95TH PERCENTILE
Prepubertal	75	80	115	120
Pubertal	80	85	120	125
Postpubertal	80	90	120	130

Table 2-4 Antihypertensive Medications and Their Use

Drug Type/Action	Drug Name	Dosage	Treatment Choice	Published Experience — Adult Type 2 Diabetes Mellitus	Published Experience — Pediatric in General	Published Experience — Pediatric Diabetes Mellitus	Recommendation — Pediatric in General	Recommendation — Pediatric Diabetes Mellitus
α/β-Blocker	Labetalol	1-3 mg/kg/day q6-12h	Special circumstances	Yes	None	None	Yes	None
α-Blocker	Prazosin	0.05-0.1 mg/kg/day q6-8h	2	Yes	No	None	Yes	Yes
β-Blocker	Propranolol	1-8 mg/kg/day q6-12h	1	Yes	Yes	None	Yes	Yes
	Atenolol	1-8 mg/kg/day q12-24h	1	Yes	Yes	None	Yes	Yes
α-Agonist	Clonidine	0.1-0.6 mg/kg/day q6h	Special circumstances	Yes	Yes	None	Yes	Yes
Calcium channel blockers	Nifedipine	0.25-2.0 mg/kg/day q4-6h	2	Yes	None	None	Yes	
	Amlodipine	2.5-10 mg/day QD			None	None	None	Yes
Angiotensin-converting enzyme inhibitors	Captopril	1.5-6.0 mg/kg/day q8h	1	Yes	Yes	Yes	Yes	Yes
	Enalapril	0.15-0.5 mg/kg/day q12-24h		Yes	Yes	Yes		
	Lisinopril	10-40 mg/day QD		Yes	No	Yes		
Angiotensin receptor blockers	Candesartan Cilexetil	8-32 mg/day QD	2	Yes	None	None	No	Yes
	Irbesartan	75-300 mg/day QD		Yes	>6 yr			
Diuretics	Furosemide	1-12 mg/kg/day q4-12h	2	Yes	Yes	None	Yes	Yes
	Hydrochlorothiazide	1-3 mg/kg/day q12h	1	Yes	Yes	None	Yes	Yes
	Spironolactone	1-3 mg/kg/day q6-12h	Special circumstances	Yes	Yes	Yes	Hirsutism	
	Triamterene	2-3 mg/kg/day q6-12h	Special circumstances					Combined with hydrochlorothiazide

However, the AAP standards focus on only cholesterol. The recommendations in Box 2-6 are a blending of the recommendations of both the ADA and AAP.

For youth with T2DM, adequate glycemic control, medical nutrition therapy, and increased physical activity are the first approaches to normalizing lipids. However, in many youth these steps are not adequate and more aggressive intervention is required. As has been the case with most other medications in this chapter, there are no evidence-based guidelines on the use of these medications in children and youth with or without diabetes. As with diabetes medications, for postpubertal youth, adult dosing schedules and monitoring are used. The statins are well tolerated, whereas the fibric acid derivatives and nicotinic acids have side effects that often lead to cessation of therapy in adolescents. For prepubertal children and midpubertal adolescents, the added concern about cardiovascular consequences often leads to increased interest in achieving glycemic control and enhancing medical nutrition therapy. However, when improvement is not seen with this approach, we have instituted pharmaceutical therapy, most commonly with the statins. Before the initiation of therapy, appropriate screening of liver (ALT, AST) and kidney function is performed and a baseline measure of creatine phosphokinase (CPK) is obtained. These laboratory tests are repeated at the visit after initiation of therapy, the visit after an increase in dosage, and if there are complaints of malaise or myalgias. Anecdotally, therapy is effective and the improvements in the lipid profile are similar to those reported in adult studies. Of note, the statins have been used to manage hyperlipidemia in children after liver or kidney transplantation. In this context, they appear to be relatively safe and efficacious. Table 2-5 lists some common hyperlipidemia medications, dosages, side effects, and contraindications.

Sexual Responsibility and Alcohol Use

There are special circumstances that merit some consideration because most children with T2DM are adolescents. Specifically, it should be noted that there is little information of the impact of metformin and other oral agents on the ova, sperm, and fetus. Therefore, it is appropriate to provide counseling to females and males regarding the avoidance of pregnancy while on oral agents. It is safe to use metformin and the other oral agents with oral contraceptives. Alcohol use is not recommended and increases the risk of lactic acidosis; therefore, excessive alcohol use, either acutely or chronically, should be avoided. As has been the case with adolescents with T1DM, frank discussions about the risks of drinking, drinking responsibly, and strategies to use in specific social situations should be initiated in a supportive, nonjudgmental manner.

Opportunities for Affecting the Extended Family

Many children with T2DM have other family members and siblings who are also at risk for diabetes; it is important that the family be made aware of the risk. Siblings of the affected child should be discussed with the parent and, when appropriate, screened for diabetes and diabetes risk. Similarly, it has been estimated that as many as 40% of adults with diabetes are unaware that they have this condition. The acceptability of screening adults in a pediatric environment and the use of a capillary glucose monitor as a screening tool may vary from locale to locale; however, we believe that the awareness is of such importance that we offer free screening to all family members. Those individuals who are found to be abnormal are then provided with guidance regarding follow-up with their primary care provider and/or referral to an adult diabetes center.

Box 2-6 Hyperlipidemia Standards for Youth With Type 2 Diabetes Mellitus

	ACCEPTABLE (mg/dL)	BORDERLINE (mg/dL)	UNACCEPTABLE (mg/dL)
Total cholesterol	≤170	170-199	≥200
Low-density lipoprotein cholesterol	≤110	110-129	≥130
High-density lipoprotein cholesterol	≥45	35-45	≤35
Triglycerides	≤150	150-199	≥200

Table 2-5 Hyperlipidemia Medications and Their Use

Medication	Starting Dose	Maximal Dose/24 hr	Dosing Schedule	Tablet/Capsule Size	Side Effects	Contraindications
Cholestyramine	5.5 g	22 g	BID	5.5 g	Gastrointestinal (GI) distress, constipation	Dysbetalipoproteinemia Triglycerides >400 mg/dL
Nicotinic acid (Niaspan)	0.5 g	2 g	HS	500, 750, 1000 mg	Flushing, hyperuricemia, GI distress	Chronic liver disease Gout, peptic ulcer disease
Gemfibrozil (Lopid)	600 mg		BID	600	GI distress, gallstones, myopathy	Severe renal or hepatic disease
Clofibrate (Atromid)	500 mg	2000 mg	BID	500 mg		
Lovastatin (Mevacor)	10 mg	40 mg	QD, BID	10, 20, 40 mg	Myopathy, increased liver enzymes	Chronic liver disease Certain drugs
Pravastatin (Pravachol)	10 mg QD	40 mg	QD	10, 20, 40 mg		
Atorvastatin (Lipitor)	10 mg QD	80 mg	QD	10, 20, 40, 80 mg		
Simvastatin (Zocor)	5-10 mg QD	80 mg	QD	5, 10, 20, 40, 80 mg		

MAJOR POINTS

Type 2 diabetes mellitus (T2DM) is now a pediatric disease with the prevalence in many locales approaching that for type 1 diabetes mellitus (T1DM). Epidemiological studies are under way to establish the true prevalence and incidence.

Children with T2DM can often be distinguished from those with T1DM by clinical findings that include (1) body mass index of greater than 85% for age and gender, (2) a strong family history of diabetes and other features of the dysmetabolic syndrome in first- and second-degree relatives, and (3) other physical or laboratory findings consistent with the dysmetabolic syndrome (e.g., hypertension, hyperinsulinemia, hyperlipidemia, acanthosis nigricans, or hyperandrogenism). Most affected children are pubertal or postpubertal at diagnosis. The majority of affected children belong to racial and ethnic minorities; however, there have been numerous reports of non-Hispanic white children with T2DM.

At diagnosis, children may span the range from no recognizable symptoms to severe diabetic ketoacidosis. The presence of ketoacidosis, the severity of the hyperglycemia, or the amount of weight lost does not differentiate between T2DM and T1DM.

The treatment of T2DM is distinctly different from that of T1DM due to a variety of social, cultural, educational, and economic issues. Compared with T1DM, more focus must be placed on changing activity and dietary habits. Accomplishing this requires more frequent visits and a behavior-based approach.

Metformin is the only oral medication currently approved for use in the treatment of diabetes in youth. Metformin doses of 1000 to 2000 mg/day divided into twice-daily dosing is often effective initial therapy when coupled with behavioral intervention.

A wide range of insulin regimens are feasible in youth with T2DM. In general, the simplest strategy that can be used to achieve control is chosen. Often this involves the use of an intermediate-acting or sustained action insulin at bedtime.

Achieving and maintaining an Hb_{A1c} of less than 7% should be the goal of therapy. Stepwise intensification of therapy, with the addition of insulin or a second oral agent, should be considered if target Hb_{A1c} is not reached within 6 months on monotherapy.

Glucose monitoring should occur a minimum of twice each day and should focus on achieving a fasting glucose level of less than 100 mg/dL and 2-hour postprandial glucose level of less than 140 mg/dL.

The other components of the dysmetabolic syndrome must be managed as well, including hypertension and hyperlipidemia. Although specific evidence-based guidelines for the management of these conditions in children with diabetes have not been established, it is reasonable to use guidelines established for adults with T2DM, especially in postpubertal adolescents.

MAJOR POINTS—Cont'd

Because most youth with T2DM are adolescents, due consideration should be given to a variety of risk-taking behaviors, including alcohol, drugs, and sexual activities that might complicate or be complicated by diabetes and diabetes medications. Appropriate counseling and/or preventive measures should be implemented.

SUGGESTED READINGS

Aaron DJ, Storti KL, Robertson RJ, et al: Longitudinal study of the number and choice of leisure time physical activities from mid to late adolescence: implications for school curricula and community recreation programs, Arch Pediatr Adolesc Med 2002;156:1075.

American Academy of Pediatrics: Physical fitness and activity in schools, Pediatrics 2000;105:1156.

American Academy of Pediatrics: Cholesterol in childhood, Pediatrics 1998;101:141.

American Academy of Pediatrics: Committee on Public Education. Children, adolescents, and television, Pediatrics 2001;107:423.

Consensus Panel: Type 2 diabetes in children and adolescents, Pediatrics 2000;105:671.

Epstein LH, Valoski AM, Vara LS, et al: Effects of decreasing sedentary behavior and increasing activity on weight changes in obese children, Health Psychol 1995;14:1.

Epstein LH: Family-based behavioral intervention for obese children, Int J Obes 1996;20(suppl 1):S14.

Fagot-Campagna A, Pettitt DJ, Engelgau MM, et al: Type 2 diabetes among North American children and adolescents: an epidemiologic review and a public health perspective, J Pediatr 2000;13:664.

Jones K, Arslanian S, McVie R, et al: Metformin improves glycemic control in children with type 2 diabetes, Diabetes 2000;49:A75.

Rosner B, Prineas RJ, Loggie JMH, et al: Blood pressure nomograms for children and adolescents by height, sex and age, in the United States, J Pediatr 1993;123:871.

National High Blood Pressure Education Program Working Group on Hypertension Control in Children and Adolescents: Update on the 1987 Task Force Report on High Blood Pressure in Children and Adolescents: A working group report for the National High Blood Pressure Education Program, Pediatrics 1996;98:649.

INTRODUCTION

During the past decade, many advances have been made regarding the etiology and molecular mechanisms of the hypoglycemic disorders, particularly hyperinsulinism (HI), the fatty acid oxidation (FAO) defects, and the glycogen storage diseases (GSDs). There has been a renewal of the debate and ongoing controversy regarding the definition of hypoglycemia. Despite these advances and discussion, little substantive data regarding the mechanisms of hypoglycemic brain damage have been presented.

This chapter is organized to review the normal physiological changes involved in glucose homeostasis. With the understanding of this process, the diagnosis of hypoglycemia is simplified. Disorders of glucose homeostasis are discussed individually, with an emphasis on neonatal hypoglycemia. A diagnostic approach to hypoglycemia is outlined, and specific therapies are discussed in each subsection. In addition, the emergency management of the hypoglycemic patient pending diagnosis is outlined.

DEFINITION OF HYPOGLYCEMIA

The definition of *hypoglycemia* is probably the most debated and least agreed-on topic among leaders in the field. Some maintain that hypoglycemia is the level of glucose that causes brain damage; others argue that it is the level of glucose above which most people maintain their glucose levels most of the time. Some have multiple definitions for hypoglycemia, such as the level required for investigation of patients and the level required for intervening and treating patients. Finally, there are those that add one further level, which is the level above which one should aim to keep the glucose in a patient being treated for a known hypoglycemic disorder. A rigid definition of hypoglycemia applicable to all occasions cannot be made.

HYPOGLYCEMIA AND BRAIN DAMAGE

What level of hypoglycemia causes brain damage? It depends on the circumstances of the hypoglycemia. It used to be thought that brain damage occurs when there is a loss of energy at a cellular level in the neurons. It was proposed, however, that abnormal excitation of neurons due to changes in the function of the receptors for excitatory amino acids, especially the *N*-methyl-D-aspartate (NMDA) receptor, is the cause of the brain damage associated with hypoglycemia. How hypoglycemia leads to local accumulation of excitatory amino acids is unclear, but the presence of either ketones or lactate during hypoglycemia appears to be protective.

The brain contains glucose-sensing (GS) and glucose-responsive (GR) neurons. The GR neurons increase firing when blood glucose levels rise, and the GS neurons increase when blood glucose levels fall. The GR neurons contain both the low-affinity ATP-sensitive potassium channel (K_{ATP} channel) *(SUR-2/Kir6.2)* and the high-affinity K_{ATP} channel *(SUR-1/Kir6.2 as found in the β cell)*. The role of these GS and GR neurons in the brain is not yet understood, but they probably play a role in the counter-regulatory hormone response to hypoglycemia.

The brain appears to need both a fuel (glucose, ketones, or lactate) plus oxygen and intact mitochondrial function to function normally. Koh et al demonstrated that neural dysfunction during hypoglycemia could be measured by brainstem auditory evoked responses or serial somatosensory evoked potentials and that the presence of ketosis during hypoglycemia prevented the abnormalities seen with hypo-

glycemia alone. Thus a patient with a disorder of gluconeogenesis such as glucose-6-phosphatase deficiency may have a blood glucose level of 30 mg/dL and have completely normal brain function because the lactate level is 10 mmol/L. On the other hand, a patient with congenital HI may also have a blood glucose level of 30 mg/dL with suppressed ketones and lactate and experience irreversible brain damage. There is no single level of blood glucose below which one can definitively state that brain damage occurs.

NORMAL GLUCOSE LEVELS

Normal glucose levels may be defined like many laboratory tests, as the mean ± 2 SDs. Some infants and children have values outside of the normal range and be healthy, whereas some have a serious underlying condition. In general, most infants and children maintain blood glucose levels between 60 and 120 mg/dL most of the time. The circumstances under which the blood sample was drawn must be taken into consideration; for example, a blood glucose level of 50 mg/dL in a toddler who has had diarrhea and vomiting for 24 hours is very different from a blood glucose level of 50 mg/dL in a toddler 3 hours after her last meal. The most common period of time that infants (specifically newborns) do not maintain their blood glucose level at greater than 60 mg/dL is the transitional period of adaptation to extrauterine life that occurs during the first 24 hours of life.

An abnormal glucose level, which is tagged by the laboratory computer as low, does not necessarily mean the patient has a disorder of glucose homeostasis. However, one must consider the possibility that the patient has a disorder of glucose homeostasis and make a determination of whether to investigate.

WORKING DEFINITION OF HYPOGLYCEMIA

The basic principle in medicine of "first do no harm" is ideally suited to those taking care of patients with abnormalities of glucose homeostasis. The price of missing a patient with a disorder of glucose homeostasis is so great that the error should be on the side of overinvestigation rather than on underdiagnosis. A classic example of this is the treatment of fever in infants younger than 6 months. Many years ago, all patients with a temperature of greater than 38.5° C underwent a septic work-up and received treatment with antibiotics until it was clear they did not have a condition requiring antibiotic treatment. It was clear that an excessive numbers of infants were treated, but the alternative of losing a child to overwhelming infection was unacceptable. A series of studies to better determine which children were at risk of sepsis were carried out prospectively, and gradually a set of guidelines were generated that allowed infants to be better assessed and avoided overtreatment. Regarding hypoglycemia, a similar problem exists. Experts agree that more studies need to be done to define hypoglycemia in terms of when brain damage occurs. Their current conclusions are that there are insufficient data and that multicenter trials are required but that these trials are impossible to conduct prospectively. Therefore one is left to make recommendations based not on hard scientific data but rather on an assessment of the literature and common sense. This generates problems for those who wish to have a definition that protects them from legal proceedings. However, under the "first do no harm" guidelines, the first concern should be for the patient and not for the law.

Hypoglycemia is defined in this chapter as a blood glucose level of less than 50 mg/dL. With this definition, children are investigated who do not have a serious underlying disorder of glucose homeostasis, but one is unlikely to miss a patient with a hypoglycemic disorder. By examining the circumstances of hypoglycemia and carrying out the appropriate studies at the time of hypoglycemia (the critical sample, Box 3-1), dangerous and invasive studies such as 24- to 48-hour fasting studies can be avoided in most infants and children with hypoglycemia. The results of studies should be interpreted compared with normative data obtained during a period of hypoglycemia rather than with random data. Many laboratory reporting systems report these biochemical results in the context of an 8 AM fasting level, which is very different from the levels of intermediary metabolites found at a time of hypoglycemia (Box 3-2). Once the etiology of hypoglycemia is determined, the therapeutic goal of maintaining glucose in the normal range can be undertaken. It is important to recognize that hypoglycemia is not a diagnosis but rather a biochemical sign of an underlying disorder. In addition, once a diagnosis of hypoglycemia has been made and treatment instigated, the goal of therapy should be to allow the child to eat in a normal pattern for age and maintain glucose levels in the normal range (>60 mg/dL at all times). In this way, if therapy fails on any given day, the patient does not plummet into the danger zone of unknown risks but rather slips into the gray zone of less-than-normal but not harmful glucose levels.

SYMPTOMS AND SIGNS OF HYPOGLYCEMIA

Symptoms of hypoglycemia can be divided into those that arise due to the body's defense mechanisms to prevent hypoglycemia (adrenergic symptoms) and those that occur as a result of neurological impairment due to neuroglycopenia (Box 3-3). It is the latter symptoms that cause most concern, because they indicate that brain function is impaired. In addition, symptoms of neuroglycopenia should trigger urgent investigation. The adrenergic symptoms are very

---

Box 3-1   Critical Sample

TEST	REQUIREMENTS
BASIC TESTS	
Complete blood cell count, electrolytes, glucose, blood gases (arterial or venous), lactate	Standard blood tubes
CRITICAL DRAW	**BLOOD TUBES**
Insulin, cortisol, growth hormone	3 mL serum
Free fatty acids, β-OH-butyrate and aceto-acetate	3 mL plasma
TOTAL AND FREE CARNITINE, ACYL-CARNITINE PROFILE	
Ammonia, lactate	1 mL plasma
C-peptide	1 mL EDTA
URINE	Urine volume required
Urine organic acids	5-10 mL urine, frozen immediately
Urine dip ketones	1-2 mL

Tests included in the critical sample should be drawn at the time of hypoglycemia (blood glucose <50 mg/dL) before correction. Sample collection requirements may vary in different institutions. The urine sample should consist of the first urine voided after the hypoglycemic episode.

Box 3-2   Normal Data for Critical Sample

TEST	NORMAL LEVELS DURING HYPOGLYCEMIA
Insulin	<2 μU/mL
Cortisol	>20 μg/dL
Growth hormone	>7-10 ng/mL
Free fatty acids	>1.5 mmol/L
β-OH-butyrate and aceto-acetate	>2 mmol/L
Lactate	<2.5 mmol/L
Ammonia	<35 μmol/L

Individual laboratories may have slightly different ranges for normal values at a time of hypoglycemia. The physician should be aware that many laboratories do not define normal values for hypoglycemia. Tests such as total and free carnitine, acyl-carnitine profile, and urine organic acids need specialist interpretation and the laboratory needs as much clinical data as possible to make a meaningful comment.

Box 3-3	Symptoms of Hypoglycemia in Infants and Children*	
ADRENERGIC SYMPTOMS	**NEUROGLYCOPENIC SYMPTOMS**	
Pallor	Headache	
Sweating	Visual disturbances	
Shakiness, trembling	Lethargy, lassitude	
Tachycardia	Difficulty with speech and thinking	
Anxiety, nervousness	Inability to concentrate	
Weakness	Mental confusion	
Hunger	Apnea (mainly in neonates)	
Nausea, vomiting	Somnolence, stupor, prolonged sleep	
	Twitching, convulsions, "epilepsy"	
	Bizarre neurological signs/personality changes	
	Loss of consciousness, coma	

*Neonates do not usually demonstrate adrenergic symptoms.

common and nonspecific and by themselves do not strongly suggest hypoglycemia. Hypoglycemia may be difficult to recognize clinically in neonates, because the children do not manifest the adrenergic symptoms very clearly. It is for this reason that centers that care for newborns have protocols for screening newborn infants at risk of becoming hypoglycemic. Infants up to 2 years of age also do not demonstrate the classic adrenergic symptoms. Both neonates and infants often present with apnea, seizures, or lethargy as the first presenting sign. It is for this reason that any neonate, infant, or child who presents to a physician with signs consistent with neuroglycopenia must have blood drawn for a glucose level, before those signs are attributed to something else. Specifically, blood must be drawn for a glucose level in all patients presenting with seizures.

PHYSIOLOGY OF GLUCOSE HOMEOSTASIS

Intrauterine Glucose Homeostasis

The intrauterine environment is one of anabolism. Growth during fetal life is the most rapid during life. The fetal-placental-maternal unit is designed to provide nutrients to the fetus, at the expense of the mother if necessary. In the normal state, there is very efficient transfer of nutrients from mother to fetus. Disruption of this supply to the fetus can result is dramatic impairment of growth and development of the fetus, which may have lasting consequences on the individual.

Glucose, amino acids, and lactate are the principal energy substrates during fetal life. Fetal glucose is almost completely derived from the mother and accounts for up to 50% of the energy use of the fetus. Fetal gluconeogenesis is normally nonexistent unless chronic and severe maternal starvation occurs. In addition, FAO and ketone utilization are minimal in the fetus. The transport of glucose to the fetus across the placenta occurs via carrier-facilitated diffusion. These glucose transporters are not insulin dependent but rather glucose concentration dependent. In times of maternal hyperglycemia, fetal glucose transport is increased and fetal hyperglycemia occurs. Likewise, in times of maternal hypoglycemia, fetal hypoglycemia occurs. Fetal glucose levels are approximately 80% those of the mother. During fetal life, increased numbers of insulin receptors are expressed. This stimulates anabolism and the deposition of glycogen in the liver, muscle, and brain. The fetal liver in a term appropriate for gestational age (AGA) infant contains relatively more glycogen than an adult liver and has up to 1% of total energy stores at birth.

Insulin is the predominant hormone in intrauterine life. The fetal β cell does not respond to acute changes in glucose concentration by changing insulin secretion; rather, it changes only in response to chronic glucose concentration changes. This imbalance of insulin secretion in response to acute glucose changes is due to an immature cyclic adenosine monophosphate (AMP)-generating system in the β cells during intrauterine life, a condition that occasionally extends into the newborn period. In addition to chronic changes in fetal glucose levels, the fetal β cell is stimulated by amino acids.

Transitional Glucose Homeostasis

The periods proceeding, during, and immediately after birth are very stressful to the fetus and, subsequently, the newborn infant. It is during this time that a smooth transition must be made from a constant glucose supply to an intermittent supply. In addition in the normally fed infant, the first breast milk contains a higher fat and lower carbohydrate mixture to which the fetus has been exposed. Temperature changes and the sudden transition from the quiet warmth of intrauterine life to the chaotic atmosphere of the normal delivery room add further stress to the newborn.

The hormonal milieu of intrauterine life is in the balance of insulin secretion with diminished glucagon and epinephrine secretion. At birth, this changes dramatically. Insulin secretion falls, and epinephrine levels surge and stimulate glucagon secretion. Growth hormone levels rise and remain high for several days. Insulin receptor numbers decrease and glucagon receptor levels increase. The cyclic AMP systems mature. This combination causes a shift from glucose utilization to glucose mobilization. Glycogen synthase is downregulated, and glycogen phosphorylase is upregulated, leading to a shift from glycogen formation to breakdown. Enzymes of gluconeogenesis are switched on, such as phosphoenolpyruvatecarboxykinase (PEPCK) and glucose-6-phosphatase. Finally, with the falling insulin levels and ingestion of high fat–containing breast milk, there is a switch from fatty acid synthesis to FAO triggered by the maturation of carnitine palmytol transferase-1 (CPT-1). All of these changes acting synergistically have the effect of mobilizing glycogen stores, triggering FAO, and generating ketone bodies for use as an alternate fuel source. This has the effect of maintaining glucose for those tissues that can only metabolize glucose for energy production. Clinically, this is manifest by a drop in blood glucose levels in the immediate newborn period. Immediate suckling and the ingestion of colostrum result in glucose levels that rise and fall again with feeding. By 12 hours of life, stability in glucose homeostasis starts to occur. The induction of the critical enzymes of gluconeogenesis and FAO leads to ketone formation, which is used by muscles to reduce glucose utilization and by liver to generate energy in the form of NADH to drive gluconeogenesis and stabilize blood glucose levels.

There is a multitude of data showing that a significant number of newborns have glucose levels less than 50 mg/dL during this phase of transition from intrauterine to extrauterine life, in particular in the interval between birth and the first two or three feedings. In the normally grown term infant, there is ample glycogen in brain astrocyte cells to buffer the abrupt changes in glucose concentration. Astrocyte glycogen reserves, laid down during intrauterine life, provide a short-term source of energy (via lactate) for neurons, so that although the blood glucose levels fall, there is an adequate intermediary metabolite supply to the neurons and brain function is not affected. These stores, however, are rapidly depleted and do not protect the infant from anything other than short-term hypoglycemia. It is postulated that this is the reason the vast majority of these infants with glucose levels less than 50 mg/dL during this transitional stage of life have no neurological impairment. However, if diminished glycogen reserves are present, such as occurs in infants born with intrauterine growth retardation (IUGR), or unavailable, such as occurs in infants born with an impairment in oxygen supply, then the period of transition may change from a merely tumultuous period to a dangerous period.

After the first 24 hours of life, the transition from intrauterine glucose regulation to extrauterine adaptation is complete. Few healthy, full-term AGA infants have hypoglycemia beyond this time. Hypoglycemia occurring beyond the first day of life should be considered abnormal.

In addition, it should be remembered that premature infants and IUGR infants are not physiologically normal infants and many have problems with glucose regulation. This occurs because they do not have the glycogen reserves of the term AGA infant; they have decreased muscle mass and gluconeogenesis from alanine may be reduced, and therefore important enzymes in glucose regulation may not be mature. Although hypoglycemia in these groups of infants may be common, it cannot be passed off as a normal variant. Persistent hypoglycemia should be prevented by feeding and intravenous glucose support, and once settled, the infants need to demonstrate they can fast for at least 8 hours while maintaining their glucose levels at greater than 60 mg/dL, before discharge.

Fasting Adaptation in Infants and Children

Fasting adaptation matures rapidly in the first days of life, and by the end of the first week, infants are able to fast for up to 18 hours. By 1 year of life, they can fast for 24 hours, and by 5 years, children may tolerate fasts of up to 36 hours. This difference in fasting tolerance comes about for two reasons. First, glucose utilization in infants, children, and adults is more related to brain weight than to body weight, and thus infants who have a greater brain-to-body ratio than adults have higher glucose utilization rates per kilogram of body weight. Second, glycogen stores and stores of gluconeogenic precursor increase with increased body size. The caloric needs of a 1-year-old are 60% of those of an adult, but the fuel stores are only 15%.

Glucose homeostasis is a finely tuned system. Throughout the day, variations in glucose levels range from 1- to 3-fold over baseline. This is in comparison to the fluctuations in ketones, which may vary 20-fold during a fast. This tight control is necessary due to the large numbers of glucose concentration–dependent glucose transporters present throughout the body.

In the immediate postprandial phase, glucose levels rise after the absorption of carbohydrate. This triggers insulin release by the β cells of the pancreas. The predominant actions of insulin are to lower the blood glucose by stimulating uptake of glucose into cells via the insulin-dependent glucose transporter Glut-4 (fat and muscle). Insulin-independent glucose transporters, Glut-1 (brain) and Glut-2 (liver and β cell), transport glucose in a concentration-dependent manner. The net effect is transport of glucose into the liver, where it is converted to glycogen by glycogen synthetase and into acetyl-coenzyme A (CoA) via glycolysis. This acetyl-CoA is converted into fatty acids and transported to adipocytes, where it is stored as fat. In muscle, glucose is stored as glycogen.

The first phase of fasting commences as the blood glucose levels fall toward 70 mg/dL and insulin secretion decreases. As insulin levels fall, inhibition of glycogenolysis, gluconeogenesis, and lipolysis is removed. Under the influence of rising glucagon levels, hepatic glycogenolysis is stimulated and glucose is released from the liver. The key enzymes involved are glucose-6-phosphatase and the glycogen debrancher enzyme. At the same time, gluconeogenesis from precursors such as alanine, glycerol, and lactate recycled from glycolysis begins to increase. However, because there are limited stores of amino acids, glucose utilization is decreased to preserve glucose for those cells that cannot utilize any other source of energy. Glycogen reserves provide glucose for about 2 to 4 hours in infants and 6 to 8 hours in adults. Lipolysis is suppressed by insulin and stimulated by growth hormone and epinephrine. With fasting, insulin is decreased and growth hormone and epinephrine are increased, resulting in increased lipolysis, which provides fatty acids for ketogenesis and glycerol for gluconeogenesis. Muscle oxidizes fatty acids to ketones and uses them for fuel and therefore conserves glucose. The brain, although unable to transport fatty acids across the blood-brain barrier, utilizes ketones generated by the liver in place of glucose. Fatty acid oxidation in liver and muscle requires three key processes, involving the carnitine cycle, β-oxidation, and ketogenesis. The energy produced by FAO helps fuel gluconeogenesis. The net effect of all of these adaptations to fasting is the preservation of glucose for those cells dependent on glucose as a fuel source, such as red blood cells, and switching to alternate fuel sources by those cells that can use alternate fuels for energy production. The changes in intermediary metabolites that occur over time with fasting in the normal child are shown in Figure 3-1.

The cause of most episodes of hypoglycemia may be correctly diagnosed when looked at in the context of the fasting system, and when the history is combined with a series of blood tests performed at the time of hypoglycemia. These blood tests are critical to the diagnosis as they allow a snapshot of the biochemical and hormonal milieu at the time of hypoglycemia (see Box 3-1). Comparison of the results of this critical draw to the "normal levels" means looking at the results compared with values expected during hypoglycemia, not the laboratory norms for age and gender (see Box 3-2). Thus the pitfall of finding an insulin level of 4 IU/L (normal fasting levels, 2 to 12 IU/L) at a time of hypoglycemia and thinking that this is within normal limits is avoided and the diagnosis of HI is not missed. "Normal" for hypoglycemia is <2 IU/L.

NEONATAL HYPOGLYCEMIA

Neonatal hypoglycemia remains a controversial area of glucose homeostasis. Most disorders causing hypoglycemia in infants and children are also manifest in the immediate neonatal period. The causes of neonatal hypoglycemia are outlined in Table 3-1. By far the most common cause of hypoglycemia in the first day of life is transitional hypoglycemia. After the first 24 hours of life, hypoglycemia that continues to occur is *not* transitional hypoglycemia. It is very important to understand that *transitional hypoglycemia* is a normal adaptation to extrauterine life and that hypoglycemia that persists beyond 24 hours of life is a pathological condition. It may not be permanent, yet it may be just as dangerous as the conditions that cause persistent hypoglycemia. This form of nonpermanent hypoglycemia is called *transient hypoglycemia*, and it tends to be due to transient regulatory problems in glucose homeostasis rather than to genetic defects. In this chapter on hypoglycemia, the causes of persistent neonatal hypoglycemia are discussed separately. This separation is not meant to imply that transient hypoglycemia is harmless but rather to highlight the differences between transitional, transient, and persistent hypoglycemia.

Transitional Hypoglycemia

Transitional hypoglycemia is by definition the hypoglycemia that occurs during the first 12 hours of life as the neonate transitions from intrauterine glucose homeostasis to extrauterine homeostasis. In addition, it should refer

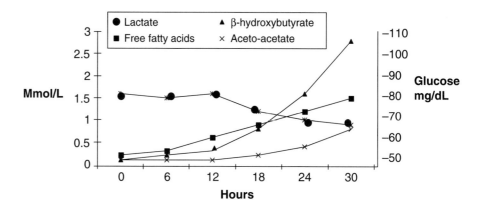

Figure 3-1 Normal Intermediary Metabolite Response to Fasting. ●, Lactate; ■, free fatty acids; ▲, β-hydroxybutyrate; X, aceto-acetate.

Table 3-1	Etiology of Hypoglycemia in Neonates, Infants and Children

Neonatal hypoglycemia
   Transitional hypoglycemia in the first 12 hours of life
   Transient hyperinsulinism
      Infants of diabetic mothers
      Glucose infusions during labor
      Perinatal stress induced hyperinsulinism
         Intrauterine growth retardation
         Postasphyxia
         Preeclampsia in mother
   Persistent genetic forms of hyperinsulinism
      Focal and diffuse hyperinsulinism secondary to *SUR1* and
         Kir6.2 defects
      Glutamate dehydrogenase hyperinsulinism
      Glucokinase hyperinsulinism
   Glycogen storage disease type 1
   Hypopituitarism
   Corticotropin (ACTH) unresponsiveness
   Adrenal insufficiency
      Adrenal hemorrhage
      Congenital adrenal hyperplasia
Hypoglycemia in infants and children
   Glycogen storage disorders (types I, III, VI, and IX)
   Glycogen synthase deficiency
   Disorders of gluconeogenesis
      Fructose-1,6-bisphosphate deficiency
      Hereditary fructose intolerance
      Phosphoenolpyruvate carboxykinase deficiency
   Disorders of fatty acid oxidation (see Table 3-2)
      Disorders of the carnitine cycle
      Disorders of beta-oxidation
      Disorders of electron transport
      Disorders of ketogenesis
   Hyperinsulinism
      Focal and diffuse hyperinsulinism secondary to *SUR1* and
         Kir6.2 defects

      Glutamate dehydrogenase hyperinsulinism
      Glucokinase hyperinsulinism
      Insulinoma
   Growth hormone deficiency
   Adrenal insufficiency
      Primary
         Addison disease
         Adrenoleukodystrophy
      Secondary
         ACTH deficiency or resistance
      Tertiary
         Hypothalamic corticotropin-releasing hormone (CRH)
            deficiency
      Steroid-induced adrenal suppression
   Non–islet cell tumor–induced hypoglycemia
   Idiopathic ketotic hypoglycemia
   Ketone utilization defects
   Iatrogenic
      Abrupt discontinuation of high-concentration intravenous
         glucose infusions
      Nissan fundoplication with gastric tube feeds
   Drugs
      Oral sulfonylureas
      β-Blockers
      Salicylates
      Pentamadine
      Quinine
   Alcohol
      Ingestion
      Skin absorption
   Acute liver failure
   Munchausen disease (by proxy)
      Insulin administration
      Oral sulfonylurea administration

only to term AGA infants. Data by Lubchenko and Bard have clearly shown that up to 30% of infants have glucose levels below 50 mg/dL in the first hours of life and that this resolves. Early feeding of breast milk or formula stimulates the enzymes involved in FAO and gluconeogenesis and replenishes glycogen stores. Management of the AGA infant with transitional hypoglycemia is early and frequent demand feeding. If after the first 12 hours of life, all preprandial glucose levels are greater than 60 mg/dL for 24 hours, no further investigations are necessary.

Transient Hypoglycemia of Infancy

Transient hypoglycemia of infancy is hypoglycemia that persists beyond 24 hours of life. This may be caused by a variety of different disorders and occurs in less than 0.5% of infants. Transient hypoglycemia is most commonly seen in preterm infants. These infants have low glycogen and fat reserves and a delay in maturity of the enzymes involved in

gluconeogenesis and FAO. They have a relatively greater brain-to-body ratio and have higher glucose utilization per kilogram of body weight. They are unable to tolerate even a 4-hour fast and need frequent feedings to maintain blood glucose at greater than 60 mg/dL. Hypoglycemia resolves in the majority of these infants once there is steady weight gain. Once the premature infant is established on bolus feeds every 3 to 4 hours and is gaining weight, he or she should have a feeding skipped; if glucose levels remain at greater than 60 mg/dL, it is most likely that the patient's glucose homeostasis has stabilized.

Infants of Diabetic Mothers

Transient elevation of insulin levels in infants of diabetic mothers (IDMs) tends to occur in diabetic women in whom glucose control was not adequate. This is often manifest in infants who weigh more than 4.5 kg at birth, but it may occur in AGA infants. During intrauterine life, high blood glucose levels in the mother result in chronically elevated glucose levels in the fetus. These chronically elevated glucose levels in the fetus stimulate chronically elevated insulin levels leading to increased fat deposition. This results in the classic fat infant with round facies and plethoric appearance. Typically, hypoglycemia in these infants take 2 to 3 days to resolve. The β cell does not immediately adjust to the rapidly falling glucose levels and continues to secrete insulin as the glucose levels fall below 70 mg/dL. Plasma free fatty acids (FFAs) and ketones are suppressed during hypoglycemia, and the infant responds to intravenous glucagon. Treatment is to maintain the blood glucose level at greater than 70 mg/dL through a combination of oral feedings and intravenous glucose infusions. A common pitfall in the management of the IDMs is to use intravenous bolus therapy without continuous dextrose infusion at 8 mg/kg/min. This causes a swinging of glucose levels from high to low and high again, and glucose instability may last for days. Maintaining the glucose between 70 mg/dL and 90 mg/dL is the optimal way to manage the IDM.

Obstetrical Intervention–Induced Hyperinsulinism

The infusion of large amounts of dextrose in the mother during the latter part of labor has been shown to induce hypoglycemia in the infant secondary to HI. This form of hypoglycemia is short lived and corrects in 2 to 4 hours. The use of β-agonists has also been shown to cause elevated cord blood insulin levels and hypoglycemia.

Transient Perinatal Stress Hyperinsulinism

It has long been recognized that infants born IUGR or after toxemia or those with perinatal asphyxia have a higher incidence of hypoglycemia persisting beyond day 2 or 3 of life. Studies by Collins et al in the 1980s and 1990s suggested that many of these infants have transient HI. This has since been confirmed, and studies have demonstrated that these infants may continue to have transient HI for up to 6 months. Some authors have suggested that glucagon deficiency is the primary etiological agent and that there is a secondary relative HI. This form of hypoglycemia is of particular danger due to the suppression of alternate fuel sources by insulin. The diagnosis of transient HI is suspected in those infants with a history of IUGR or perinatal stress. In addition, the findings of a glucose utilization rate of greater than 8 mg/kg/min, measurable insulin levels at the time of hypoglycemia, suppressed FFAs and ketones, and a glycemic response (>30 mg/dL) to the intravenous injection of 1 mg of glucagon at the time of hypoglycemia confirm the diagnosis.

Treatment of transient HI is to maintain the blood glucose at greater than 70 mg/dL with intravenous infusions of

glucose plus oral feedings. Diazoxide at 10 mg/kg/day effectively treats most cases, but rarely 15 mg/kg/day is required. If diazoxide does not result in a rapid resolution of hypoglycemia, one must consider the possibility that the HI is one of the more severe genetic varieties. Diazoxide reaches full effect in 5 days. Once the patient is off all intravenous fluids, a fasting study must be done to demonstrate that the infant can maintain the blood glucose at greater than 70 mg/dL for at least 12 hours before discharge. A fasting study done when the infant has been off diazoxide for 1 week, by 6 months of age, confirms the resolution of HI and confirms that it was a transient problem. At this age, a infant should fast for 18 hours with a normal intermediary metabolite response (Box 3-2).

GLYCOGEN STORAGE DISORDERS

Glycogenolysis, the term used to describe the breakdown of glycogen to glucose, is the first defense against hypoglycemia in the fasting state. Once infants start to extend their feeding interval, glycogenolysis takes on a very important role in glucose homeostasis. It is for this reason that the most severe forms of GSD do not present in the immediate newborn period but rather as the infant becomes older. Not all disorders of glycogen metabolism cause hypoglycemia; some are manifest as muscle weakness and cardiomyopathy, rather than having an effect on glucose homeostasis. This section is confined to those forms of GSD with hypoglycemia as a manifestation, including GSD-I, -III, -VI, and -IX and what some refer to as GSD-0, or glycogen synthase deficiency.

Glucose-6-phosphatase Deficiency (GSD-Ia)

Glucose-6-phosphatase deficiency, or GSD-Ia, occurs due to a deficiency of the enzyme glucose-6-phosphatase. This is an autosomal recessive disorder caused by mutations in the *G6Pase* gene, located on chromosome 17. It occurs in approximately 1:100,000 children. Although it causes severe hypoglycemia from infancy on, more cases are diagnosed after 1 year of age with failure to thrive, protuberant abdomen due to massive hepatomegaly, and metabolic acidosis. The striking feature of GSD-Ia is the apparent lack of symptoms due to hypoglycemia and the remarkable normality of development despite severe hypoglycemia. This disorder typifies why a single value of glucose does not predict whether brain damage will occur. Patients with GSD-Ia have elevated levels of lactate, which the brain readily uses as fuel during the prolonged and severe episodes of hypoglycemia. Although the hypoglycemia does not cause brain damage, it does stimulate counterregulatory hormone responses, and levels of cortisol, GH, and epinephrine are elevated. This causes constant stimulation of glycogenolysis and gluconeogenesis. The effect of this is to push liver metabolism of glucose into glycolysis and the formation of lactate. Elevated lactate levels cause metabolic acidosis, which in its severe form triggers hyperventilation. In addition, there is constant lipolysis, resulting in elevated triglycerides and hyperlipidemia (blood samples described as creamy are often reported). Sequestration of phosphate in the form of glucose-6-phosphate results in depletion of cellular ATP. This results in increased uric acid formation as a result of adenosine degradation, which together with the competition at a renal tubule level for excretion with lactate results in hyperuricemia. Thus the classic clinical presentation of GSD-Ia is short stature with a protuberant abdomen, associated with hypoglycemia, lactic acidosis, hyperlipidemia, hyperuricemia, and mildly elevated liver enzymes. Platelet adhesiveness is reduced, causing easy bruising. Despite massive liver enlargement (sometimes so large it is missed unless the examiner starts at the iliac crest), the spleen is rarely enlarged and there is rarely portal hypertension.

Long-term complications of GSD-Ia include a diabetes-like nephropathy (focal glomerular sclerosis), nephrocalcinosis, and proteinuria leading to end-stage renal failure. From the age of 10 years on, transformation of benign nodules in the liver to malignancy may occur. Osteoporosis, secondary to chronic acidosis, is a problem in the later decades.

Diagnosis is made by the finding of lactic acidosis associated with hypoglycemia, marked elevation of triglycerides and uric acid, and minimal elevation of liver function tests. In contrast to the normal rise in blood glucose, in response to glucagon in the immediate postprandial phase, patients with GSD-Ia have no rise in glucose but rather a brisk rise in lactate. Diagnosis can now be made by genetic testing or by enzyme analysis performed on liver tissue obtained by biopsy.

Treatment of GSD-Ia focuses on two aspects: (1) avoidance of fasting for more than 3 to 4 hours and (2) avoidance of the use of excessive fructose and lactose, which must first be metabolized by glucose-6-phosphatase in the liver, for the glucose so generated to be liberated from the hepatocyte. The emphasis has shifted to avoidance of fasting, and this can be achieved by feedings every 3 hours during the day and continuous dextrose infusions via nasogastric tube overnight. Once children reach the age of 1 year, uncooked cornstarch can be added to the regimen in doses of 1 g/kg to enable fasts of up to 4 hours to safely occur and of 2 g/kg for a 6-hour fast. Continuous nocturnal glucose infusions may be very dangerous to the patients should the infusion abruptly stop by accident. Under these circumstances, hypoglycemia rapidly ensues and, due to the suppression of lactate, there is inadequate time for lactate levels to rise; the patient is found seizing or dead in bed. It is a remarkable feature of GSD-Ia that the patient may never have symptomatic hypoglycemia until treatment is begun and may never experience hypoglycemic brain damage until treatment is begun. However, treatment clearly improves the lactic acidosis, enabling better linear growth and prevention of osteoporosis. In addition, treatment causes the liver to return to near normal size and decreases the risk of hepatic adenomas, lowers triglyceride and urate levels, is thought to prevent or delay the onset of renal complications, and induces a sense of well-being to the patient.

Glucose-6-phosphatase Deficiency (GSD-Ib)

Hepatic glucose-6-phosphatase is known to be a multicomponent enzyme system with several components that together convert glucose-6-phosphate (G-6-P) into glucose and phosphate. This reaction occurs in the endoplasmic reticulum (ER) of the hepatocyte and requires at least three translocase enzymes. T1 transports G-6-P into the ER, T2 transports the phosphate out of the ER, and T3 transports the free glucose out of the ER. GSD-Ib is due to T1 deficiency and is identical to GSD-Ia with the addition of neutrophil dysfunction. This causes an immune deficiency secondary to neutropenia and is manifest as oral ulceration, skin abscesses, and chronic inflammatory bowel disease. Management of the hypoglycemia is identical to GSD-Ia, but the neutropenia remains a problem. Granulocyte colony-stimulating factor has been successfully used to treat the neutropenia. GSD-Ic is due to T2 deficiency and a problem with the transport of phosphate out of the ER.

Debrancher Enzyme Deficiency (GSD-III)

Amylo-1,6-glucosidase deficiency results in the inability to degrade glycogen past its 1:4/1:6 branch points (hence called debrancher deficiency). Only approximately 10% of glycogen stores are accessible before a branch point comes up. Once a branch point is reached, glycogenolysis cannot proceed and hypoglycemia ensues. Elevated lactate levels do not occur because glycolysis may proceed completely without a buildup of lactate. Deposition of glycogen in the liver causes massive hepatomegaly, associated with marked elevations of liver enzymes with failure to thrive. Because gluconeogenesis can occur effectively, hypoglycemia is not as severe as GSD-Ia and occurs only after more prolonged fasting. There is not such an overdrive of counterregulatory hormones and so lipolysis is not constantly switched on and hyperlipidemia is not a feature. Ketonuria occurs with prolonged fasting.

Long-term complications include severe muscle weakness and death from cardiomyopathy in those with muscle involvement. Cirrhosis of the liver may occur, leading to liver failure.

The diagnosis is suspect in children with failure to thrive and massive hepatomegaly. Unlike patients with GSD-Ia, those with GSD-III have marked elevation of AST and ALT. There is no elevation of lactate with hypoglycemia and there is a rise in glucose in response to the fed glucagon stimulation test, but not in the fasted glucagon stimulation test (after a 6- to 8-hour fast). Diagnosis may be made by enzymatic studies on liver biopsy or in white blood cells. In addition to liver problems, about 33% to 50% patients have a myopathy resulting in muscle weakness and cardiomyopathy. These children develop elevations in creatine kinase (CK) from 3 or 4 years on.

Treatment for the nonmyopathic form is frequent feeding and avoidance of overnight fasting by continuous glucose nasogastric feeding or nocturnal uncooked cornstarch therapy. For those with myopathy, high-protein diet acts as a source of gluconeogenic substrate and may prevent the severe muscle wasting and cardiomyopathy.

Liver Phosphorylase (GSD-VI) and Phosphorylase-Kinase (GSD-IX) Deficiency

These two forms of GSD are milder than forms GSD-Ia, -Ib, and GSD-III and difficult to differentiate. The phosphorylase system is responsible for breaking down the straight chains of glycogen until the debrancher step. Once past the branch point, the phosphorylase system continues to cleave glucose-1-phosphate moieties from the glycogen chain. Deficiency in either phosphorylase or its kinase results in the inability to break down glycogen. Despite this, hypoglycemia is not prevalent and occurs only with prolonged fasting. Hepatomegaly is the predominant feature. Patients with these forms of GSD do very well; their hepatomegaly responds well to frequent feeding and avoidance of overnight fasting. Patients get better spontaneously by puberty. Growth retardation is rarely found.

Glycogen Synthase Deficiency (GSD-0)

Glycogen synthase deficiency is the rarest of the hypoglycemic GSDs. The genetic etiology of this condition has been elucidated and patients have been found with mutations in the liver glycogen synthase gene. There are few reports, but patients have fasting-induced hypoglycemia and hyperketonemia. In addition, they may present with hyperglycemia or glycosuria postprandially. The postprandial hyperglycemia occurs as a result of the inability of the liver to store glucose as glycogen. Lactate levels may rise as glucose undergoes glycolysis as its main pathway of disposal.

The glucagon stimulation test in the fasted state shows no increase in glucose with a rise in lactate. Treatment was initially described with a high-protein diet, but the simple avoidance of fasting may be adequate therapy.

DISORDERS OF GLUCONEOGENESIS

Disorders of gluconeogenesis are rare and cause hypoglycemia after the initial stages of fasting are complete and glycogen reserves are depleted. Typically, the hypoglycemia is associated with acidosis, both lactic and ketoacidosis. Although there are many steps involved in gluconeogenesis, most of the enzyme deficiencies do not have hypoglycemia as their primary defect (Figure 3-2). Much has been written about hypoglycemia in galactosemia, in practice hypoglycemia is rarely a presenting symptom of galactosemia and most likely occurs only in relation to sepsis or acute liver failure associated with galactosemia. Similarly, pyruvate carboxlyase (PC) would appear to hold the potential to have significant hypoglycemia, yet this is a minor part of PC deficiency. Severe lactic acidosis and hyperammonemia, with coma and hypotonia, are the most common presenting features. PEPCK is also extremely rare cause of hypoglycemia.

Fructose-1,6-bisphosphatase Deficiency

Fructose-1,6-bisphosphatase (FDPase) deficiency was first described by Baker and Weingrad in the early 1970s. This enzyme catalyzes the irreversible reaction of fructose-1,6-bisphosphate to fructose-6-phosphate. The absence of this enzyme prevents gluconeogenesis from fructose, lactate, and amino acids such as alanine. Classically, FDPase may present in the newborn period with severe neonatal hypoglycemia, respiratory distress, and coma associated with marked lactic acidosis and ketosis. There may be hepatomegaly. Approximately 50% of patients, with milder disease, first present in later life after periods of prolonged fasting or intercurrent illness. Between episodes of decompensation, the lactic acidosis resolves and hepatomegaly may be subtle. Differentiation from GSD-Ia is made based on the glucagon stimulation test, which in the fed state in FDPase causes a rise in glucose, in contrast to GSD-Ia, in which glucose does not rise but lactate does.

Presentation in the newborn period is usually associated with the most severe deficiencies. Treatment of newborns requires correction of hypoglycemia with glucose infusion rates of at least 8 to 10 mg/kg/min. Bicarbonate, in very large doses, may be required to correct the lactic acidosis. Insulin infusions may occasionally be required to suppress gluconeogenesis if the lactic acidosis does not resolve. Older infants and children with milder forms often

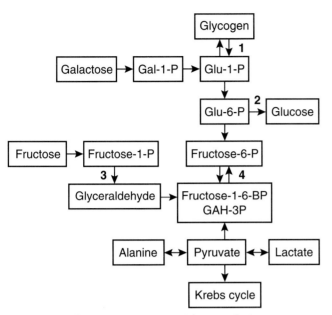

Figure 3-2   The Important Steps in Glycogenolysis, Gluconeogenesis, and the Metabolism of Fructose. Glu, glucose; Gal, galactose; P, phosphate; GAH, glyceraldehyde; BP, bisphosphate; 1, debrancher enzyme (GSD-III); 2, glucose-6-phosphatase (GSD-I); 3, fructoaldolase (HFI); 4, FDPase.

respond to intravenous glucose and do not require large amounts of bicarbonate or insulin. Long-term management consists of the avoidance of prolonged fasting and reducing fructose in the diet. During periods of intercurrent illness, either nasogastric glucose or intravenous glucose infusion at 8 mg/kg/min should be administered to prevent decompensation.

Hereditary Fructose Intolerance

Hereditary fructose intolerance (HFI) has been described as an idiosyncratic reaction to fructose. It is an autosomal recessive condition occurring in approximately 1:20,000 people, and two mutations are commonly identified. Affected patients classically demonstrate a total avoidance of fructose due to learned behavior that ingestion of certain foods and beverages causes discomfort. On exposure to fructose, levels of fructose-1-phosphate rapidly accumulate in cells lining the gastrointestinal tract and in hepatocytes. This causes a rapid depletion of phosphate resulting in an acute shortage of adenosine triphosphate (ATP), causing a cellular energy failure. In the gut, this becomes manifest as vomiting and diarrhea and abdominal pain, and in the liver, as hypoglycemia, possibly leading to acute liver failure. Renal failure may follow. The episode of hypoglycemia may be short lived and self-resolving when only small quantities of fructose are ingested.

Patients with HFI do not present until fructose exposure in the diet occurs. This often happens from 4 months of age

on. Fructose is found as the main sugar in fruit, honey, and many sweet vegetables. As a disaccharide, it is found in table sugar (sucrose) in combination with glucose. Many years ago, intravenous preparations of fructose were common, but not so now. This is fortunate because infants and children who receive intravenous fructose, unless in controlled circumstances such as a fructose challenge test, may develop profound hepatorenal failure. Infants rapidly learn to avoid fructose and, as adults, rarely get dental caries due to sugar avoidance. A history of symptoms of hypoglycemia and abdominal discomfort induced by feeding should alert one to the possibility of HFI. Treatment is the removal of fructose from the diet and intravenous infusion of glucose to support the patient until the fructose is cleared from the system. Long-term outcome is good provided there is strict avoidance of fructose in the diet.

FATTY ACID OXIDATION DISORDERS

One of the most critical steps in fasting adaptation is the liberation of fatty acids from lipid stores, and transport to the liver, where they undergo FAO. The liver, by exporting ketones generated from FAs to the brain, contributes to the decreased need for glucose during fasting. In addition, skeletal and cardiac muscle, by utilizing fatty acids for energy production, minimize the overall body requirement for glucose. The combination of ketone utilization by the brain and muscle is responsible for 80% of total body energy needs during fasting. In addition, FAO provides the energy for gluconeogenesis and the provision of glucose for those cells unable to utilize other fuel sources. Hence this system is very important.

Classically, disorders of FAO present at a later stage of fasting adaptation than either disorders of glycogenolysis or gluconeogenesis. In general, they also tend to present in infants and children at an older age as feeding intervals become more prolonged. The first manifestation of an FAO disorder in previously healthy infants and children may occur when they become exposed to the metabolic stress of their first intercurrent illness. The FAO disorders cause not only hypoglycemia but also cardiac and skeletal muscle abnormalities (Table 3-2). Many of these disorders have all three abnormalities, and some manifest only as hypoglycemia.

Disorders of FAO are inherited in an autosomal recessive manner. Recently, with the adoption of extended newborn screening by tandem mass spectroscopy, most affected patients are detected at birth before developing signs and symptoms. This modern technology has many advantages as well as some disadvantages. Parents do not appreciate the severity of the illness, and physicians assume that patients

Table 3-2   Clinical Features of Disorders of Fatty Acid Oxidation

Enzyme/Transport Deficiency	Hepatic (Predominantly Hypoglycemia)	Cardiac	Skeletal Muscle Manifestations	
			Acute Rhabdomyolysis	Chronic Myopathy
Carnitine Cycle Defects				
Carnitine transporter (CTD)	X	X		X
Carnitine palmityl transferase-1 (CPT-1)	X			
Carnitine/acyl-carnitine transferase-2 (CPT-2)	X	X		X
Carnitine palmityl transferase-2 (CPT-2)	X	X	X	X
β-Oxidation Defects				
Acyl-CoA Dehydrogenases				
Very long-chain (VLCAD)	X	X		X
Medium-chain (MCAD)	X			
Short-chain (SCAD)				X
3-Hydroxyacyl-CoA Dehydrogenases				
Long-chain (LCHAD)	X	X	X	X
Short-chain (SCHAD)				X
Medium-chain ketoacyl-CoA thiolase			X	
2,4-Dienoyl-CoA reductase (DER)				
Electron Transport Defects				
Electron transfer flavoprotein (ETF)X	X	X	X	X
ETF dehydrogenase (ETF-DH)	X	X	X	X
Ketone Synthesis				
HMG-CoA synthase				X
HMG-CoA lyase				

CoA, coenzyme A; HMG, 3-hydroxy-3-methylglutaryl.
*In addition patients with the severe ETF disorders may have a "fishy" odor.

presenting later in life could not have an FAO disorder, because there is newborn screening. However, as is known for hypothyroidism, newborn screening is fallible and physicians must be aware of the signs and symptoms of the FAO disorders.

Hypoglycemia

Most of the disorders of FAO have hypoglycemia and hepatic dysfunction as a component of the condition. The exceptions to this are short-chain acyl-CoA dehydrogenase deficiency (SCAD) and short-chain 3-hydroxyacyl-CoA dehydrogenase deficiency (SCHAD). Medium-chain acyl-CoA dehydrogenase deficiency (MCAD), by far the most common FAO defect, is typical of the hepatic manifestations. After a period of metabolic stress such as fasting in an infant or a child who was previously well, oxidation of medium-chain fatty acids by the mitochondrial β-oxidation systems is blocked. As a result, about 12 to 15 hours into a fasting stress, there is an inability to produce ketones and glucose levels fall. Hypoglycemia is associated with elevated

FFAs but inappropriately low ketone levels in the plasma. Patients, if untreated, develop lethargy, coma, and seizures and may die. This is in part due to the hypoglycemia but also due to the toxicity of FFAs, elevation of ammonia due to impairment of the urea cycle, and acute liver dysfunction. Mortality and morbidity rates from the first metabolic crises in MCAD may be as high as 25%. Liver enlargement during the acute episode is common due to fat deposition; this resolves with resolution of the acute decompensation. In the past, many patients with MCAD were confused with Reye syndrome. MCAD deficiency is suggested by a family history of sudden infant death syndrome or acute life-threatening events in a sibling.

The diagnosis of MCAD (and other FAO disorders) is best made at the time of presentation. The critical sample at the time of hypoglycemia reveals elevated fatty acids, low plasma ketones, and absent urine ketones (but they may be as high as moderate depending on the hydration status of the patient and the form of FAO). There is acidosis, including lactic acid elevation in some forms, and abnormal liver function tests. Plasma urate is elevated, and ammonia may also be elevated. The acyl-carnitine profile is diagnostic in many instances, except primary carnitine deficiency and CPT-1. Urine organic acids and urine acyl-glycines also provide clues to the metabolic perturbation.

Treatment of hypoglycemia is to provide glucose infusion of at least 8 mg/kg/min to suppress lipolysis and correct the hypoglycemia. A characteristic of the FAO disorders is that the patient looks sicker than the level of glucose would suggest and does not respond as quickly to intravenous glucose infusion as one would expect. Supportive treatment of coma, dehydration, and seizures is also required. The hyperammonemia usually corrects with glucose administration.

Cardiomyopathy

Primary carnitine deficiency causes the most severe manifestations of cardiomyopathy, presenting as congestive heart failure or acute ventricular arrhythmias. Echocardiography shows in some forms of FAO defects as a dilated cardiomyopathy and in others a hypertrophic cardiomyopathy. The cardiomyopathy may present in an isolated manner but more often is part of an acute metabolic decompensation. Initial provision of glucose via intravenous infusion is generally not sufficient to reverse the cardiomyopathy, and inotropic support is often required. In acute decompensation, it is often the cardiomyopathy that is fatal.

Skeletal Muscle

Skeletal muscle problems may be acute or chronic. Acute episodes of rhabdomyolysis have been reported in CPT-2, long-chain 3-hydroxyacyl-CoA dehydrogenase deficiency (LCHAD), and SCHAD deficiency. In these cases, elevations of creatine phosphokinase (CPK) causing renal failure may occur during fasting stress or secondary to intercurrent illness. Between episodes, there may be chronic elevation of CPK or CPK may return to normal. Acyl-carnitine and urine organic acid tests should be performed in all patients with rhabdomyolysis.

Chronic muscle weakness occurs in many of the FAO disorders and may present from infancy to later in life. Optimal metabolic control may help the prevention of progression of the myopathy, but in some cases it may be progressive and cause death.

Miscellaneous Signs and Symptoms

Malformations may be found at birth in patients with electron transfer abnormalities such as severe multiple acyl-CoA dehydrogenase deficiencies (MADD, formerly known as glutaric aciduria type 2) and CPT-2. These may include brain malformations and renal abnormalities.

Renal tubular acidosis occurs in CPT-1 and is usually transient during acute decompensation. Patients with MADD may have a fishy smell to the urine. Neurodevelopmental delay is seen in SCAD patients who have no evidence of a history of acute decompensation. In many of the remainder of the FAO defects, developmental delay occurs as a result of an acute metabolic decompensation.

Treatment of the Fatty Acid Oxidation Disorders

Treatment of the FAO defects consists primarily of meticulous attention to the prevention of fasting stress. Patients must understand the potential risks associated with intercurrent illness and be able to manage sick days. Frequent feedings of fluid rich in carbohydrates is essential during intercurrent illness. It is important to note that if one waits for hypoglycemia to develop in patients with known FAO disorders, it may be too late to prevent metabolic decompensation. Carnitine therapy is recommended only for those with primary carnitine deficiency, although some have recommended it for many of the disorders of FAO. Restriction of fat in the diet has been recommended for very long-chain 3-hydroxyacyl-CoA dehydrogenase (VLCAD), LCHAD, and carnitine translocase deficiency, with supplemental medium-chain triglycerides, which bypass the need for the carnitine cycle. Treatment of rhabdomyolysis, in addition to intravenous glucose, requires forced alkaline diuresis and, if renal failure occurs, dialysis. Cardiac failure may be treated with diuretics and inotropic support.

Outcome

Patients with MCAD, the most common FAO defect, in general do very well, and once the diagnosis is made, they should have a good outcome. Some of the disorders, however, such as carnitine translocase, LCHAD, severe neonatal CPT-2, and the severe form of MADD, have a poor prognosis even with intervention. Patients with primary carnitine deficiency usually do well once carnitine therapy is commenced.

DISORDERS OF HORMONAL REGULATION OF GLUCOSE METABOLISM

Hypoglycemia as a result of hormonal imbalance may be divided into several subtypes. Hyperinsulinism due to genetic defects in the regulatory pathways of insulin secretion is by far the most common hormonal cause of hypoglycemia.

Deficiencies in multiple anterior pituitary hormones may also cause hypoglycemia. Isolated growth hormone (GH) deficiency or isolated cortisol deficiency causes a less severe hypoglycemia than multiple pituitary hormone deficiencies.

Hypopituitarism

Up to 20% of patients with congenital hypopituitarism have significant hypoglycemia from birth. In some cases, the hypoglycemia is very severe with such increased glucose requirement that oral feeding is unable to maintain glucose levels greater than 60 mg/dL. Patients sometimes require glucose infusion rates of 10 to 15 mg/kg body weight/min. This sort of increased glucose utilization can make hypopituitarism difficult to differentiate from congenital HI. Clinically, there may be a history of persistent jaundice. The physical examination may reveal micropenis in males, central cleft lip and/or palate, and eye abnormalities such as septo-optic dysplasia or be completely normal. In rare cases, the jaundice has progressed to a severe form of hepatitis; there have been reports of cirrhosis from long-term untreated hypopituitarism. Genetic defects in genes such as *PIT-1* or *PROP-1* may cause multiple anterior pituitary hormone deficiencies. In older children, hypopituitarism may be caused by tumors such as craniopharyngioma or glioma, by trauma causing transection of the pituitary stalk, by infiltration such as histiocytosis, by tuberculosis, or by autoimmune hypophysitis.

Deficiency of corticotropin (ACTH) leading to cortisol insufficiency results in impaired gluconeogenesis. Deficiency of GH plays a role in the increased glucose utilization rates due to a relative excess of insulin over counterregulatory hormones. Lipolysis is impaired and ketogenesis reduced. It is for this reason that newborns with a combination of cortisol insufficiency (secondary to ACTH deficiency) and GH deficiency are often hypoketotic, whereas older children with GH deficiency alone are more likely to be ketotic.

The critical sample at a time of hypoglycemia may be helpful in ruling out GH and cortisol deficiency. This is because in those with GH or cortisol sufficiency, elevated levels occur about 20 to 30 minutes after the hypoglycemia first occurs as part of the counterregulatory hormone response. Hence, GH levels of greater than 7 ng/dL and cortisol levels of greater than 20 µg/dL rule out hypopituitarism. If elevated levels are not seen at the time of hypoglycemia, then provocative studies of cortisol response to ACTH or corticotropin releasing factor (CRF) and GH stimulation tests should be undertaken. Free T_4 levels should be measured because thyroid-stimulating hormone levels in hypopituitarism may be inappropriately normal despite low free T_4. In addition to the confusion caused by finding an increased glucose infusion requirement, the glucagon stimulation test may show a rise of greater than 30 mg/dL at the time of hypoglycemia. These two features can make hypopituitarism difficult to differentiate from HI.

Treatment is to provide glucose via the oral or intravenous route to keep the blood glucose greater than 60 mg/dL. In addition, GH therapy should be instituted (0.3 mg/kg/wk divided daily or, rarely, twice daily) and cortisol replacement by mouth dosed every 8 hours (12-15 mg/m²/day). Some infants require greater than physiological replacement doses of GH and cortisol to prevent hypoglycemia. Thyroid replacement must not be forgotten, especially if the focus is on the prevention of hypoglycemia.

Isolated Cortisol Deficiency

In newborns, isolated cortisol deficiency is almost always part of a more complex congenital adrenal hyperplasia (CAH) syndrome. Female infants are virilized as a result of the most common form of CAH, 21-hydroxylase deficiency, but male infants may not be detected so easily. In addition to cortisol deficiency, aldosterone deficiency causes salt-losing crises in 50% of affected patients. This is usually manifest as weight loss, dehydration, and collapse. Hypoglycemia associated with hyperkalemia should lead one to suspect adrenal insufficiency, and a cause such as CAH should be sought (see Chapter 10).

In older children, cortisol insufficiency is more commonly secondary to autoimmune adrenal disease (Addison disease) and rarely secondary to adrenoleukodystrophy (ALD). Although ALD is X-linked, it can cause adrenal insufficiency in females. In both forms of primary adrenal insufficiency, there is both glucocorticoid and mineralocorticoid loss and hypoglycemia is associated with hyperkalemia and hyponatremia. Patients may be pigmented secondary to markedly elevated ACTH levels.

Initial treatment with hydrocortisone at rates of 50 to 100 mg/m²/day intravenous glucose for hypoglycemia and normal saline for hyperkalemia and hyponatremia stabilizes the patient. Once the patient has recovered from the acute decompensation, oral hydrocortisone at 15 mg/m² body surface area and oral mineralocorticoid are indicated.

Isolated Growth Hormone Deficiency

Isolated GH deficiency may cause hypoglycemia both in the newborn period and later in life. It should be suspected in patients with ketotic hypoglycemia who are not growing well. It often presents only after prolonged fasting with intercurrent illness. Random GH measurements are rarely of use in diagnosing GH deficiency, and one should screen for GH deficiency by measuring insulin-like growth factor-I (IGF-I) and IGF binding protein 3 (IGFBP-3). Treatment is GH replacement, and in those with hypoglycemia as a presenting feature, a fasting study should be done on GH to demonstrate resolution of hypoglycemia.

It is important to note that isolated GH deficiency and isolated cortisol deficiency may mimic idiopathic ketotic hypoglycemia and that both should be ruled out before making the diagnosis of idiopathic ketotic hypoglycemia.

Congenital Hyperinsulinism

Congenital HI is the most common and most severe form of persistent neonatal hypoglycemia. It is a genetically heterogeneous disorder with four genes identified to date. *SUR-1* and *Kir6.2* encode a hetero-octomeric protein called the sulfonylurea receptor. This is a K_{ATP} channel that plays a pivotal role in insulin secretion. *Glud-1* encodes the enzyme glutamate dehydrogenase (GDH), an enzyme responsible for the oxidation of glutamate to α-ketoglutarate and a key player in amino acid–stimulated insulin release. The fourth gene, *glucokinase (GK),* encodes the enzyme that, in β cells, is the rate-limiting step for glucose entry and glycolysis. Thus it acts as the glucose sensor of the β cells, and as its activity increases, the metabolic flux of the β cell increases and insulin is secreted (Figure 3-3).

K_{ATP} Channel Hyperinsulinism

K_{ATP} channel HI is the most common form of HI. It is what was formerly known as persistent hyperinsulinemic hypoglycemia of infancy (PHHI), or nesidioblastosis. Originally thought to be an autosomal recessively inherited condition, it is now known to be inherited in three different manners. Two forms of K_{ATP} channel HI cause diffuse disease of the pancreas and occur as a result of autosomal recessive or dominant mutations in *SUR-1*. Only recessive mutations in

Kir6.2 have been identified to date. A third mode of transmission is responsible for the focal form of K_{ATP} channel HI. Loss of heterozygosity of chromosome 11, in addition to inheritance of a paternal mutation in the K_{ATP} channel genes, causes a focal area of the pancreas to proliferate and secrete insulin in a dysregulated manner, whereas the remainder of the pancreas is completely normal. Unlike diffuse K_{ATP} channel HI, focal K_{ATP} channel HI may be cured by surgical resection of the affected region.

Clinically, the dominant form of K_{ATP} channel HI is milder than the other two forms. Patients often do not present in infancy; presentations as late as adult life have been reported. Patients with dominant K_{ATP} channel HI present with fasting-induced hypoglycemia; this may be manifest as seizures or lethargy following a prolonged fast. At the time of hypoglycemia, insulin levels are elevated, FFAs and ketones are suppressed, and IGFBP-1 levels suppressed. There is an inappropriate rise in the blood sugar following the administration of glucagon during hypoglycemia. Patients may be responsive to diazoxide, but if diazoxide fails to control hypoglycemia, 98% pancreatectomy is indicated.

Diffuse and focal K_{ATP} channel HI present in a similar manner; it is very difficult to differentiate clinically between the two. Sixty percent of patients present in the newborn period with severe hypoglycemia. They may be large for gestational age (LGA) and mimic the infant of the diabetic mother. They often have a high glucose requirement of up to 25 to 30 mg/kg body weight/min. Untreated, they may experience seizures, apnea, and death. About 30% of patients present in the first year of life; they often have a history of being born AGA and often have some hypoglycemia in the neonatal period that was passed off as "normal variation." As they become older and their feeding interval increases and they start to sleep through the night, they begin to develop symptoms of lethargy, irritability, excessive hunger, and even seizures. The diagnosis is suspected in infants with an increased glucose requirement to prevent hypoglycemia. Like those with dominant K_{ATP} channel HI, at the time of hypoglycemia, insulin levels are elevated, FFAs and ketones are suppressed, and IGFBP-1 levels are suppressed. There is an inappropriate rise in the blood sugar following the administration of glucagon during hypoglycemia. Cortisol and GH levels are elevated; if not, stimulation tests to rule out hypopituitarism should be performed.

Initial treatment of the acute episode of hypoglycemia is to rapidly correct the blood glucose to greater than 70 mg/dL. This is achieved with an intravenous bolus of 2 mL/kg body weight of 10% dextrose (200 mg/kg body weight of glucose) followed by an infusion of at least 8 mg/kg body weight/min of glucose (5 mL of 10% dextrose/kg body weight/hr). If hypoglycemia persists after 15 minutes, the glucose infusion rate should be increased by 50% and blood

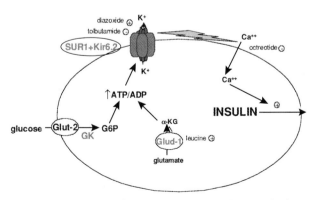

Figure 3-3 Pathways of β-cell insulin secretion showing the four congenital HI genes (circled).

glucose checked again after 15 minutes and until greater than 70 mg/dL. Diazoxide (15 mg/kg body weight/day), a K_{ATP} channel opener, is rarely effective in K_{ATP} channel HI, because it is the protein on which it acts that is dysfunctional. Octreotide, an analogue of native somatostatin, in doses of up to 20 μg/kg body weight/day has been effective in controlling blood glucose. Its use, however, is confounded by tachyphylaxis. It may be given via subcutaneous injection every 6 to 8 hours or via continuous subcutaneous infusion by pump. It may also be given intravenously via continuous infusion. Nifedipine has been reported to be effective in several case reports, but in practice, it rarely works.

For more than half of patients with K_{ATP} channel HI, medical therapy fails and surgery is indicated. It is at this point that the management of patients with HI becomes critical. The surgical therapies for focal and diffuse disease are radically different and the outcomes are also different. Focal HI may be cured by partial resection of the affected pancreas, leaving behind often as much as 80% of the pancreas. On the other hand, patients with diffuse disease require a 98% pancreatectomy. The outcome of this is diabetes or persistent hypoglycemia. In the majority of diffuse cases, the postoperative hypoglycemia is easier to control than it is preoperatively, but rarely a total pancreatectomy is required to prevent severe hypoglycemia and brain damage. To successfully differentiate focal from diffuse disease and to complete a successful operation, a team of highly specialized members including interventional radiologists, histopathologists, and surgeons is vital. Identification of patients with focal disease may be achieved by studying the responses to a series of acute insulin response tests. Those in whom focal disease is suspected require localizing procedures. Currently, the two approaches are transhepatic portal venous sampling (THPVS) and pancreatic arterial stimulation with calcium and venous sampling of insulin (PASVS). These procedures are carried out in an interventional radiology suite, under general anesthesia, with meticulous attention to maintaining the glucose levels just above hypoglycemia. At surgery, biopsy samples from the head, body, and tail of the pancreas are studied under frozen section; if they confirm focal HI, a search is made for the focal lesion. This is a painstaking operation and may take 8 to 10 hours in the most difficult cases.

Before discharge after surgery, all focal patients should be fasted to hypoglycemia or to ketosis to demonstrate a cure. The long-term risk of diabetes in patients with partial pancreatectomy is very low.

Glutamate Dehydrogenase Hyperinsulinism (GDH HI)

Patients with GDH HI tend not to present in the newborn period but rather in the first few months of life. They usu-

ally are not LGA. Symptoms may first occur when foods high in protein are introduced to the diet, such as when weaning from breast milk to formula milk, introducing solids, or first fasting the child overnight. In the past, patients with GDH HI might have been said to have leucine-sensitive hypoglycemia because it was noted that some patients with HI were triggered by protein in the diet. The hallmark of GDH HI is that in addition to the classic biochemical features of HI, they also have hyperammonemia without elevations in glutamine. It is this feature that sets them apart from patients with urea cycle defects. Not only is the glutamine level not elevated, but also they seem to be asymptomatic to the elevation of ammonia. In addition, the ammonia levels do not fluctuate with protein intake, nor are they suppressible with high glucose infusions.

Clinically, patients with GDH HI have both fasting-induced hypoglycemia and postprandial hypoglycemia. Formal fasting studies reveal an abnormally short fasting duration, but surprisingly they may mount a normal ketone response during the fast. The glucagon stimulation test results are abnormal, demonstrating a rise in glucose at a time of hypoglycemia. The patients are most often responsive to diazoxide, which improves not only fasting glucose levels but also the protein-induced hypoglycemia. Rarely, a low-protein diet may be indicated.

Mutations in *Glud-1* are dominant, but there is a high rate of spontaneous mutations. Although there are hot spots for mutations on *Glud-1*, mutations have been found all over the gene. These mutations are activating mutations and are expressed in the β cell, liver, and brain. In the β cell, they act by decreasing the ability of guanosine triphosphate (GTP) to inhibit GDH. As a result, leucine stimulates GDH to oxidize glutamate to α-ketoglutarate and the release of ammonia. This enters the Krebs' cycle and generates ATP, which stimulates insulin release via the K_{ATP} channel. In the liver, the decreased glutamate levels impair the ability to generate *n*-acetylglutamate (NAG). NAG is a key allosteric activator of carbamoyl-phosphate synthetase, the first step in the urea cycle. Hence, patients have leucine-stimulated hypoglycemia and persistent elevated ammonia levels, and because glutamate levels are low, they have low glutamine levels.

Glucokinase Hyperinsulinism (GK HI)

To date, only a few families with activating mutations in *GK* have been described. Most patients present outside of the neonatal period with fasting-induced hypoglycemia. They do not have increased glucose requirement, and insulin levels are suppressed when blood glucose drops to about 30 to 40 mg/dL. They respond well to diazoxide.

Acquired Hyperinsulinism

Hyperinsulinism occurring after the age of 2 or 3 is often a result of an insulinoma. Patients with insulinoma have symptoms that are the same as those with congenital HI. They tend to be older and do not have elevated ammonia levels. Hypoglycemia is primarily induced by prolonged periods of fasting and often is progressive over years. The key biochemical differentiation between patients with congenital HI and insulinoma is the levels of proinsulin. In the normal patient and patients with congenital HI, proinsulin levels are less than 10% of insulin levels. Insulinoma patients may have levels greater than 40%. Patients with insulinoma are often diazoxide responsive at first but eventually require surgery. Both PASVS and THPVS accurately localize insulinomas. Abdominal computed tomography or magnetic resonance imaging rarely identifies the lesion. A much more sensitive technique is either intraoperative or endoscopic ultrasonography; this is in contrast to focal K_{ATP} channel HI, in which these standard radiological techniques do not identify lesions.

Surgical resection is curative. Lesions are mostly benign adenomas, but malignant insulinomas have been described in children as young as 13 years. Consideration must be given to the possibility that the patient may have a multiple endocrine neoplasia syndrome (MEN 1), and a careful family history should be taken.

Factitious Hyperinsulinism

In rare instances, factious HI has been detected. This can occur as part of the complex syndrome of Munchausen disease by proxy in which a caregiver administers oral insulin secretagogues to mimic HI. Routine toxic screens of the urine does not detect this, and if it is suspected, a sample of the suspected drug should be given to the laboratory to determine if it is in the patient's blood. In this case, insulin, C-peptide, and proinsulin levels are elevated, but the proinsulin-to-insulin ratio may be normal. In the instance of surreptitious insulin administration, insulin levels are very high and C-peptide and proinsulin levels are low. An exception to this is the novel insulin analogues such as aspart (Novolog; Novo Nordisk) or lispro (Humalog; Eli Lilly). In these circumstances, some of the high sensitive monoclonal insulin assays do not detect the insulin at all and the patient behaves as if there was HI but levels of insulin, C-peptide, and proinsulin are suppressed. Special insulin assays are available from the manufacturer to detect these insulins.

Treatment of sulfonylurea overdose may require 18 to 24 hours of glucose infusion, or longer. In rare circumstances, intravenous glucagon infusions of 1 mg/day may be required. The treatment of insulin overdose is similar. It is important to note that the pharmacokinetics of insulin change when massive overdoses are given; in particular, the duration of action becomes much greater.

IDIOPATHIC KETOTIC HYPOGLYCEMIA

Idiopathic ketotic hypoglycemia (IKH) is a poorly understood and often abused diagnosis. In essence, it refers to children who have an abnormally shortened fasting tolerance with apparently normal intermediary metabolite and hormonal response to fasting in whom all other diagnoses have been ruled out. Any infant, child, or adult, if fasted long enough, develops ketosis, and glucose levels fall to the hypoglycemic range. Whether one calls this state of hypoglycemia IKH is debated. In general, I prefer to separate those children in whom ketosis and hypoglycemia occur after 24 hours of fasting from those with hypoglycemia and ketosis triggered in an abnormally short time. It is this latter group who have IKH and require supervision. For the former, if there is a clear-cut history that a child (age 2-5 years) has gone greater than 24 hours with no oral intake, has large ketones in the urine, has a normal examination, and has a normal past medical history, then no further testing is necessary unless further episodes occur.

The pathophysiology of IKH is thought to be due to decreased substrates for gluconeogenesis and FAO. The children tend to be thin and have lower muscle mass than those not affected. Alanine levels after an overnight fast have been shown to be lower than normal. Because this is such an important gluconeogenic amino acid, it is thought that this is an important component of IKH.

IKH generally occurs in infants and children between the ages of 18 months to 5 years. Occasionally, patients as young as 9 months may be diagnosed with IKH, and it may persist as late as 10 years. However, when one sees patients at the extremes of the age range, one must be particularly suspicious of an alternate diagnosis. Classically, patients with IKH present during an episode of intercurrent illness associated with poor oral intake, vomiting, or diarrhea. They may be excessively dehydrated, limp, and lethargic. Very rarely are they comatose or have a seizure. The clinical examination should be normal other than signs of the intercurrent illness; there is no evidence of hepatomegaly. The critical sample at the time of hypoglycemia demonstrates elevated FFAs, elevated ketones, lactate that may be elevated if there is an associated dehydration but otherwise is normal, suppressed insulin and C-peptide, and large ketones in the urine. Plasma acyl-carnitine and urine organic acids reflect ketosis and do not have the characteristics of the FAO defects. A glucagon stimulation test does not cause the glucose to rise.

Treatment of the acute episode is to raise the blood glucose to greater than 70 mg/dL, once the critical blood sample has been taken, with a 2 mL/kg body weight bolus of 10% dextrose and then a continuous dextrose infusion. Long-term care is to avoid fasting of greater than 12 hours by giving a bedtime snack. If the patient has further episodes despite following the guidelines of avoiding prolonged fasting, even if all the laboratory tests of the critical sample are normal, careful consideration should be given to an alternative diagnosis. In particular, MCAD, SCHAD, ketone utilization defects (see Fatty Acid Oxidation Disorders), glycogen synthase deficiency (GSD-VI or -IX), and isolated GH or cortisol deficiency should be considered. In particular, children who develop IKH in the absence of intercurrent illness and within 12 hours of last eating should be particularly carefully investigated.

IATROGENIC HYPOGLYCEMIA

There are sometimes incidences when medical management of a patient results in hypoglycemia. The following are some examples of iatrogenic hypoglycemia.

Acute interruptions of intravenous glucose infusions may trigger hypoglycemia. This is particularly seen in patients on total parenteral nutrition (TPN) with higher dextrose content, and it occurs when either the line is blocked, accidentally removed, or shut off suddenly. Insulin secretion induced by the high glucose infusion rate cannot stop quickly enough, and a rebound hypoglycemia occurs. Patients on nocturnal TPN who cannot feed often require a slow weaning from TPN in the morning rather than an abrupt cessation.

Premature infants who have been on *continuous nasogastric feeding* for a long time sometimes have difficulty in transitioning to bolus feeds. Switching from continuous to 2-hourly or 3-hourly feedings may precipitate hypoglycemia. In this case, a good technique is to add bolus feedings on top of a reduced-rate continuous feeding and to gradually decrease the basal rate and increase the bolus feeding. Once the infant is on all bolus feedings, a fast to determine whether the infant can keep the blood glucose level at greater than 60 mg/dL for 8 hours should be done before discharge.

Certain drugs are known to be associated with hypoglycemia. Propranolol has been implicated as a cause of drug-induced hypoglycemia, although its mechanism is unknown. Salicylates have caused hypoglycemic deaths after the ingestion of large quantities. Hypoglycemia is thought to occur due to the uncoupling of oxidative phosphorylation and the subsequent increased glucose utilization that occurs. Pentamidine causing hypoglycemia during the treatment of infections such as pneumocystitis in patients with human immunodeficiency virus infection has been reported. Hypoglycemia secondary to HI has been reported as a consequence of either Bordetella vaccine or the disease itself. This, however, is an extremely rare side effect. Patients undergoing treatment of malaria with quinine may also have a secondary HI state due to stimulation of insulin secretion.

Nissan Fundoplication With Gastric Tube Feeding

The use of Nissan fundoplication and gastric tube feedings to treat severe reflux is one of the main causes of iatrogenic hypoglycemia. Because this procedure is often done in patients who have previously sustained severe brain damage, the signs or symptoms, such as postprandial seizures, may not be noticed. In the past, the potential to develop hypoglycemia as a complication of the operation has rarely been explained in obtaining the consent of the parents; however, it is clear that late dumping hypoglycemia may occur in more than 25% of patients who have this procedure done.

The classic symptoms of acute-onset pallor, shakiness, and sweatiness, followed by neuroglycopenic symptoms such as lethargy and seizures, occur 60 to 90 minutes after a liquid feeding through the gastric tube. It almost always proceeded by an acute rise in the blood glucose to greater than 160 mg/dL between 15 and 60 minutes after the feeding. It is important to note that the symptoms of late dumping often occur in the absence of classic early dumping. Classic early dumping occurs as a result of a high osmotic load reaching the small intestine, drawing water into the gut, and causing sudden hypotension, tachycardia, sweatiness, and pallor associated with acute diarrhea.

The diagnosis of late dumping is made by finding hypoglycemia 1 to 2 hours after a bolus feeding, yet it is not present after a slow weaning from a continuous feeding. Most children with late dumping can fast for 24 hours or longer. The diagnosis may be confused with HI because the children may have elevated insulin levels, suppressed FFAs and ketone levels, and possibly even a positive glycemic response to glucagon. The key is that unlike patients with HI, late dumping patients have normal prolonged fasting. Treatment is difficult, and many agents have been used in the past, including octreotide, diazoxide, and nifedipine. The most successful treatment is a combination of a complex-carbohydrate formula with acarbose in doses of 12.5 to 75 mg/feeding. Acarbose competes with the disaccharides in the small intestine for the disaccharidases and prevents the rapid absorption of glucose that triggers the high glucose that precedes the fall.

MISCELLANEOUS CAUSES OF HYPOGLYCEMIA

Acute Liver Failure

Acute liver failure from any etiology may cause hypoglycemia. The liver is the key organ in glucose homeostasis. It stores glycogen to buffer the postprandial fall in glucose. It is the site of gluconeogenesis and FAO, supplying glucose and ketones to the rest of the body. Acute liver failure may occur due to drug toxicity, poisoning, trauma, tumor, cirrhosis, infection, and metabolic disease such as tyrosinosis and galactosemia. The diagnosis of liver failure is usually obvious and must be nearly complete to cause hypoglycemia. The treatment is to provide glucose at a rate of 4 to 8 mg/kg body weight/min.

Reactive Hypoglycemia

Reactive hypoglycemia is a term used commonly in the past for hypoglycemia that occurs after meals but is not fasting induced. It commonly occurs in adolescent girls, rarely in boys. Patients complain of symptoms such as dizziness, nausea, headache, paleness, hunger, and irritability relieved by food. Most have not had the classic Whipple triad (symptoms of hypoglycemia associated with measured hypoglycemia that resolve with the administration of glucose). Most have a family history of "hypoglycemia." Many have had an oral glucose tolerance test (OGTT) that demonstrates glucose may fall into the 50s or 60s several hours after a meal. It cannot be emphasized too strongly that there is no place for an OGTT in the investigation of hypoglycemia. Up to 25% of normal children have a downward swing in blood glucose on an OGTT.

Most disorders of glucose homeostasis are precipitated by fasting, not by feeding. There are only three forms of hypoglycemia that might present with hypoglycemia within 1 to 3 hours after a meal but not after a 12-hour overnight fast. These exceptions to the rule that all childhood hypoglycemia is fasting induced are (1) GDH hyperinsulinism, in which protein ingestion triggers hypoglycemia; (2) Nissan fundoplication–induced late dumping; and (3) hereditary fructose intolerance in which drinking a fructose load triggers sudden and severe hypoglycemia.

Alcohol-Induced Hypoglycemia

Unlike adults, in whom hypoglycemia is associated with chronic alcoholism, in children, alcohol-induced hypoglycemia comes about as a result of acute ingestion or absorption of alcohol. Sources of alcohol in children include mouthwash, rubbing alcohol on the skin, and tippling in parents' glasses when they are not looking. Alcohol impairs gluconeogenesis, inhibits hepatic uptake of lactate, and inhibits hypoglycemia-stimulated GH and cortisol release. Thus, in a typical scenario, the child drinks alcohol and does not wake up the next morning, being found comatose in bed.

The diagnosis of alcohol-induced hypoglycemia is made by finding alcohol in the urine or blood of affected patients. FFAs and ketones may be moderately elevated with a shift toward increased β-hydroxybutyrate reflecting the abnormal NADH/NAD ratio often found in these children. There may be an increased anion gap. Intravenous infusions of glucose to correct the hypoglycemia are usually sufficient to treat the child; however, if cerebral edema has occurred, dexamethasone may be required. Mortality in pediatric alcohol-induced coma is significant.

Hypoglycorrhachia

Although not strictly a hypoglycemic disorder, hypoglycorrhachia is a disorder of low cerebrospinal fluid glucose in the presence of normal blood glucose. It is very rare, and it is difficult to diagnose. A defect in *Glut-1*, the brain glucose transporter, results in impairment of glucose transport across the blood-brain barrier and into neurons. The result is seizures and brain damage. Most cases have been diagnosed due to the recognition of low cerebrospinal fluid glucose in a lumbar puncture performed to detect meningitis. Treatment using the ketogenic diet has been proposed. This is thought to work by providing alternate fuels such as ketones, which can cross the blood-brain barrier, enter cells, and be used for energy production.

Nonpancreatic Tumor Hypoglycemia

Certain non-insulin–secreting tumors may be associated with hypoglycemia, in particular large retroperitoneal tumors, such as Wilm's tumor and hepatoblastoma. Initially it was proposed that extraction of glucose across the tumor vascular bed was responsible for the hypoglycemia. Subsequently, it became apparent that an insulin-like factor was likely involved. Classical biochemical findings at the time of hypoglycemia are decreased free fatty acids, increased glucose utilization, and impaired glucose production. Insulin-like growth factor (IGF)-II has been demonstrated in the sera of affected patients. Interestingly, it is "big IGF-II" (a large molecular form of IGF-II), and both serum and tumor contain a large proportion of this form of IGF-II. "Big IGF-II" stimulates the IGF-I receptor and cross activates the insulin receptor causing hypoglycemia. Stimulation of the IGF-I receptor causes downregulation of growth hormone secretion. This reduces IGFBP-3 secretion, which, in turn, lessens the binding capacity of free IGFs and thus increases the potential of the abnormal and dysregulated production of big IGF-II to cause hypoglycemia. Treatment with growth hormone causes increased IGFBP-3, which reduces the free IGF pool and thereby decreases hypoglycemia on a temporary basis until definitive treatment is completed. Removal of the tumor by surgical resection or by chemotherapy/ radiotherapy is often required to resolve the hypoglycemia completely.

Rarely Hodgkin's disease has been described to cause hypoglycemia because of insulin receptor antibodies that bind and stimulate the receptor, mimicking the effects of insulin.

DIAGNOSTIC APPROACH TO THE PATIENT WITH HYPOGLYCEMIA

Most cases of hypoglycemia present in emergency situations. Often, there is no time for a considered and thoughtful approach to the patient, so it is important to be prepared. The greatest difficulty faced by physicians is having the correct tubes for blood draws for when low glucose is detected. The best situation is to have a set of tubes ready for the specialized tests. This delay of 30 seconds to draw blood before administering a glucose bolus may avoid hospitalization, including a dangerous fasting study that could precipitate a metabolic crisis. Box 3-1 lists the tests required, the minimal sample volumes, and the type of tubes required to collect the samples.

History

A critical part of the diagnostic process is to determine the history of the event. The timing of the hypoglycemia in relation to duration of fasting is a key element in the diagnostic process. Hypoglycemia occurring 12 to 18 hours into an intercurrent illness with poor oral intake may suggest an FAO disorder in a previously well child. On the other hand, the same situation in a poorly growing boy with a history of neonatal hypoglycemia and micropenis might suggest hypopituitarism or GH deficiency. A history of being born LGA and having hypoglycemia from the newborn period are suggestive of HI. The clinician should ask if there any precipitating factors, such as weaning from breast feeding (consider HI), first overnight fast (consider HI or FDPase), first bottle of juice (consider HFI), or a party in the house the night before with half-empty glasses of alcohol left out (consider alcohol ingestion). Is there a family history of sudden infant death or

acute life-threatening events? (Consider FAO disorders.) Has the child been growing well? (Consider GH deficiency or GSD-1.) All of these questions may be asked after the child has been treated as long as the critical samples have been drawn; then additional studies may be carried out as necessary.

Physical Examination

Many patients with hypoglycemia have a normal physical examination. This may often be a clue as to what the patients does not have rather than to what he or she does have. There are some signs that point to a specific disorder. LGA infants suggests HI, either being an IDM or having a genetic HI. A careful search for midline malformations, including the optic nerves, may yield a clue to hypopituitarism. Examination of the abdomen may reveal hepatomegaly suggestive of the GSD, if severe, or FAO disorders, if more subtle. Hyperpigmentation may be noted in primary adrenal insufficiency; however, patients may present in crisis without this sign. Abnormal neurological signs may indicate adrenal leukodystrophy. Short stature with increased weight for height is seen in GH deficiency. Evidence of a myopathy may be suggestive of an FAO disorder, as may cardiac failure due to cardiomyopathy.

Laboratory Studies

The critical blood draw is the key to diagnosis. Many of these tests are not immediately available, so it is useful to have a diagnostic algorithm based on some simple tests (Figure 3-4). The first step is to assess whether there is acidosis associated with hypoglycemia. If there is, then it must be determined if this is ketoacidosis or lactic acidosis. Hypoglycemia and lactic acidosis are suggestive of disorders of gluconeogenesis and GSD-1, whereas hypoglycemia and ketosis are suggestive of GSD-III, -IV, or -IX, of hypopituitarism, or of isolated GH or cortisol deficiency. In the absence of these disorders and with a consistent history, IKH can be considered. In the absence of acidosis, the FFA-to-ketone ratio must be considered. Low FFA and ketone levels suggest that HI is due to a genetic defect, an insulinoma, or factitious HI. It would also be consistent with hypopituitarism in the newborn period. High FFA and low ketone levels are strongly suggestive of an FAO disorder. As the tests for FFAs and ketones may take weeks to get results, in the face of hypoglycemia and no acidosis, the glucagon stimulation test could be administered. In patients with HI, there is a rise of greater than 30 mg/dL at a time of hypoglycemia, whereas in disorders of FAO, there is no such rise.

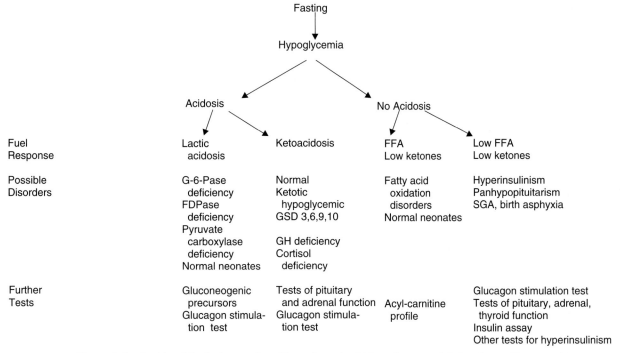

Figure 3-4   An Algorithmic Approach to Hypoglycemia. FDPase, fructose-1,6-diphosphatase; FFA, free fatty acids; G-6-Pase, glucose 6-phosphatase; GH, growth hormone; GSD, glycogen storage disorder; SGA, small for gestational age. (From Thornton PS, Finegold DN, Stanley CA, Sperling MA: Pediatric Endocrinology, 2nd edition, WB Saunders, p. 381, © 2002).

ACUTE MANAGEMENT OF HYPOGLYCEMIA

In the acute situation, the goal is to get the blood glucose level to greater than 70 mg/dL as soon as the critical sample has been drawn or the glucagon stimulation test has been completed. This is usually achieved with a minibolus of 2 mL of 10% dextrose/kg body weight (200 mg glucose/kg) by intravenous push. This must be followed by a continuous infusion of glucose at 8 mg/kg body weight/min, which is approximately 5 mL of 10% dextrose/kg body weight/hr. The blood glucose should be checked 15 minutes after the bolus and, if less than 50 mg/dL, a second bolus should be given and the infusion rate increased by 50% to 7.5 mL/kg body weight/hr. Careful attention must be paid to electrolyte balance and to the possibility of fluid overload. If high rates of glucose infusion are required, such as occurs in HI, a higher concentration of glucose should be administered through a central line instead of the boluses.

In rare circumstance when the patient is seizing and the glucose level is not recordable or is less than 20 mg/dL, a bolus of 5 mL of 10% dextrose/kg body weight (500 mg of glucose/kg body weight) should be given.

Once the patient is stabilized, the glucose level should be measured initially hourly and then less frequently as appropriate. The patient should not be discharged to home until a complete investigation is performed or an arrangement is made to keep the patient safe until a full evaluation is complete.

MAJOR POINTS

Hypoglycemia is a biochemical sign, not a diagnosis.
Hypoglycemia causes brain damage.
The definition of hypoglycemia is a plasma glucose level of less than 50 mg/dL.
Whipple triad includes the (1) symptoms of hypoglycemia associated with (2) a true measured plasma glucose of less than 50 mg/dL and (3) resolution of symptoms after correction of the glucose level to the normal range. For a diagnosis of hypoglycemia, all three conditions must be present.
Hypoglycemia does not always cause brain damage because the brain can utilize alternate fuels such as lactate and β-hydroxybutyrate.
Whenever a patient with hypoglycemia is seen, the following question must be asked: "Do I know for absolute certainty why this patient has hypoglycemia?" If the answer is no, then the clinician must perform a critical blood draw (Box 3-1) before treatment if it is at all reasonably possible.

Continued

MAJOR POINTS—Cont'd

The presence or absence of acidosis is a key point in the diagnosis of the cause of hypoglycemia. Always calculate the anion gap.

Transitional hypoglycemia is a physiological condition that occurs in many normal-term newborns in the first 12 hours of life.

Hypoglycemia in infants born small or large for gestational age, prematurely, or after fetal distress is *not* transitional hypoglycemia and must be treated and the etiology sought if it persists for longer than 3 days.

Any neonate with hypoglycemia lasting longer than 3 days should have a fasting study to demonstrate normal fasting tolerance before discharge.

By 3 days of life, a normal infant can go at least 8 hours with food and not develop hypoglycemia.

Any hypoglycemia occurring during a glucose infusion of greater than 6 to 8 mg/kg/min is *absolutely* abnormal and must be investigated.

Persistent hypoglycemia in the newborn period is most commonly caused by hyperinsulinism.

A glucose response to glucagon of greater than 30 mg/dL most strongly suggests hyperinsulinism as the cause of the hypoglycemia.

Hyperinsulinism is known to be caused by defects in at least four genes: *Sur1*, *Kir6.2*, *Glud-1*, and *glucokinase (GK)*.

Most cases of K_{ATP} channel hyperinsulinism (*Sur1* and *Kir6.2* defects) fail medical therapy and require surgery.

Pancreatic surgery should be done in centers with multidisciplinary teams experienced in differentiating focal from diffuse K_{ATP} HI. Focal K_{ATP} may be cured by partial pancreatectomy, whereas diffuse K_{ATP} HI requires near-total pancreatectomy.

Newborn males with a small penis and hypoglycemia should suggest hypopituitarism.

Hypopituitarism is at the bottom of the list of causes of prolonged jaundice in the newborn but at the top of the list of causes of prolonged jaundice and hypoglycemia.

Hypopituitarism is *the* cause of prolonged jaundice, hypoglycemia, and small penis in the newborn male.

Children with glucose-6-phophatase deficiency often present with hepatomegaly and short stature rather than with hypoglycemia.

Children with glycogen synthase deficiency may present with hyperglycemia and hypoglycemia in the same patient.

Hypoglycemia and muscle (cardiac or peripheral) abnormalities should make the clinician consider fatty acid oxidation defects and mitochondrial disorders.

Nissen fundoplication with gastric tube insertion does cause hypoglycemia, although it is not always mentioned on the consent form.

The use of the oral glucose tolerance test in the evaluation of hypoglycemia is at the end of the list of things to do, not at the top.

SELECTED READINGS

Hypoglycemia in General

Bier DM, Leake RD, Haymond MW, et al: Measurement of "true" glucose production rates in infancy and childhood with 6,6-dideuteroglucose, Diabetes 1977;26:1016.

Cornblath M, Hawdon JM, Williams AF, et al: Controversies regarding definition of neonatal hypoglycemia: suggested operational thresholds, Pediatrics 2000;105:1141.

Koh THHG, Eyre JA, Aynsley-Green A: Neonatal hypoglycemia—the controversy regarding definition, Arch Dis Child 1988;63:1386.

Koh THHG, Aynsley-Green A, Tarbit M, et al: Neural dysfunction during hypoglycemia, Arch Dis Child 1998;63:1353.

Lubchenko LO, Bard N: Incidence of hypoglycemia in newborn infants by birth weight and gestational age. Pediatrics 1971;67:831.

Hyperinsulinism

Aynsley-Green A, Hussain K, Hall J, et al: Practical management of hyperinsulinism in infancy, Arch Dis Child 2000;82:F98.

Collins JE, Leonard JV, Teal D, et al: Hyperinsulinaemic hypoglycaemia in small for dates babies, Arch Dis Childhood 1990;65:1118.

Ferry RJ, Kelly A, Grimberg A, et al: Calcium-stimulated insulin secretion in diffuse and focal forms of congenital hyperinsulinism, J Pediatr 2000;137:239.

Glaser B, Thornton PS, Otonkoski T, et al: Genetics of neonatal hyperinsulinism, Arch Dis Child 2000;82:F79.

Grimberg A, Ferry RJ, Kelly A, et al: Dysregulation of insulin secretion in children with congenital hyperinsulinism due to sulfonylurea receptor mutations, Diabetes 2001;50:322.

Levitt-Katz LE, Satin-Smith M, Collett-Solberg P, et al: Insulin like growth factor binding protein-1 levels in the diagnosis of hypoglycemia caused by hyperinsulinism, J Pediatr 1997;131:193.

Glycogen Storage Disease

Chen YT, Burchell A: Glycogen storage diseases. In Scriver CR, Beaudet AL, Sly WS, et al, editors: The Metabolic and Molecular Basis of Inherited Disease, 7th ed, New York, 1995, McGraw-Hill, pp 935-966.

Lei KJ, Pan CJ, Shelly LL, et al: Identification of mutations in the gene for glucose-6-phosphatase, the enzyme deficient in glycogen storage disease type 1A, J Clin Invest 1994;93:1994.

McCawley L, Korchak HM, Douglas SD, et al: In vivo and in vivo effects of granulocyte colony stimulating factors (GCSF) on neutrophils (PMN) in glycogen storage disease type 1B: GCSF therapy corrects the neutropenia and the defects in respiratory burst activity and calcium mobilization, Pediatr Res 1994;35:84.

Orho M, Bosshard NU, Buist NRM, et al: Mutations in the liver glycogen synthase gene in children with hypoglycemia due to glycogen storage disease type O, Clin Invest 1998;102:507.

Wolfsdorf JI, Keller RJ, Landy H, et al: Glucose therapy for glycogenosis type I in infants: comparison of intermittent uncooked cornstarch and continuous overnight glucose feedings, J Inherit Metab Dis 1997;20:559.

Gluconeogenesis

Baker L, Weingrad AI: Fasting hypoglycemia in metabolic acidosis associated with deficiency of hepatic fructose I,6 bisphosphatase activity, Lancet 1970;2:13.

Fatty Acid Oxidation

Roe CR, Coates PM: Acyl-CoA dihydrogenase deficiencies. In Scriver CR, Beaudet AL, Sly WS, et al, editors: The Metabolic and Molecular Basis of Inherited Disease, 7th ed, New York, 1995, McGraw-Hill, chapter 45.

Miscellaneous

Agus MS, Levitt Katz L, Satin-Smith M, et al: Non islet cell tumor associated with hypoglycemia in a child: Successful long-term therapy with growth hormone, J Pediatr 1995;127:403.

Ng D, Ferry RJ, Kelly A, et al: Acarbose treatment of post-prandial hypoglycemia in children following a Nissen fundoplication, Pediatr Res 2000;47:135.

Mark V, Teale JD: Drug-induced hypoglycemia. Endocrinol Metab Clin North Am 1999;28:555.

SEXUAL DEVELOPMENT

CHAPTER 4

Normal Pubertal Development

PETER A. LEE

HOWARD E. KULIN

INTRODUCTION

Puberty is the stage of life when the reproductive system matures together with completion of somatic growth and sexual maturity. Although the mechanisms that drive this process are not completely understood, the primary influences emanate from the central nervous system. The involved neuroendocrine systems focus on the pulsatile gonadotropin-releasing hormone (GnRH) release by GnRH neurons in the arcuate nucleus of the hypothalamus. Neurotransmitters that exert inhibitory or stimulatory influences include acetylcholine, catecholamines, γ-aminobutyric acid, opioid peptides, prostaglandins, and serotonin. Peripheral factors that influence GnRH activity include steroid and peptide hormones, body mass and composition, nutritional factors, and natural or synthetic environmental substances.

PHYSIOLOGY OF PUBERTY

The physiological control system for the onset of puberty first becomes operative during fetal life, is then restrained, and finally amplifies so that GnRH from the hypothalamus stimulates gonadotropin release from the pituitary. The gonadotropins, luteinizing hormone (LH) and follicle-stimulating hormone (FSH), in turn stimulate the gonad, resulting in the secretion of sex steroids and gamete formation.

The release of GnRH is episodic throughout life, but pulsations become more apparent in association with sleep at the onset of puberty. The amplitude and frequency of release attain a characteristic pattern for males and females, the latter varying with and controlling the menstrual cycle. The hypothalamic-pituitary-gonadal (HPG) axis remains operative in early infancy, and then becomes relatively, but not completely, quiescent during childhood.

By midgestation, high levels of LH and FSH are produced in response to GnRH, with secretion becoming attenuated as gestation proceeds. At birth, there is a very brief rise of gonadotropins, similar to other pituitary peptide hormones, with a rapid decline over the next few days. Within the first few weeks of life, there is a rise of circulating levels of LH and FSH signaling the neonatal period of increased HPG activity. Levels peak sometime between 6 and 12 weeks, subsequently waning over the following months.

Throughout early childhood, there is quiescent HPG activity, although both the pituitary and gonad are capable of response if stimulated. Thus, the restraint during early childhood is at the level of the central nervous system with suppressive influences on the hypothalamus. During this period, inhibitory influences apparently overcome the stimulatory influences, followed by a reversal beginning at the onset of puberty.

Interestingly, this reversal of neural stimuli begins in midchildhood, some few years before most of the physical changes that signal the clinical event of puberty. The gonadotropin rise from mid to late prepubertal childhood is also larger than the increment during the years of the physical and reproductive changes of puberty. Thus, the gonadotropin increment of puberty occurs over several years with the initial changes beginning between ages 5 and 7 years.

Suprahypothalamic sites, the limbic system, and higher cortical centers influence both production and release of GnRH by neurons within the hypothalamus. Inhibitory and stimulatory factors, primarily neurotransmitters, affect the GnRH-secreting neurons, which are concentrated within the arcuate nucleus in the medial basal hypothalamus and control GnRH release. GnRH is secreted into the hypothalamic-hypophyseal portal system, thereby reaching receptors on the gonadotropes, the LH- and FSH-secreting cells of the pituitary. These cells respond to increased episodic GnRH stimulation with augmented gonadotropin, particularly LH synthesis and release of similar periodicity. LH and FSH are released into the portal system, and reach the gonad via the systemic circulation.

The ovary, in response to gonadotropins, increase androstenedione synthesis (stimulated by FSH) by the granulosa cells. Androstenedione is a primary substrate for the LH-stimulated synthesis of estradiol in the theca cells. In the testes, LH plays a primary role in the stimulation of testosterone synthesis by the Leydig cells, while the primary role of FSH appears to involve spermatogenesis, in part via an inverse relationship with inhibin B.

The feedback interaction between the hypothalamic-pituitary unit and the gonad undergoes changes during puberty, with the system being highly sensitive in the midchildhood and early pubertal period. A correct regulation of this set point is particularly important for follicular maturity, allowing appropriate amounts of FSH, and for the development of oocyte release through positive feedback via the ovulatory LH surge.

HORMONE CHANGES OF PUBERTY

Hormone Changes: Gonadotropins

Both LH and FSH progressively rise well before the first physical changes of puberty become apparent. However, because of pulsatile secretion, because of considerable interindividual variation, and because different gonadotropin assays measure different molecular variations, it is often not possible to ascertain prepubertal from pubertal

levels with a single plasma sample. Because the prepubertal range overlaps the pubertal range for both LH and FSH, a blood level verifies puberty only if it is above the prepubertal limit. In addition, because prepubertal individuals secrete relatively greater amounts of FSH than LH and the rise of FSH with puberty is less, overlap between prepubertal and postpubertal FSH measurements are considerable. However, the ratio of LH to FSH may be useful, with a ratio of less than 1 (LH < FSH) being consistent with the prepubertal state, whereas a ratio of greater than 1 (LH > FSH) suggests puberty. Urinary gonadotropin assessments, which provide an integrated measure of pulsatile secretion but require sample preparation, are less readily available but provide better discrimination of pubertal versus prepubertal states. Sequential increments in urinary gonadotropins provide confirmation of the pubertal process.

A commonly used test for detecting the transition to a pubertal HPG axis is the rise of LH and FSH after stimulation by either GnRH or a GnRH analogue. A pubertal response is characterized by a rise of LH greater than that seen among prepubertal children, because FSH responses do not necessarily differ, particularly among girls. Interpretation of GnRH stimulation tests requires that the ranges of prepubertal and pubertal responses be known for the particular gonadotropin assays that are used.

Hormone Changes: Sex Steroids

Circulating sex steroids are of gonadal and adrenal origin. Increased adrenal sex steroid production, primarily androgens, known as *adrenarche,* begins well before the rise of gonadal steroids and physical puberty changes. Dehydroepiandrosterone sulfate (DHEAS) levels provide the best hormonal marker of adrenarche because this androgen has a prolonged half-life and, hence, more constant circulating levels.

The primary sex steroid from the testes is testosterone, with the initial rise in circulating levels marking *gonadarche,* before physical pubertal changes occur. Testosterone levels are secreted in a diurnal pattern, so that higher levels are found early in the day. Estradiol is the primary estrogen from the ovaries; however, levels fluctuate considerably and most commercially available assays are not sensitive enough to detect the earliest rises. Because progesterone is secreted primarily by the corpus luteum during the luteal phase, there are minimal changes in circulating levels during puberty until after ovulation has begun.

Control of gonadal steroidogenesis occurs primarily by episodic stimulation of gonadotropins. LH is the primary stimulator of Leydig cell testosterone production. Increased adrenal sex steroid production results from a shift in steroidogenic enzyme expression and greater expression of sex steroid pathways. The stimulus for this shift is unknown, but it appears not to be primarily under corticotropin (ACTH) control.

In general, the profiles of the rise of sex steroids during puberty are gradual. Mean levels of sex steroids and intermediate metabolites rise with successive Tanner stages, with testosterone among males and estradiol among females being particularly pertinent. Marked elevation of progesterone among females does not occur until after menarche, when progesterone and estradiol levels, as well as intermediate metabolites, vary during the menstrual cycle.

Other sex steroids that increase during puberty among both genders include androstenedione, dehydroepiandrosterone (DHEA), DHEAS, estrone, and 17-hydroxyprogesterone; these steroids are primarily of adrenal origin but also are secreted by the gonad. Sex steroid–binding protein levels also rise. Free testosterone levels gradually rise among both genders, whereas the percent of total testosterone that is free (unbound) decreases. Dihydrotestosterone levels rise among males throughout puberty; levels are low in females.

PHYSICAL CHANGES CHARACTERISTIC OF PUBERTY

Puberty is defined as when physical changes begin, reflecting underlying hormonal stimulation. Traditionally, the onset of breast development or sexual hair has been considered the marker for the onset of puberty among girls and genital growth constitutes the marker for boys. Because the changes of puberty may be very gradual and slowly progressive, the precise age of onset of a given event may be difficult to document.

Early, minimal but detectable breast development does not necessarily herald the onset of progressive pubertal change. Likewise, although androgen stimulates the growth of sexual hair among both males and females, the presence of a few, coarse, pigmented pubic or axillary hairs (*pubarche*) does not necessarily indicate activation of the HPG axis. Sexual hair growth may result from increasing adrenal androgen synthesis (adrenarche), an event that antecedes puberty. Adrenarche can be documented hormonally by measuring levels of DHEAS, DHEA, or androstenedione. Early or timely adrenarche alone can cause pubic hair development.

The physical development pattern among males and females occurs in an expected sequence. Tanner staging criteria for breast, pubic hair, and male genital development are universally used, with five Tanner stages for each criteria (Tanner stage 1 is prepubertal and Tanner stage 5 is adult). Other changes during puberty include increased linear

growth, weight gain, axillary hair growth, menarche and the attainment of regular menses, skin changes, onset of adult-type body odor, and acne of varying severity.

Pubertal gynecomastia, a common occurrence in more than two thirds of boys, typically appears at midpuberty. Other midpubertal events include the attainment of sperm production accompanied by ejaculation. Mature sperm counts are not found until late adolescence. Changes in voice pitch, the onset of axillary hair, accelerated height and weight gain, and the onset of acne are also typically midpubertal. The development of facial and chest hair and the extension of coarse hair beyond the pubic region onto the abdomen and thighs are later pubertal events and may progress well after the completion of puberty. Density and distribution of hair are related more to genetic factors than to circulating androgen levels.

SECULAR CHANGES IN THE AGE OF PUBERTY

The most reliable milestone of female puberty is the age of onset of menses, menarche, and this event has been used to ascertain secular changes in puberty. In northern Europe, it has been documented that the average age of menarche decreased by 2 to 3 months per decade from 1840 for more than a century. In developed countries, it appears that this trend is not continuing or, if so, it has continued at a considerably diminished rate because the mean age has been 12 years for the past three decades.

Data have been interpreted to indicate that the age of onset of the initial changes of puberty still may be progressing to younger ages. However, such an interpretation is not well substantiated in the United States or Europe. It may be that there has been a gradual trend to an earlier age of onset, but if so, the tempo of puberty has slowed, because the age of menarche and the completion of puberty, as noted later, appears unchanged. It is possible that earliest changes are not always indicative of actual upregulation of the pituitary axis but rather are a response to mildly increased circulating levels of sex steroids, which are not gonadotropin dependent. Such increases may be a consequence of metabolic changes related to increased body size for age with a greater proportion of body fat. It has also been suggested that sex steroid imitators, "endocrine disruptors," may accumulate in the body as a consequence of ingestion of food additives or other environmental factors and may stimulate sex steroid–mediated physical changes.

If the secular trend toward earlier puberty is continuing, albeit at a much slower rate, it is likely a consequence of better nutrition, increased body mass, better socioeconomic conditions, less disease, and different mental and psychological input, all factors that have long been thought to relate to this trend.

NORMAL AGE OF PUBERTY

The most recent U.S. data concerning the age of puberty are from the Third National Health and Nutrition Evaluation Survey (NHANES III), which included pubertal staging from age 8.0 to 17.9 years in a large cohort of males and females consisting of 25% whites, 35% African Americans, 35% Mexican Americans, and 4% of other ethnicity. This survey involved a cross section of the populations from all of the United States except Hawaii, included the civilian, noninstitutionalized population, and did not exclude those with chronic medical conditions.

Previous studies on the age of puberty in the United States have been limited. Among the few reports, most are from very limited population samples. A large series, the National Health Examination Survey III (NHES III), collected data from 1966 to 1970 and included 6150 males and females but did not begin until age 12 years, precluding documentation of early pubertal events. Data were collected to age 17 years and included visual assessment of pubertal development. This survey, as well as NHES II (1963-1965), recorded the age of menarche. The Pediatric Research in Office Settings (PROS), an office-based research network, reported data collected in 1992 and 1993 from 17,077 girls aged 3 through 12 years. Data included an assignment of Tanner staging and age of menarche, col-

lected from 65 pediatric practices at health supervision or problem-related office visits. Although this study reported significant differences in the age of the onset of puberty among black girls, compared with white girls, the interpretation that puberty overall was beginning earlier may be unfounded because the differences appear to be primarily a consequence of racial differences.

The median ages of entry by white, black, and Mexican American females into pubertal stages from the NHANES III are outlined in Table 4-1; data for males are given in Table 4-2 although Tanner genital stages from NHANES III are not consistent with previously reported data. Racial differences among males have not yet been completely defined but must be taken into consideration when assessing pubertal development.

Girls

Although there are no physical markers that absolutely indicate the progressive pubertal activation of the hypothalamic-pituitary-ovarian axis, the onset of breast development remains the best indicator. Until recently, normative puberty studies reflected the majority white population of the United States. Current data verify that the onset of pubic hair as well as breast development occurs, on the average, earlier among African American females than among other racial-ethnic groups. The most recent data

Table 4-1   Median Pubertal Stages Among Females (NHANES III)

	White	Black	Mexican American
Breast (Br) stage			
2	10.4	9.5	9.8
3	11.8	10.8	11.4
4	13.3	12.2	13.1
5	15.5	13.9	14.7
Approximate early limit (2.5 percentile) of entry			
Br2	8.0	6.6	6.8
PH2	8.0	6.7	7.4
Pubic hair (PH) stage			
2	10.6	9.4	10.4
3	11.8	10.6	11.7
4	13.0	11.9	13.2
5	16.3	14.7	16.3
Menarche	12.6	12.1	12.3

Source: Sun SS, Schubert CM, Chumlea WC, et al: National estimates of the timing of sexual maturation and racial differences among US children. Pediatrics 2002;110:911.

Table 4-2   Median Age of Attainment of Tanner Stages of Puberty Among Males (NHANES III)

	White	Black	Mexican American
Pubic hair (PH) stage			
PH2	12.0	11.2	12.3
PH3	12.7	12.5	13.1
PH4	13.6	13.7	14.1
PH5	15.7	15.3	15.8
Approximate age for 2.5 percentile			
PH2	9.5	8.2	9.3
Genital (G) stage			
G2	11.1	10.8	11.1
G3	12.6	12.0	13.0
G4	15.3	15.1	15.4
G5	16.6	16.4	16.9

Sources: Sun SS, Schubert CM, Chumlea WC, et al: National estimates of the timing of sexual maturation and racial differences among US children. Pediatrics 2002;110:911; and Herman-Giddens ME, Wang L, Koch G: Secondary sexual characteristics in boys: estimates from the National Health and Nutrition Examination Survey III, 1988-1994, Arch Pediatr Adolesc Med 2001;155:1022.

(NHANES III) suggest that the median age for the onset of breast development (see Table 4-1) is 10.4 years for white girls, 9.5 years for black girls, and 9.8 years for Mexican American girls. Extrapolation of these data back to younger ages indicates that 2.5% of white girls have the onset of breast development before the age of 8.0 years, whereas about 17% of black girls and 15% of Mexican American girls do so. The median age of onset of pubic hair development (see Table 4-1) for black girls is 9.4 years compared with 10.6 years among non-Hispanic whites and 10.4 years among Mexican Americans.

The mean age for the population as a whole, not considering racial differences, may be interpreted to suggest an earlier onset of breast development, but this appears to be primarily a consequence of racial differences. Overall evidence suggests that the early age limit of onset extends to somewhat younger ages. Two SDs below the mean of pubertal onset among all girls is 7.5 years, rather than 8 years as previously considered.

The usual sequence of pubertal events is outlined in Box 4-1. NHANES III data are consistent with previous information indicating that the average age for completion of puberty (adult breast development) is 14.0 years. Coupled with the stable age of menarche, a skewed onset of breast development to a somewhat earlier age for all girls suggests onset of breast development at a somewhat earlier age. Because earlier onset is not likely to accompany a slower tempo of puberty, the best interpretation of the data would seem to be racial differences rather than significantly earlier onset. It is possible that the initial physical changes of puberty, the first evidence of breast development, do not reflect actual pubertal onset involving the upregulation of the HPG axis. It may be the result of minimal increased hormone stimulation, perhaps related to changes in body mass index or to minimal increases in circulating estrogens independent of persistent gonadotropin stimulation or as a consequence of other hormone-like stimulators. In addition, because the PROS data were collected in primary care office settings, with multiple observers, there may have been considerable variability in judgment for assignment of breast stage 2.

Boys

The physical finding that best reflects the activation of the hypothalamic-pituitary-testicular (HPT) axis in the male is testicular enlargement. Pubertal testicular growth precedes all other physical changes of male puberty but requires actual measurement of testis length or volume. Testicular volume, other than the alteration of the appearance of scrotal fullness, is not a traditional criterion for the assignment

---

Box 4-1 Usual Sequence of Attainment of Pubertal Milestones

FEMALES

Tanner stage 2 breast development (breast budding, broadened areolae, elevated contour)
Tanner stage 2 pubic hair development (coarse, pigmented, initially labial)
Peak linear growth acceleration
Greatest rate of weight gain
Tanner stage 3 breast development (breast and areolar enlargement)
Tanner stage 3 pubic hair (extension onto mons pubis)
Onset of axillary hair growth
Onset of acne
Menarche
Tanner stage 4 breast development (typically secondary mound of tissue)
Tanner stage 4 pubic hair (adult density but not distribution)
Tanner stage 5 breast development (adult contours with size variation)
Regular menstrual cycles
Tanner stage 5 pubic hair development (adult distribution and density)

MALES

Testicular growth (volume >3 mL)
Tanner stage 2 genital development (scrotal maturation and penile growth in length)
Tanner stage 2 pubic hair development (coarse, pigmented hair, both scrotal and at base of penis)
Tanner stage 3 genital development (further penis, scrotum, and testicular growth)
Tanner stage 3 pubic hair (adult density around genitals)
Peak linear growth acceleration
Onset of pubertal gynecomastia
Greatest rate of weight gain
Onset of axillary hair growth
Change in voice pitch
Onset of acne
Spermarche (sperm first seen in morning urinary void)
Tanner stage 4 genital development (further penile growth in length and breadth)
Tanner stage 4 pubic hair (adult density but not distribution)
Onset of facial hair growth
Tanner stage 5 pubic hair development (adult density with distribution extending beyond genitals)
Tanner stage 5 genital development (within normal range of adult size)

of Tanner stage 2 genital development. Although all Tanner staging is in part subjective, the differentiation of Tanner genital stage 2 from stage 1 may be the most difficult and inaccurate of these parameters. There is a published suggestion of a modification of stage 2 to include testicular volume, which has clinical advantages.

The most recent data concerning male Tanner staging are also from NHANES III. Unfortunately, Tanner 2 genital staging recorded for this survey is at markedly earlier ages compared with previous data, so that it almost appears that different criteria were used. There is considerable variation in size and appearance of genitalia among prepubertal boys and for the same boy at different points in time during late childhood. NHANES III data were collected by multiple observers involving a single examination of each participant. This technique may lead to a significant margin of error.

Comparative data of studies over more than three decades (Table 4-3) indicate that mean age at entry into Tanner genital stage 2 may trend toward younger ages, whereas attainment of stage 5 does not. With the lack of consistent data, it seems reasonable to use the traditional early limit of 9 years for boys, not as a verified date for normal onset of genital stage 2 but as a guideline for consideration of assessment of early puberty. More data are required before an age of onset of puberty among males can be verified and before it can be ascertained whether there is an earlier onset of Tanner stage 2 genital development currently occurring among boys.

Onset of pubic hair development, although an objective criterion, may not be a consequence of HPT axis pubertal upregulation. NHANES III data indicate that the early limit and mean age of the onset of Tanner stage 2 pubic hair development are similar to those previously used for white boys, about 9.3 years and 12.0 years, respectively. The onset of sexual hair growth among African American males begins 9 to 10 months earlier (median, 11.2 years) and progresses

earlier than among whites and Mexican Americans. Median age of onset among Mexican Americans is 12.3 years. Data concerning the usual sequence of male puberty are outlined in Box 4-1.

The NHANES III data concerning the age of attainment of both Tanner stage 5 genital and pubic hair development completion of puberty are similar to older data. Median age of entry into Tanner stage 5 pubic hair development is 15.7, 15.3, and 15.8 years for whites, blacks, and Mexican Americans, respectively. For Tanner genital stage 5, the median respective ages are 16.0, 15.0, and 15.8 years. These data do not suggest that puberty is being completed earlier. Therefore, similar to the situation among girls, if puberty is beginning earlier, it is not being completed earlier.

PRACTICAL APPROACH TO THE AGE OF PUBERTY

Tables 4-1 and 4-2 are based on the best available data and may be used as general guidelines to determine whether puberty is occurring at an appropriate age and rate. If a child has clear pubertal changes with verified progression at an age that is at the lower limit for normal, consideration for referral to a pediatric endocrinologist to rule out central precocious puberty or an abnormal cause of pubertal development is appropriate. Likewise, if puberty has not yet clearly begun at the upper age limit, referral for assessment of causes of pubertal delay should occur.

Pubertal Growth

Except during infancy, there is no other period when growth rates are greater than during puberty. Pubertal growth can be considered in three phases: (1) a period of minimal growth velocity just before the time when sex steroid levels (primarily estradiol in both genders) rise and

Table 4-3 Age (years) of Onset of Tanner Genital Stages 2 and 5

Tanner Stage 2	Tanner Stage 5	Data Collection	Race	Reference(s)
12.2	15.5	1969-1974	White*	Lee, 1980
11.4	15.2	1980s	White*	Biro et al, 1995
11.3	14.6	1985-1993/1969-1974	White*	Roche et al, 1995; Harlan et al, 1979
10.1	15.9		White	Herman-Giddens et al, 2001; Sun et al, 2002
9.6	15.3		Black	Herman-Giddens et al, 2001; Sun et al, 2002
10.4	16.4		Mexican American	Herman-Giddens et al, 2001; Sun et al, 2002

*More than 95%.

provide a primary stimulus for growth, (2) the time of most rapid growth or peak height velocity that occurs earlier in girls than in boys, and (3) a final growth phase with progressive deceleration.

Among girls, growth acceleration is actually the first manifestation of increasing estradiol, and it begins before Tanner stage 2 breast development appears. Among most girls, peak height velocity occurs during breast stage 3, before menarche. After menarche, most girls are in the third or decelerating phase of pubertal growth. Because the pubertal growth spurt occurs later among boys than among girls, boys are taller at the onset of peak height velocity. In the majority of boys, pubertal growth continues after Tanner stage 5 development has been attained.

In addition to sex steroids, the growth spurt is dependent on a normal hormonal milieu including an euthyroid status, increased growth hormone (GH) secretion, and insulin-like growth factor-I (IGF-I) levels. GH levels double during puberty, primarily by an increase in GH pulse amplitude. IGF-I levels are highest during puberty and rise in response to increasing estradiol and GH.

A key role of estradiol for pubertal growth and skeletal maturation is suggested by growth patterns in patients with specific conditions in which estrogen effect is blocked. Data suggest that estrogen, specifically estradiol, is a dominant stimulator of the increased skeletal maturity associated with puberty and is necessary to attain skeletal maturity, whereas testosterone appears to have a separate role in bone lengthening.

Skeletal Age (Bone Age)

There is a specific pattern of skeletal maturity and ossification related to age and gender. Females in general have a skeletal maturity about 2 years advanced in relation to males; that is, the ossification pattern of a skeletal age of 7 years for a boy is similar to 9 years for a girl. Skeletal maturity is an indicator of biological maturity, with events of puberty being more closely correlated with bone age than with chronological age. The variation of bone age in relation to chronological age is defined in standard deviations, with the limits of bone age for chronological age being +2 SDs. Bone age is determined from radiographs, most commonly of the hand and wrist.

The onset of puberty correlates better with bone age than with chronological age. For example, because the mean age of onset of Tanner stage 2 breast development is 10.5 to 11.0 years, a female can be expected to exhibit this pubertal stage when she attains a bone age of 10.5 to 11.0 years, whether her chronological ages is 9 or 13 years at that time. Puberty among males can be expected to begin at about the time of attainment of a skeletal age of 11.5 to 12.5 years.

Shift in Body Composition

Significant differences in body composition between males and females occur during pubertal growth. These are largely hormonally driven, with the predominant androgen effect among males stimulating the greater proportion of lean body mass including skeletal mass than among females, with females attaining a greater relative percentage of body fat. Skeletal differences include relative greater hip-to-waist growth among females. Androgen-stimulated fat distribution is typically central, whereas female distribution is around the pelvis. The peptide hormone leptin is produced in adipose tissue, has metabolic effects, and appears to be related to gonadotropin secretion. Whether leptin levels among humans are a reflection of body composition changes leading to pubertal gonadotropin secretion, have a role in the induction of puberty, or both is unclear.

Bone Density

Puberty is a period critical for the acquisition of normal bone density. Peak increases in bone density occur during the first 3 years of life and during puberty. During childhood years, there is a correlation of bone mineral density (BMD) with weight, height, and age and later with pubertal stage, particularly for axial BMD. Although Tanner staging is a strong determinant for girls, weight is a major determinant for boys. The mean age for acceleration of accrual of increased density is 10 years for girls and 13 years for boys. Key factors during puberty include activity, calcium intake, weight, and hormone levels. Excessive exercise is associated with reduced bone density, but exercise intervention programs with increased physical activity in the typical pubertal girl have a positive effect. Normal hormone levels for stage and adequate calcium intake are crucial. During puberty, there is a progressive increase in total body bone mineral content and lean body mass and a progressive decrease in body fat.

PSYCHOLOGICAL FACTORS AND SEXUAL BEHAVIOR

Adolescence is the period during which humans develop the capacity for reproduction and a greater interest in sexual activity. Crucial identity formation takes places at this stage, involving changing roles at the expense of emotional conflict. Early adolescence is commonly accompanied by need to affirm self-esteem, intense feelings of anxiety and depression, and marked sensitivity to shame and humiliation. These tasks, at a time of physical changes and increasing sex drive, tend to accentuate concerns about sexual activity, especially masturbation, adequacy of physical sexual development, and sexual identity.

In modern society, adolescents may engage in sexual stimulatory behavior alone or with peers that may involve same-sex peers, particularly during early puberty. There is evidence that both masturbation and sexual activities involving others currently begin at an earlier age than occurred several decades ago.

At the present time, physical maturity and readiness for sexual activity occur years before generally social acceptability. This construct is in contrast to events during most of the history of mankind, when the age of sexual maturity was also the age when marriage and reproductive life began. As a consequence of multiple factors in the past few centuries, physical maturity has occurred at younger ages, whereas the age of expected and desired marriage and reproduction has occurred later in life. This pattern has led to conflicts among families and in relation to social and religious mores. Typical adolescents are physically capable and interested in sexual activity long before they have attained adult psychological sexual maturity.

Most youth at the onset of physical pubertal changes begin to establish interpersonal relationships with those of the opposite sex. Mid-adolescence is characterized by an interest in dating, involvement in peer groups with both genders, and an interest in the meaning of life, which may be expressed in religious activities and advocacy for causes and in becoming active in various service projects. By late adolescence, maturity begins to reach the point at which one becomes capable of a mature love relationship with one partner.

By mid-adolescence, a sense of gender identity is intensified. Masculine and feminine concepts, attitudes, and expected behavior are formed for each individual and for his or her peers. A perception of attitudes about overt sexual behavior develops based on the values and norms acquired. Peer norms, or what is perceived as peer norms, have a powerful influence on the behavior that subsequently develops. The age at which an individual becomes sexually active does not correlate with the attainment of any specific milestone of physical development but is profoundly affected by socioeconomic status, educational attainment of family members, goal orientation, and religious conviction. Substance abuse, peer pressure, media messages, communication with parents, overall discipline in the home, and age of sexual activity or first pregnancy of parents all have an impact on the outcome.

Most teenagers cope with adolescent challenges and resolve issues involving dependency/independence with the family, peer-group versus family loyalty, privacy versus sharing thoughts with peers, and the formation of gender roles and sexual object choice. They should be encouraged to be realistic about risk-taking behaviors and the behavioral freedoms. Adolescence involves much more than the hormonal and physical changes of puberty; messages and guidance from family, peers, other adults, media, and the general mores of the culture may be powerful positive or negative effects.

How rising hormone levels act to influence adolescent behavior remains an enigma. The best studies to date use a hormone deplete/hormone replete model during which sex steroids can be administered to adolescents deficient in such substances. Using a double-blind protocol, surprisingly few effects of sex steroids were found on adolescent behavior, including sexual behavior. In contrast to considering adolescents the "victims of raging hormones," puberty may well be a time of "social dampening." That is, social factors rather than hormone influences are likely the predominant forces dictating behavior in the adolescent.

MAJOR POINTS

Puberty occurs when there is resurgence of pituitary gonadotropin release, driven by an increase in episodic hypothalamic gonadotropin-releasing hormone (GnRH) stimulation. Neural stimulatory factors on the hypothalamus outweigh the inhibitory influences that are predominant during childhood.

Pubertal gonadotropins can be documented by random serum or urinary luteinizing hormone and follicle-stimulating hormone levels or by a pubertal luteinizing hormone response to GnRH stimulation above the prepubertal range. (Normal ranges vary depending on the particular assay used.)

The first physical growth of breast and pubic hair (evidence of sex steroid effects) does not necessarily indicate that the hypothalamic-pituitary-gonadal axis has become activated.

If secular changes toward an earlier onset of puberty are continuing, it is at a very slow rate. Ascertainment of such change is difficult because there are no readily available markers of pubertal onset.

SUGGESTED READINGS

Biro FM, Lucky AW, Huster GA, et al: Pubertal staging in boys, J Pediatr 1995;127:100.

Boot AM, de Ridder MA, Pols HA, et al: Bone mineral density in children and adolescents: relation to puberty, calcium intake, and physical activity, J Clin Endocrinol Metab 1997;82:57.

Chumlea WC, Schubert CM, Roche AF, et al: Age at menarche and racial comparisons in U.S. girls, Pediatrics 2003;111:110.

de Muinck Keizer-Schrama SMP, Mul D: Trends in pubertal development in Europe, Hum Reprod Update 2001;7:287.

DeRidder CM, Thijssen JHH, Bruning PF, et al: Body fat mass, body fat distribution, and pubertal development: a longitudinal study of physical and hormonal sexual maturation of girls, J Clin Endocrinol Metab 1992;75:442.

Herman-Giddens ME, Wang L, Koch G: Secondary sexual characteristics in boys: estimates from the National Health and Nutrition Examination Survey III, 1988-1994, Arch Pediatr Adolesc Med 2001;155:1022.

Herman-Giddens ME, Slora EJ, Wasserman RC, et al: Secondary sexual characteristics and menses in young girls seen in office practice: a study from the Pediatric Research in Office Settings Network, Pediatrics 1997;99:505.

Juul A, Bang P, Hertel NT, et al: Serum insulin-like growth factor-I in 1030 healthy children, adolescents, and adults: relation to age, sex, stage of puberty, testicular size, and body mass index, J Clin Endocrinol Metab 1994;78:744.

Harlan WR, Grillo GP, Cornoni-Huntley J, et al: Secondary sex characteristics of boys 12 to 17 years of age: the U.S. Health Examination Survey, J Pediatr 1979;95:293.

Kulin HE, Finkelstein JW, Susman E, et al: The role of sex hormones on the control of behavior during human puberty. In Bourguignon JP, Plant TM, editors: The Onset of Puberty in Perspective, Amsterdam, 2000, Elsevier Science.

Kulin HE, Bell PM, Santen RJ, et al: Integration of pulsatile gonadotropin secretion by timed urinary measurements: an accurate and sensitive 3-hour test, J Clin Endocrinol Metab 1975;40:783.

Lee PA: Pubertal neuroendocrine maturation: early differentiation and stages of development, Adolesc Pediatr Gynecol 1988;1:3.

Lee PA: Normal ages of pubertal events among American males and females, J Adolesc Health Care 1980;1:26.

Lee PA, Witchel SF: The influence of estrogen on growth, Curr Opin Pediatr 1997;9:431.

Neely EK, Hintz RL, Wilson DM, et al: Normal ranges of immunochemiluminometric gonadotropin assays, J Pediatr 1995;127:40.

Okasha M, McCarron P, McEwen J, et al: Age at menarche: secular trends and association with adult anthropometric measures, Ann Hum Biol 2001;28:68.

Ponder SW, McCormick DP, Fawcett HD, et al: Spinal bone mineral density in children aged 5.00 through 11.99 years, Am J Dis Child 1990;144:1346.

Roche AF, Wellens R, Attie KM, et al: The timing of sexual maturation in a group of US white youths, J Pediatr Endocrinol Metab 1995;8:11.

Rubin K, Schirduan V, Gendreau P, et al: Predictors of axial and peripheral bone mineral density in healthy children and adolescents, with special attention to the role of puberty, J Pediatr 1993;123:863.

Sun SS, Schubert CM, Chumlea WC, et al: National estimates of the timing of sexual maturation and racial differences among U.S. children, Pediatrics 2002;110:911.

Susman EJ, Finkelstein JW, Chinchilli VM, et al: The effect of sex hormone replacement therapy on behavior problems and moods in adolescents with delayed puberty, J Pediatr 1998;133:521.

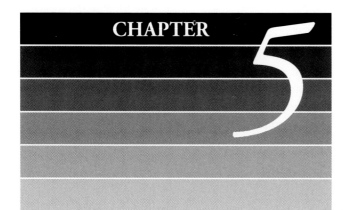

CHAPTER 5

Early Pubertal Development

PETER A. LEE

INTRODUCTION

The differential diagnosis of early pubertal development, including distinguishing early variants of puberty without rapid progression from precocious puberty, may be difficult at initial presentation. Although precocious puberty progresses at an accelerated rate, the initial history and physical examination among most children presenting with this complaint are often inconclusive. To ascertain whether puberty is excessive for age requires careful initial assessment, including, if indicated, basal hormonal and skeletal age estimation and longitudinal observation for progression.

AGE CRITERIA INSUFFICIENT

Previously, precocious puberty was diagnosed when physical pubertal changes became apparent at an age younger than the lower limit for the onset of such changes (8 years among females and 9.0-9.5 years among males in the United States). It now appears that these traditional limits may be based on inadequate or outdated data that did not consider racial differences or that a small portion of the population is experiencing an earlier onset of puberty. The current use of a particular age limit to assign the diagnosis of precocious puberty is inappropriate, unless the child presents already having progressed with clearly advanced pubertal development and growth for age. There also is evidence that children who have earlier onset of puberty generally progress more slowly, making it essential that it be ascertained whether changes represent normal early puberty or changes that fall beyond the normal range. Racial differences exist, with earlier onset among African American children. Further, in some instances, it is difficult to ascertain a clear demarcation between Tanner stages 1 and 2 on initial examination of genital stage for boys or

73

of breast stage among girls, particularly among those who have a full chest.

Data concerning current normal age ranges for pubertal development are still being collected, but Tables 4-1 and 4-2 can serve as a guideline for judging whether pubertal changes are early. However, it is essential to remember that there is overlap between the age of onset of pubertal changes that may herald early, slowly progressive but normal puberty and disproportionately progressive precocious puberty indicative of pathology.

Box 5-1 lists categories of early pubertal development that represent a continuum. These categories are not static; therefore, that which is initially considered a benign variant

of normal may progress into a more advanced category, or a case of nonprogressive precocious puberty, may regress to a less advanced category. Premature adrenarche and thelarche present with isolated early sexual hair growth and breast development. Both have long been recognized and considered variants of normal development. These changes occur at an age younger than the norm without pubertal activation of the hypothalamic-pituitary-gonadal (HPG) axis.

EARLY ANDROGEN-STIMULATED CHANGES

The presence of pubic hair during childhood (premature pubarche) unassociated with other significant pubertal change has been considered a variant of normal. Usually this reflects premature adrenarche, the early onset of a pubertal process that is distinct from the activation of the HPG axis. Adrenarche designates the onset of increased androgen production from the adrenal gland, which may be documented hormonally as young as 6 years of age. Premature adrenarche occurs when androgen production from the adrenal is sufficient to stimulate sexual hair growth that may be accompanied by other mild androgen-mediated changes (acne, oily skin, adult-type body odor, and axillary hair). Generally, this is not associated with a significant growth spurt or advancement in skeletal maturation. However, these early changes may be the initial presenting evidence of more than early adrenarche, such as disorders of androgen metabolism that become manifest later with more signs of hyperandrogenism. Thus, when a child presents with sexual hair at a young age for race and gender, basal hormonal levels should be documented to verify that levels are in the range expected after early adrenarche. Onset during infancy, extremely rapid progression of adrenarche, or the presence of other evidence of virilization such as clitoromegaly could indicate an androgen-producing lesion or congenital adrenal hyperplasia. The management of such patients is outlined in the section concerning early androgen-stimulated changes. Parents should be cautioned to watch such children as they progress through puberty for any evidence suggesting hormonal imbalance.

EARLY ESTROGEN-STIMULATED CHANGES

Infants and young girls who have detectable pubertal breast development with no or minimal other evidence of pubertal change may have premature thelarche. This entity is generally considered to be the consequence of extrasensitive end-organ (breast tissue) response to prepubertal estrogen

---

Box 5-1 Categories of Early Pubertal Development

VARIANTS OF NORMAL

Premature Adrenarche

May manifest by premature pubarche (sexual hair)
Independent of gonadal pubertal change
Must be differentiated from disorders of androgen metabolism

Premature Thelarche

Not a consequence of pubertal hormonal stimulation
Breast development not associated with other significant pubertal changes
May be initial presentation of other forms of early pubertal development

Nonprogressive Early Puberty

Early onset but slowly progressive pubertal changes
Later milestones occur generally within normal age ranges
Growth and skeletal maturity occur in synchrony so height is not compromised

PRECOCIOUS PUBERTY

Central Precocious Puberty

Early onset and rapid progression of pubertal changes
A consequence of early activation of hypothalamic-pituitary-gonadal (HPG) axis
May result in dramatically accelerated development for age and loss of stature of growth potential

Peripheral Precocious Puberty

Significant early pubertal changes occurring as a consequence of hormonal stimulation other than via pubertal activation of the HPG axis
Underlying etiology should be sought and treatment involves that indicated for underlying cause
May result in significant untimely maturity and growth compromise

levels including increased aromatase activity or to minimally elevated prepubertal estrogen secretion but not the consequence of early centrally activated pubertal ovarian hormonal secretion. As such, it is considered a benign condition, with subsequent puberty occurring in a normal fashion. However, this may also be the *initial manifestation* of the early onset of physical puberty that progresses slowly so that later milestones are attained at expected ages and statural growth dynamics are not altered. This entity is referred to as *nonprogressive precocious puberty* and requires no treatment. Female patients with nonprogressive early puberty who are untreated achieve normal adult heights that exceed the heights of untreated patients with progressive precocious puberty. It is important not to misdiagnose and treat this entity as central precocious puberty (CPP) to avoid unnecessary extra medical attention and cost and the detrimental effects of labeling the child with an abnormal condition. Conversely, the diagnosis of nonprogressive early puberty necessitates subsequent observations to verify the diagnosis and ensure that puberty is progressing slowly.

Breast development in girls may also be the first finding of *progressive precocious puberty.* If so, progression of pubertal changes becomes apparent in the weeks or months after breast enlargement is first noted. Progressive precocious puberty may be either central or peripheral, which represent different entities.

PROGRESSIVE ESTROGEN-STIMULATED CHANGES

With continued stimulation by estrogen, the development of girls advance so that not only does breast and genital development progress, but also body composition and configuration, skeletal growth, and facial characteristics attain a more mature appearance. This is associated with a marked acceleration of growth and advanced epiphyseal maturation. These changes occur with estrogen stimulation alone. These changes may be accompanied by changes, such as sexual hair, stimulated by androgens of either ovarian or adrenal origin. Such progressive changes at a young age constitute precocious puberty, which may be either centrally or peripherally mediated.

PROGRESSIVE ANDROGEN-STIMULATED CHANGES

As noted earlier, low levels of androgen stimulate the onset of sexual hair growth among prepubertal boys. Additional pubertal changes, such as penis growth, scrotal maturation, and accelerated somatic growth, require greater amounts of androgen. Progressive changes clearly excessive for age should be considered precocious puberty. On physical examination, it is important to determine whether testicular growth is occurring. Enlargement of the testes suggests that CPP is occurring or that a rare mutation such as a luteinizing hormone (LH) receptor–activating mutation has occurred. The absence of testicular enlargement suggests that the androgens are derived from another source, either the adrenals or an exogenous exposure. Early pubertal changes accompanied by accelerated linear growth and a rapid skeletal maturity rate are consistent with precocious puberty. The assessment of such changes must investigate whether early puberty is occurring with pubertal activation of the HPA axis (CPP) or is the consequence of sex steroid effect independent of gonadotropin secretion (peripheral precocious puberty [PPP]).

PRECOCIOUS PUBERTY

As noted earlier, the criteria for the diagnosis of precocious puberty are complex and specific age limits for the onset of physical changes are insufficient. As also noted, at presentation with initial physical changes, it may be unclear whether the actual onset of pubertal activity of the HPG axis is occurring.

Precocious puberty among both males and females is accompanied by growth acceleration. This growth acceleration is a consequence of sex steroid stimulation of skeletal growth. Estrogen is apparently the most potent stimulus in both sexes, the source of the estrogen among boys being primarily via peripheral conversion from testosterone. Immature bones mature rapidly, with estrogen exposure resulting in the typical pattern among children with precocious puberty of growth acceleration but with a disproportionate advance in skeletal age. This diminished growth relative to the rate of skeletal maturation results in the loss of height potential. Some causes of precocious puberty may not be associated with growth acceleration, as occur among former oncology patients who may have concomitant precocious puberty and growth hormone deficiency or in the rare situation described later involving hypothyroidism.

Central Precocious Puberty

CPP occurs more frequently among females than males; PPP is more unusual among females than among males. CPP may be a consequence of a known or an identifiable underlying central nervous system (CNS) disturbance or may be associated with no apparent abnormality (idiopathic) (Box 5-2). Among girls, most are idiopathic, whereas males with CPP more frequently have a known or

Box 5-2   Etiology of Central (Gonadotropin-Releasing Hormone–Dependent) Precocious Puberty

IDIOPATHIC

Sporadic or familial
  More frequent among females than males
  Not uncommonly found among children moving from
    underdeveloped countries

CENTRAL NERVOUS SYSTEM DERANGEMENTS

Hypothalamic hamartomas
  Redundant hypothalamic tissue containing gonadotropin-
    releasing hormone–secreting neurons
  Isolated from usual central nervous system inhibitory
    effects
Congenital aberrations/anomalies
  May be associated neurological or mental defects
  Myelomeningocele
  Septo-optic dysplasia
  Hydrocephalus (may be reversible)
Central nervous system space-occupying lesion
  Arachnoid cysts
  Astrocytomas
  Craniopharyngiomas
  Ependymomas
  Ectopic pinealomas
  Gliomas
  Optic gliomas (associated with neurofibromatosis type 1)
  Pituitary adenomas
  Tumors associated with tuberous sclerosis
Central nervous system damage secondary to
  Chemotherapy
  Inflammation (encephalitis/meningitis)
  Irradiation
  Surgery
  Trauma

SECONDARY TO CHRONIC EXCESSIVE SEX STEROID EXPOSURE

Peripheral precocious puberty
Congenital adrenal hyperplasia

demonstrable CNS abnormality. CNS problems associated with precocious puberty include redundant or excessive hypothalamic tissue (hypothalamic hamartoma), other congenital malformations such as arachnoid cysts, tumors (optic gliomas, hypothalamic astrocytoma), and CNS injury from trauma, infections, or anoxia. CNS lesions stimulate and upregulate intermittent gonadotropin-releasing hormone (GnRH) secretory bursts to alter the prepubertal balance between stimulatory and inhibitory influences. CPP may occur among children who have received radiation therapy and chemotherapy for childhood malignancies that reduce inhibitory influences on the hypothalamus. This group also may develop growth hormone deficiency and

may not present with the typical findings of CPP, since growth acceleration may not be present. CPP may also occur as a consequence of CNS maturation secondary to marked sex steroid stimulation from other sources such as sex steroid–producing tumors or undiagnosed or inadequately treated congenital adrenal hyperplasia; such exposure during prepubertal years appears to mature the HPG axis. Change to a better environment or rapid weight gain in a poorly nourished or otherwise deprived individual may also be associated with early pubertal maturation.

Peripheral Precocious Puberty

PPP occurs after sex steroid stimulation that is independent of HPG axis activity and gonadotropin secretion. In PPP, the same clinical findings—accelerated growth, breast and genital development among girls, and virilization of genitalia among boys with varying sexual hair development—may occur. Among boys with PPP, testicular growth is minimal because such growth requires gonadotropin stimulation. Therefore, boys with considerable phallic enlargement but small testes are suspected to have a form of PPP. In PPP, as with CPP, pubertal changes can progress rapidly. Among girls, vaginal bleeding can occur, although ovulation would not be expected. Endometrial sloughing may be due to excessive or fluctuating estrogen secretion with a sudden decrease in estrogen effect. The pattern of bleeding is often erratic but may be quite regular.

Ovarian, Testicular, and Adrenal Sex Steroid–Secreting Tumors

These tumors are rare. Sex steroid levels are often, but not always, greatly elevated, with the profile of the estrogen or androgen levels suggesting excessive ovarian, testicular, or adrenal cortical secretion. Ovarian tumors may be identified by a unilateral mass on examination or ultrasonography. Estrogen-secreting ovarian tumors are usually associated with rapid changes of estrogen-responsive tissues and asymmetrical ovarian enlargement. Testicular tumors should present with testicular asymmetry, with the larger testis being or containing a firm mass. This can be easily confirmed with ultrasonography. Leydig cell tumors of the testis are associated with testosterone levels in or above the adult male range, rapidly progressing androgen-stimulated changes, and testicular asymmetry, sometimes with the portion of the involved testis being firmer on palpation. Adrenal tumors may present as an abdominal mass or asymmetrical adrenal enlargement detected by abdominopelvic sonography. Adrenal steroid–producing tumors may also produce excessive glucocorticoids and present as part of the Cushing syndrome, secrete only excessive androgens, or, extremely rarely, estrogen and androgen or estrogen alone.

Male and female patients may then present with precocious puberty—females with hyperandrogenism, or males with evidence of estrogen excess, primarily gynecomastia. It should be noted that unilateral or bilateral intrascrotal masses may represent hyperplasia of adrenal rest tissue among boys with undiagnosed, untreated, or inadequately treated congenital adrenal hyperplasia.

Exogenous Hormones

Sex steroids or gonadotropins are an unlikely but potential cause of PPP. Estrogen should not be present in foods and cosmetics produced in the United States. Topical androgens available as either prescription drugs or unregulated androgens may cause significant virilization in the prepubertal child. More than a single exposure is generally necessary for medications containing sex steroids to cause changes.

Among males, but not females, *chorionic gonadotropin secretion of tumor origin* causes PPP. Tumors may be CNS, mediastinal, or hepatic. Human chorionic gonadotropin (hCG) binds to the LH receptor to stimulate Leydig cell differentiation and testosterone secretion, resulting in precocious puberty. The LH effect of hCG alone does not result in pubertal changes among females because both LH and follicle-stimulating hormone (FSH) are necessary for follicular development and estrogen secretion. Although PPP generally presents in males without testicular enlargement or with a testicular mass, the instances that result from gonadotropin receptor stimulation, such as hCG or TSH stimulation of the FSH receptor, present with bilateral testicular growth.

The McCune-Albright Syndrome, Ovarian Cysts, and Male-Limited Gonadotropin-Independent Precocious Puberty (Luteinizing Receptor–Activating Mutations)

These are autonomous causes of precocious puberty. The *McCune-Albright syndrome* classically included a triad of autonomous endocrinopathies (most commonly, precocious puberty), polyostotic fibrous dysplasia, and café au lait skin macules. However, only one or two of these findings may occur. Ovarian steroidogenesis is stimulated by an activating G protein mutation in the cyclic adenosine monophosphate (cAMP) system resulting in activation of cAMP without gonadotropin stimulation. This postconception somatic mutation affects cells of the ovaries among patients with this diagnosis. This results in estrogen secretion, which may be intermittent, stimulating pubertal changes and withdrawal uterine bleeding. Other associated endocrinopathies, all as a consequence of autonomous secretion, include thyrotoxicosis, excessive glucocorticoid production resulting in Cushing syndrome, and growth hormone excess resulting in gigantism or acromegaly. Each of the endocrine glands or tissues affected in this condition have an early somatic mutation resulting in a constitutively activated G protein.

Ovarian cysts may autonomously secrete estrogen and cause usually nonsustained PPP but also occur in association with CPP and premature thelarche in the normal prepubertal child. Functional cysts are a rare consequence of normal prepubertal ovarian follicular development. When a follicle continues to grow rather than following the usual pattern in children of limited growth and regression, such an estrogen-secreting cyst may develop. The etiology may include sporadically increased gonadotropin stimulation during childhood. The presence of a cyst is neither indicative of pathology nor diagnostic of a significant abnormality. In the absence of other demonstrable pathology, an ovarian cyst may be the cause of unsustained PPP.

Male-limited gonadotropin-independent precocious puberty (LH receptor–activating mutations) is associated with testicular steroidogenesis and spermatogenesis, even though gonadotropin levels are low or suppressed. The stimulation results from activation of the LH receptor. Inherited in an autosomal dominant fashion, the onset is at a very young age, and presentation is with growth acceleration with genital, including testicular, growth. This form of PPP is a consequence of activating mutations of the LH receptor resulting in G protein activation and increased cAMP production with Leydig cell testosterone secretion. Basal and GnRH-stimulated gonadotropin levels are prepubertal or suppressed, whereas testosterone levels are elevated. Over time, the pubertal hypothalamic-testicular axis becomes activated, leading to secondary CPP.

Chronic Primary Hypothyroidism

Pubertal changes suggestive of precocious puberty occur very rarely among patients with *chronic primary hypothyroidism*. Physical findings include testicular enlargement among boys and breast development, sometimes with galactorrhea, among girls. Full pubertal development does not occur. Multicystic ovaries commonly occur. Growth rates may not be accelerated but may actually be diminished. Skeletal age may be delayed rather than advanced because of the thyroid hormone deficiency. The pathophysiology of this disorder appears to involve occupation of the FSH receptor by TSH when present in high excess. Elevated prolactin secretion, which occurs in chronic primary hypothyroidism, may be contributing to the breast changes. When the hypothyroidism is treated with thyroid hormone and TSH levels are suppressed into the physiologic range, premature sexual development regresses.

Congenital Adrenal Hyperplasia

Excessive adrenal androgen production in *congenital adrenal hyperplasia* is a cause of PPP among males. The typical presentation includes advanced genital, somatic, and skeletal growth and maturation but without an increase in the testicular volume. However, as noted, boys may have enlargement of scrotal contents, which may be intratesticular or extratesticular hyperplasia of adrenal rest tissue that may be present unilaterally or bilaterally. Congenital adrenal hyperplasia occurs among both males and females, but the androgen-stimulated changes present as inappropriate virilization rather than as precocious puberty among females. However, among both females and males, if there is chronic exposure to increased sex steroids, as with delayed diagnosis of congenital adrenal hyperplasia or inadequate therapy, secondary CPP may occur.

DIFFERENTIAL DIAGNOSIS

Assessment of Early Breast Development Among Girls

Early breast development may be evidence of premature thelarche (normal prepubertal variant), nonprogressive precocious puberty (normal pubertal variant), or CPP (progressive GnRH-driven precocious puberty) or the consequence of estrogen exposure from any nonphysiological source (PPP).

An algorithm is presented for the assessment of a girl with a presenting complaint of breast development (Figure 5-1).

Medical History

As background to the assessment outlined in Figure 5-1, general evaluation should be aimed at determining whether significant changes are occurring and searching for clues concerning underlying abnormalities. A detailed history of the age when pubertal changes were first noted and progression of any pubertal characteristics should be carefully sought. The history should include possible exposure to sex steroids or other medications, age of puberty of family members, and current or previous medical conditions, particularly involving the neurological system, skin, or thyroid gland. The presence of and odor of any vaginal discharge should be noted. Growth rates should be determined from heights at previous ages to ascertain whether there has been acceleration. Available previous heights and weights should

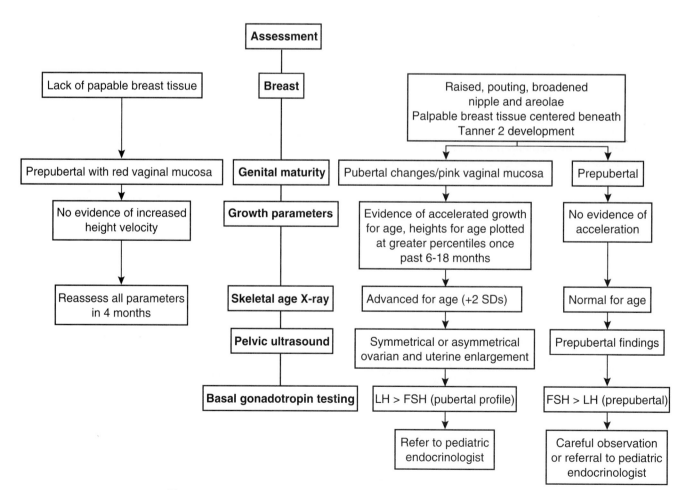

Figure 5-1   Algorithm concerning presenting complaint of breast development.

be plotted on a growth chart, as well as growth rates calculated over intervals of 6 months or longer. After infancy, a growth rate greater than the prepubertal rate of 5 to 6 cm/yr is consistent with a pubertal growth rate.

Physical Examination

The physical examination should first determine whether actual breast development is present or adipose tissue has been mistaken for glandular breast tissue (see Figure 5-1). Unless clear breast budding is present with pouting of the areolae, protruding nipples, or a palpable disc of firm breast tissue centered beneath, it may be difficult to ascertain whether breast development has actually begun. This may be a particular problem in the stocky or heavy girl because adipose tissue develops in the breast area with a contour that appears to be breasts. Often areolar diameter and pigmentation are helpful because they increase with estrogen exposure, but with obesity, the areolae may become stretched and increase in diameter as a consequence of the extra subcutaneous tissue. When on palpation, the tissue is less dense beneath the areolae, it is unlikely that pubertal breast tissue growth has begun.

As part of the full general examination, pertinent findings include height, weight, arm span, upper/lower segment ratio, funduscopic examination, visual fields by confrontation, thyroid gland, and skin for texture and pigmentation. The genitalia should be carefully inspected. The presence and distribution of pubic hair and the relative size of the labia minora should be noted; the latter may be an index of estrogen stimulation. Although it is often initially unnecessary to palpate the vulva and introitus, inspection of the vaginal mucosa provides information concerning estrogen effect. The greater the estrogen effect, the thicker is the mucosal layer and the pinker is the appearance. A red vaginal mucosa is consistent with no estrogen stimulation, whereas a pink, moist mucosa suggests estrogen effect. Local irritation or infection may, however, invalidate this observation.

Laboratory Studies

Initial laboratory studies are based on the physical and growth rate findings. If only questionable or minimal breast tissue is present, follow-up is much more important than laboratory testing. Minimal testing includes LH and FSH levels, and if there is a suggestion of growth acceleration, a skeletal age radiograph provides documentation of maturity. LH and FSH levels, however, may overlap the prepubertal–pubertal range and thus are helpful only if they are clearly elevated above the prepubertal range. The use of the more sensitive third generation assays enables distinction of a low prepubertal value from a pubertal value. LH/FSH ratios may be more helpful, because a ratio of less than 1 is

suggestive of prepubertal secretion, whereas a ratio of greater than 1 suggests pubertal secretion.

Testosterone levels are useful in assessment among males, although some commercially available assays may have poor sensitivity. The routine estradiol assays are usually not sensitive enough to be particularly useful; sensitive assays are potentially very useful but not generally available.

Ultrasonography

Among girls, abdominal-pelvic sonography may be useful to ascertain to the effects of stimulation by pubertal hormones. Variations in the size and symmetry of the ovaries, adrenal glands, and the uterus may suggest the underlying etiology. In CPP, ovarian and uterine volume should be symmetrically increased. Ovarian tumors generally present with unilateral enlargement and asymmetry. Cysts may be identified among prepubertal girls, those with premature thelarche, CPP, or PPP. Significant estrogen effect, whether as a consequence of CPP or PPP, stimulates uterine growth and endometrial thickening, indicated by the endometrial stripe visualized on ultrasonography. Adrenal size in the diagnosis of mild adrenal hyperplasia is seldom helpful, although rare adrenal tumors can be thereby visualized.

More thorough laboratory testing is usually more appropriately ordered after referral to a pediatric endocrinologist. If the results of the evaluation outlined in Figure 5-1 suggest that CPP may be occurring, subsequent laboratory testing is usually directed toward differentiating central (gonadotropin-dependent) from peripheral (gonadotropin-independent) precocious puberty.

Gonadotropin-Releasing Hormone or Gonadotropin-Releasing Hormone Analogue Stimulation Testing

If findings are suggestive of full precocious puberty or the screening tests suggest CPP, GnRH or GnRH analogue (GnRHa) stimulation testing is indicated to determine if responses are consistent with pubertal gonadotropin secretion. This diagnostic test is the sine qua non for the diagnosis for CPP. A clearly pubertal gonadotropin response is indicative of pubertal activation of the hypothalamic-pituitary axis. Such testing involves an acute intravenous or subcutaneous administration of GnRH or GnRHa with measurement of gonadotropins before and at timed intervals after the injection. Doses of GnRH may range from 25 to 50 μg/m^2, although most commonly 100 μg is administered. When GnRHa is given, the subcutaneous preparation of leuprolide acetate may be used at a dose of 20 μg/kg given subcutaneously.

The child with CPP has a response pattern after GnRH or GnRHa stimulation similar to the usual pubertal response with a significant rise of gonadotropins, particularly

LH, of much greater magnitude than in the prepubertal child. The actual magnitude of the rise in gonadotropins depends on the assay used. The more sensitive assays result in lower levels for basal and stimulated values, so the relative increase after stimulation may not be useful. Generally, for the third-generation assays, the stimulated LH values during prepuberty peak at 6 μU/L or below, whereas the pubertal response is much greater than 6, with values usually ranging from 10 to 40 and occasionally as high as 60. Prepubertal females have a substantial rise of FSH compared with prepubertal males. The increment in FSH response with pubertal maturation is considerably less than for LH; therefore, the FSH response is less helpful. Using the newer assays, FSH commonly increases to a range of 7 to 25 μU/L among prepubertal girls, which overlaps with the response in pubertal girls.

Other screening tests may include but are not limited to thyroid function tests, prolactin, adrenal androgens (androstenedione, dehydroepiandrosterone [DHEA], and DHEA sulfate [DHEAS]), and, among boys, quantitative hCG.

Central Nervous System Magnetic Resonance Imaging

Magnetic resonance imaging (MRI) of the CNS with particular attention to the hypothalamus and pituitary region should be considered only after gonadotropin-dependent precocious puberty has been diagnosed, unless there are neurological abnormalities. Such studies are indicated for most males and females presenting with CPP. It has been debated whether girls older than 5 years have less risk of CNS lesions and less need for CNS MRI assessment, but there remains a risk of a lesions with no abnormal neurological findings. It has been suggested that markedly elevated estradiol levels and lack of pubic hair at presentation suggest a greater risk.

Assessment of Mild Androgen Effects Among Boys and Girls

Girls may present with only androgen-stimulated findings—pubic hair, axillary hair, acne, oily skin, and, in unusual instances, clitoromegaly. Assessment should be focused on potential causes of androgen excess rather than the differential of full female precocious puberty (Figure 5-2). Causes of androgen excess in childhood include premature adrenarche, excessive adrenal androgen synthesis including mild adrenal hyperplasia, gonadal excess (initial manifestation of ovarian hyperandrogenism), and, rarely, adrenal and gonadal androgen-secreting tumors.

Hyperandrogenism among females may progress to include hirsutism, excessive acne, clitoromegaly, voice change, an accelerated growth rate or tall stature, excessive muscle development, and a masculine habitus. A common cause of virilization among prepubertal girls is the mild forms of the congenital virilizing adrenal hyperplasia, especially 21-hydroxylase deficiency. As noted earlier, unexplained mild virilization during late prepubertal years may herald ovarian hyperandrogenism. Other causes are very rare and include androgen-producing tumors. Adrenal tumors are adenomas or carcinomas; ovarian tumors include arrhenoblastomas, choriocarcinomas, dysgerminomas, and teratomas. Hormone production and malignancy vary for these tumors. It should also be noted that, although rare, clitoral enlargement may result from abnormal tissue, such as a neurofibroma, rather than virilization.

Screening tests for androgen excess include testosterone, androstenedione, DHEA, DHEAS, and 17-hydroxyprogesterone for the most common form of adrenal hyperplasia, a common cause of PPP among boys. Among males, the spectrum of findings extends from minimal sexual hair to full androgen-stimulated changes (Figure 5-3). Males who present with virilization and evidence of testicular growth should be evaluated for precocious puberty, as outlined in the next section.

Assessment of Boys With Early Pubertal Changes, With or Without Testicular Enlargement

The approach for the assessment of males presenting with early pubertal changes is outlined in Figure 5-3. Males with gonadotropin-dependent precocious puberty have testicular growth consistent with other pubertal changes comparable to that which occurs during normal pubertal development. As noted earlier, categories of gonadotropin-independent precocious puberty (PPP) among boys are not a consequence of pituitary LH-stimulated testicular testosterone production. When puberty is gonadotropin driven, bilateral testicular growth occurs (see Figure 5-3). Males presenting with CPP have bilateral testicular enlargement, whereas most with PPP do not. Exceptions include male-limited gonadotropin-independent precocious puberty, hCG-secreting tumors, and primary hypothyroidism.

History

Boys with precocious puberty may present with a history of noticeable weight gain, a dramatic increase in muscle mass, accelerated linear growth, deepening of the voice, and more mature facies, as well as genital changes and sexual hair. The history should document changes in growth and pubertal progression, as well as evidence of neurological problems, prior medical conditions and their treatment, especially radiotherapy or chemotherapy, and signs and symptoms of hypothyroidism. Family history of the onset of pubertal maturation is also essential.

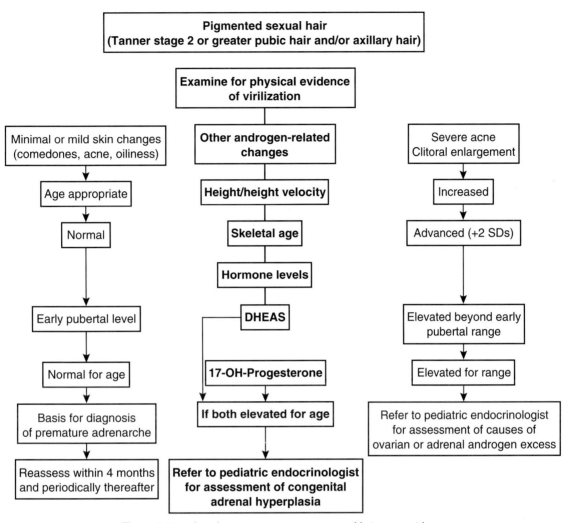

Figure 5-2 Algorithm concerning premature sexual hair among girls.

Physical Findings

Emphasis should be placed on the funduscopic, neurological, and skin examination and a careful genital examination. Tanner staging of genital size and pubic hair should be assigned with careful palpation and a measurement of testicular volume and symmetry. Generally, a testis less than 2 cm in longitudinal axis is considered to be of prepubertal size, whereas a testis longer than 2.5 cm is pubertal.

The size and symmetry of the testes among boys presenting with precocious puberty provide a diagnostic clue that guides the assessment (see Figure 5-3).

Laboratory Studies

Initial assessment includes LH, FSH, and testosterone levels. A testosterone level greater than the prepubertal range (>10 ng/dL) verifies pubertal levels of androgens. However, unless gonadotropin levels are above the prepubertal range with the LH higher than the FSH level, differentiation between CPP and PPP cannot be made. As noted earlier, other tests may include thyroid function tests to rule out this rare cause of PPP, 17-hydroxyprogesterone as a screen for the most common form of adrenal hyperplasia, adrenal androgens (androstenedione, DHEA, or DHEAS to document status of adrenarche or to rule out adrenal androgen excess), and hCG.

If physical examination and growth data indicate accelerated growth, the skeletal age should be documented. This provides a reference to judge subsequent progression, may verify previous excessive stimulation, and allows an assessment of diminished and future growth potential.

Central Nervous System Magnetic Resonance Imaging

Although it may be controversial whether all girls with CPP should have an MRI of the CNS, it is unequivocally indicated for all males because the proportion of males with CPP who have demonstrable CNS abnormalities is high.

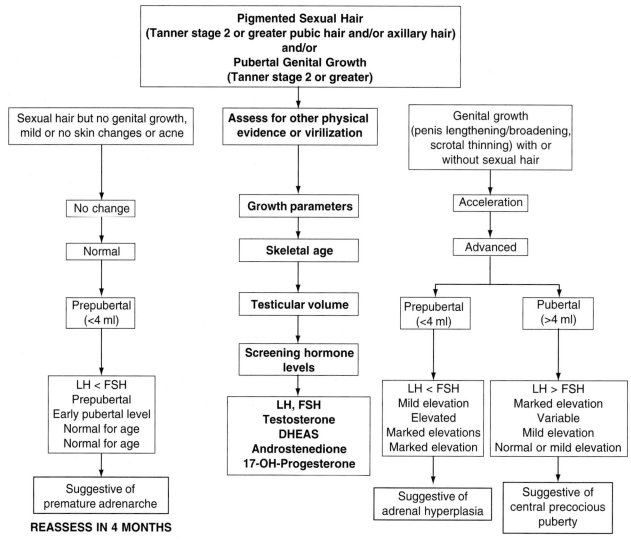

Figure 5-3   Early onset of pubertal changes among boys.

NATURAL HISTORY OF CENTRAL PRECOCIOUS PUBERTY

All aspects of pubertal development progress with early physical maturity, leading initially to tall stature during childhood but then to premature attainment of foreshortened adult height on achieving reproductive and sexual maturity. Biological maturity is accompanied by a shift in body composition and increased bone density for age. Although serious psychological problems are not characteristic during or after precocious puberty, there may be social or psychological adjustment problems. These are primarily a consequence of being taller and more mature appearing, perhaps stressing peer acceptance and resulting in adults anticipating and expecting greater maturity, sophistication,

and an adolescent demeanor. Although children may physically be quite mature, their cognitive and social development is age appropriate, and their perceptions, particularly concerning sexuality, are not advanced. The disparity between their physical appearance and their age may make them at particular risk for sexual abuse.

MANAGEMENT OF AND TREATMENT FOR CENTRAL PRECOCIOUS PUBERTY

Whether therapy is instituted to arrest pubertal progression, children with CPP and their parents should have a fundamental understanding of the physiological process. The child should be told at his or her level of understanding that the normal process of becoming a man or woman like his or her parent sometimes begins too early and progresses too quickly.

Treatment should be considered if it is judged appropriate to halt untimely pubertal maturation, including menstruation, and to reverse the consequences of the accelerated growth rate and skeletal maturation. Concerns about psychological and social stress as a consequence of earlier development than peers and the prediction of diminished adult height and disproportionately shortened limbs may be considered indications for therapy. The effects on growth and skeletal maturation are mediated by estradiol in both females and males (in males, testosterone is aromatized to estradiol). Acceleration of skeletal maturation in relation to height gain limit adult height potential. Such children, growing at accelerated rates during childhood, become tall during childhood but complete growth prematurely to ultimately be short as adults.

GnRHa therapy has revolutionized the treatment of CPP. Pituitary gonadotropin secretion responds to the pulsatile delivery of GnRH, which is extremely short-lived. The administration of long-acting GnRHa downregulates its receptors and diminishes secretion of LH and FSH. Suppression of gonadotropin secretion removes excessive sex steroid stimulation, allowing pubertal maturation, including cessation of menses, to regress or stop progressing. The suppression of sex steroid secretion causes a deceleration in growth rate and bone maturation to a prepubertal rate, leading to an appearance and height more appropriate for age and an improved adult height prediction. Rate of accrual of bone density would be expected to decrease with therapy, so if bone density before therapy was advanced for age, it may shift toward normal. With early treatment, physical appearance and height normalize for age, and further pubertal development is postponed until the appropriate age. With delay in treatment until a more advanced stage of puberty, pubertal maturation and growth acceleration are suppressed, but the child may continue to appear mature for age and the improvement in final height may be more limited.

GnRHa are the treatment of choice for CPP when it has been decided that temporary interruption of the puberty is appropriate. The goal is to use a dosage sufficient to completely suppress gonadotropin secretion and halt the progression of puberty based on the dosage that would suppress +2 SDs of the patient population—0.3 mg/kg/28 days of leuprolide acetate depot is recommended.

It is important that the child understands that she or he is not ill but that his or her body has begun changing into a man or woman too soon and that the treatment is given to stop this process and allow them to develop more similarly to their peers. It is also appropriate to offer assurance that the treatment will be stopped at the age when puberty

is supposed to happen and that the child develops the same as everyone else. Psychological counseling should include sex education geared to the level of understanding of the patient and a discussion of the pathophysiology of the etiological diagnosis, providing both the patient and the parents with all available information if desired.

Monitoring Treatment of Precocious Puberty

Verification of complete suppression of gonadotropin secretion is necessary to maximize desired results. Decreased gonadotropin secretion is the first discernible evidence of downregulation by GnRHa. Although a short-term stimulatory phase occurs, within 1 week LH and FSH levels should be low, both at baseline and after GnRH stimulation, and sex steroids suppressed.

If there had been significant proliferation of the endometrium before therapy, one episode of withdrawal bleeding may occur as a consequence of the diminishing estradiol levels with initiation of therapy. Thereafter, withdrawal bleeding during therapy is indicative of inadequate suppression.

During therapy, pubertal changes should not progress and may regress. Tanner staging may regress or remain unchanged, although on physical examination, the glandular breast tissue is less estrogenized. Growth rates decelerate and generally become appropriate for a prepubertal child of the same gender and the skeletal age stops advancing as rapidly. Thereafter, skeletal age advances approximately 1 year per year until the skeletal age typical of puberty is reached (about 10.5 years for females and 12.5 years for males). After skeletal maturity reaches this point, it advances at a slow rate so that the change in skeletal age is less than the advance in chronological age, resulting in an increased predicted adult height. Predicted adult height increases, to a greater extent among males than females treated with GnRH. Monitoring treatment of precocious puberty ensures that desired results are occurring: cessation of physical pubertal progression and menses, slowing of skeletal age maturation rate, and growth at a prepubertal growth rate.

Because adrenarche, the pubertal increase in adrenal androgen secretion, is independent of the HPG axis, it is not affected by GnRHa therapy. Adrenal androgen production and pubic hair growth can be expected to gradually increase as occurs throughout normal puberty.

Although patients have complained about weight gain on GnRHa therapy, the overall data do not support marked weight gain. With the decrease of sex steroids, it would not be unexpected to find changes in body composition toward relatively greater fatty tissues and less lean body mass, although this has not been documented. Girls and boys with precocious puberty tend to be heavy with relatively increased lean body mass for age. Body mass index does not increase during therapy, but there may be a relative increase in fatty tissue. Before therapy, body mass index (BMI) was increased for age (standard deviation score [SDS] 1.1 ± 0.1) but not for bone age (SDS 0.1 ± 0.1). At end of treatment, BMI in within the normal range: 0.9 ± 0.1 for age and 0.6 ± 0.1 for bone age. This may be related to increase in lean body mass pretreatment, whereas it is not clear what body composition shifts occur with treatment.

It is pertinent to consider the effect of GnRHa for CPP on bone mineral density (BMD) because puberty is a key period of significant accrual of BMD. Before therapy, BMD has been found to be increased for chronological age but appropriate for skeletal age among patients with CPP. Evidence during therapy suggests that minimal accrual occurs, but BMD does not become subnormal for age because levels are advanced for age as a consequence of CPP.

Outcome After Gonadotropin-Releasing Hormone Analogue Therapy for Central Precocious Puberty

Discontinuation of therapy is followed promptly with resumption of pubertal gonadotropin secretion. Physical changes of puberty resume within months of discontinuation. Among females, menses begin or resume on the average between 12 and 18 months, overall within 2.5 years. Ovulation has been documented and pregnancy has occurred after treatment. Among males, normal sperm production has been documented.

GnRH therapy not only reclaims lost height potential but also precludes further diminished height potential. The best height outcomes are found for those starting on therapy before age 6 years and, among girls, for those discontinuing therapy at skeletal age of 12.0 to 12.5 years. Adult height is better among males than among females and is positively correlated with height at onset of therapy, height at end of therapy, duration of treatment, and target height. Continued growth after discontinuation of therapy has generally been disappointing. Females have no post-treatment growth spurt, so adult height is less than predicted adult height at the time therapy is discontinued. Males do have a period of growth acceleration after the end of therapy, resulting in a relatively greater height gain. Adult height is within target height range (the genetic estimate of expected height calculated based on parents' heights) with final adult height SDS being close to 0 for males and 0.5 SD greater among males than among females. Thus, final adult heights are greater than predicted height at the onset of therapy.

Body proportions among untreated children with precocious puberty are affected by the early skeletal maturity of long bones resulting in progressively shorter arms and legs

in relation to total height. Arm span is shorter and upper-to-lower segment ratios (the head and truck or sitting height compared with leg length) are less than the usual ratio, which approximates 1.0 after growth is complete. Thus, without treatment, individuals are not only shorter but also have altered body proportions. These proportions are normalized among patients with CPP who have been treated with GnRHa.

BMD after therapy had been found to be normal among both genders. Males have been found to have normal area and volumetric BMD. Females have normal bone density SDS for the lumber spine and the femoral neck. BMD after treatment with GnRHa in patients with progressive CPP does not differ from that in a slowly progressive group without treatment or adolescent females without precocious puberty.

GnRHa therapy is the treatment of choice for children with CPP. It should be considered for patients who have early, progressive pubertal development, accelerated growth and skeletal maturity, and pubertal gonadotropin secretion. Therapy should be monitored to verify full suppression of gonadotropin secretion, which will be followed by cessation of pubertal changes and deceleration of skeletal maturity and growth rates. After appropriate therapy, reproductive function as evidenced by ovulation, spermatogenesis and pregnancy, BMD and adult height can be expected to be normal.

MANAGEMENT OF AND TREATMENT FOR PERIPHERAL PRECOCIOUS PUBERTY

If there is a specific treatable underlying cause, such as congenital adrenal hyperplasia, or an ovarian, testicular, or adrenal tumor, the therapy indicated for that condition also decreases sex steroids. If primary hypothyroidism is present, appropriate thyroid replacement therapy suppresses thyroid-releasing hormone and thyroid-stimulating hormone (TSH) hypersecretion; concomitantly the stimuli for pubertal development and pubertal characteristics regress.

The autonomous secretion of sex steroids caused by activating mutations in the McCune-Albright syndrome and in male-limited gonadotropin-independent precocious puberty is difficult to effectively treat. Treatment is aimed at diminishing the synthesis or metabolic effects of the sex steroid. Because the etiology is independent of pubertal gonadotropin secretion, treatment with GnRHa is inappropriate and ineffective, unless or until secondary CPP occurs. Aromatase inhibitors (including litrazole at 2.5 mg/kg/day) may be effective in suppressing estrogen synthesis. Medroxyprogesterone has been used to treat precocious puberty in the McCune-Albright syndrome with varying success. Caution should be used in treating patients with severe bony lesions because the lesions may be exacerbated by the hypocalcemic effect of the drug. Ovarian cysts usually spontaneously regress within a few months. After a cyst has been documented by ultrasonography, surgical resection should not be considered unless there is evidence of an impending surgical emergency. If all evidence indicates that the pubertal change is being stimulated by the autonomously functioning but self-limiting cyst, treatment is watchful waiting. A repeat pelvic sonogram within 2 to 3 months can be expected to verify regression of the cyst, usually making further treatment unnecessary.

MAJOR POINTS

Minimal breast maturation is a signal that careful observation is indicated, whereas early onset and rapid progression require prompt further assessment.

Children with premature thelarche or premature pubarche should be carefully followed to verify that they do have these diagnoses of variants of normal development. Girls with premature thelarche may subsequently manifest precocious puberty, whereas premature pubarche among children, which is usually a consequence of premature adrenarche, may actually be the first manifestation of ovarian or adrenal hyperandrogen states.

Early onset of physical changes of puberty that progresses slowly so that later milestones attained at expected ages and statural growth dynamics are not altered should be considered a variant of normal or nonprogressive precocious puberty and requires no treatment.

Central precocious puberty is defined as early onset of puberty involving early onset and progression of physical changes of puberty, verification of pubertal gonadotropin secretion, accelerated growth, and skeletal maturity rate.

Gonadotropin-releasing hormone analogue therapy should be considered for children with central precocious puberty who have progressive puberty and are developing in an untimely fashion with accelerated growth and skeletal age. The best height outcomes are found for those starting on therapy before age 6 years and, among girls, for those discontinuing therapy at a skeletal age of 12.0 to 12.5 years.

Children with progressive precocious puberty who do not have gonadotropin-stimulated development should be carefully assessed for etiologies of peripheral precocious puberty.

The size and symmetry of the testes among boys presenting with precocious puberty provide a diagnostic clue that guides the assessment.

SUGGESTED READINGS

Anasti JN, Flack MR, Froelich J, et al: A potential novel mechanism for precocious puberty in juvenile hypothyroidism, J Clin Endocrinol Metab 1995;80:276.

Arrigo T, Cisternino M, Galluzzi F, et al: Analysis of the factors affecting auxological response to GnRH agonist treatment and final height outcome in girls with idiopathic central precocious puberty, Eur J Endocrinol 1999;141:140.

Bertelloni S, Baroncelli GI, Ferdeghini M, et al: Final height. gonadal function and bone mineral density of adolescent males with central precocious puberty after therapy with gonadotropin-releasing hormone analogues, Eur J Pediatr 2000;159:369.

Boot AM, de Muinck Keizer-Schrama S, Pol HA, et al: Bone mineral density and body composition before and during treatment with gonadotropin-releasing hormone agonist in children with central precocious and early puberty, J Clin Endocrinol Metab 1998;83:370.

Chalumeau M, Chemaitilly W, Trivin C, et al: Central precocious puberty: an evidence-based diagnosis tree to predict central precocious nervous system abnormalities, Pediatrics 2002;109:61.

Galluzzi F, Salti R, Bindi G, et al: Adult height comparison between boys and girls with precocious puberty after long-term gonadotrophin-releasing hormone analogue therapy, Acta Paediatr 1998;87:521.

Heger S, Partsch CJ, Sippell WG: Long-term outcome after depot gonadotropin-releasing hormone agonist treatment of central precocious puberty: final height, body proportions, body composition, bone mineral density, and reproductive function, J Clin Endocrinol Metab 1999;84:4583.

Herman-Giddens ME, Slora EJ, Wasserman RC, et al: Secondary sexual characteristics and menses in young girls seen in office practice: a study from the Pediatric Research in Office Settings Network, Pediatrics 1997;99:505.

Jensen A-MB, Brocks V, Holm K, et al: Central precocious puberty in girls: internal genitalia before, during and after treatment with long-acting gonadotropin-releasing hormone analogues, J Pediatr 1998;132:105.

Kaplowitz PB, Oberfield SE: Reexamination of the age limit for defining when puberty is precocious in girls in the United States: implications for evaluation and treatment, Pediatrics 1999;104:936.

Klein KO, Baron J, Barnes KM, et al: Use of an ultrasensitive recombinant cell bioassay to determine estrogen levels in girls with precocious puberty treated with a luteinizing hormone-releasing hormone agonist, J Clin Endocrinol Metab 1998;83:2387.

Lazar L, Pertzelan A, Weintrob N, et al: Sexual precocity in boys: accelerated versus slowly progressive puberty gonadotropin-suppressive therapy and final height, J Clin Endocrinol Metab 2001;86:4127.

Leger JL, Reynaud R, Czernichow P: Do all girls with apparent idiopathic precocious puberty require gonadotropin-releasing hormone agonist treatment? J Pediatr 2000;137:819.

Lee PA: Central precocious puberty: an overview of diagnosis, treatment, and outcome, Endocrinol Metab Clin North Am 1999;28:901.

Marti-Henneberg C, Vizmonso B: The duration of puberty in girls is related to the timing of its onset, J Pediatr 1997;131:618.

Mul D, de Muinck Keizer-Schrama SM, Oostdijk W, et al: Auxological and biochemical evaluation of pubertal suppression with the GnRH agonist leuprolide acetate in early and precocious puberty, Horm Res 1999;51:270.

Palmert MR, Malin HV, Boepplle PA: Unsustained or slowly progressive puberty in young girls: initial presentation and long-term follow-up of 20 untreated patients, J Clin Endocrinol Metab 1999;84:415.

Palmert MR, Mansfield MJ, Crowley WF Jr, et al: Is obesity an outcome of gonadotropin-releasing hormone agonist administration? Analysis of growth and body composition in 110 patients with central precocious puberty, J Clin Endocrinol Metab 1999;84:4480.

Pasquino AM, Pucarelli I, Segni M, et al: Adult height in girls with central precocious puberty treated with gonadotropin-releasing hormone analogues and growth hormone, J Clin Endocrinol Metab 1999;84:449.

Virdis R, Street M, Zampoli M, et al: Precocious puberty in girls adopted from developing countries, Arch Dis Child 1998;78:152.

CHAPTER 6

Delayed Puberty

MADHUSMITA MISRA

MARY M. LEE

INTRODUCTION

The onset of puberty is marked by increasing secretion of sex steroids in response to central activation of the hypothalamic-pituitary-gonadal (HPG) axis. The timing of this process is variable but is strongly influenced by genetic factors. Puberty is considered delayed when the first manifestations of secondary sexual characteristics or the attainment of sexual maturity occur at an age that is 2.5 SDs later than the population mean. In girls, this is defined as lack of breast budding *(thelarche)* at 13 years of age or immature breast development and failure to start periods *(menarche)* at age 15. The absence of menarche at age 16 with normal breast and pubic hair development is more appropriately designated *primary amenorrhea*. In boys, puberty is delayed if testicular enlargement (>4 ml) or pubic hair is not present by 14 years of age. Puberty is also considered abnormal if it progresses at a slow pace after starting at an appropriate age. The mean duration from the onset of puberty to menarche is 2.4 ± 1.1 years, and from onset to achievement of adult testicular volume, 3.2 ± 1.8 years. An unusually slow progression or "stalled or arrested" pubertal maturation merits comprehensive assessment to exclude pathology. In girls, it is important to determine whether the signs of puberty are completely absent or incomplete with discordance in pubic hair and breast development. Individuals with androgen insensitivity syndrome, for example, may have well-developed breasts with absent or scant pubic and axillary hair.

DIFFERENTIAL DIAGNOSIS

Delayed puberty can be caused by deficient hypothalamic and/or pituitary function (low gonadotropins and low sex

---

Box 6-1   Causes of Pubertal Delay

HYPOGONADOTROPIC HYPOGONADISM

Constitutional delay in growth and development
Idiopathic hypogonadotropic hypogonadism
Kallmann syndrome (*KAL-1* gene mutations)
Adrenal hypoplasia congenita (*DAX-1* gene mutations)
Mutations in the genes for follicle-stimulating hormone
    (FSH), luteinizing hormone (LH), and the
        gonadotropin-releasing hormone (GnRH) receptor
Mutations in prohormone convertase, homeobox, and
    PROP-1 genes
Structural
    Septo-optic dysplasia
    Hypothalamic and pituitary tumors
    Head trauma, radiation, surgery
    Central nervous system infections, infiltrative diseases
Prader-Willi and Lawrence-Moon-Biedl syndromes
Lifestyle and body composition: undernutrition, anorexia
    nervosa, intense exercise
Chronic diseases: inflammatory bowel disease, hepatic and
    renal diseases, malignancies, iron overload

HYPERGONADOTROPIC HYPOGONADISM
Males

    Klinefelter syndrome
    Gonadal dysgenesis
    Testicular regression syndrome
    Bilateral orchitis, testicular surgery, radiation,
        chemotherapy
    Abnormalities in testosterone synthesis
    5α-Reductase deficiency
    Inactivating mutations of LH and FSH receptor genes
    Androgen-insensitivity syndromes
    Noonan syndrome

Females

    Turner syndrome, gonadal dysgenesis (complete or partial)
    Idiopathic primary or premature ovarian failure
    Surgical oophorectomy, radiation, or chemotherapy
    Inactivating mutations of LH and FSH receptor genes
    Androgen insensitivity

EUGONADAL CAUSES

Partial or complete noncanalization of the vagina,
    imperforate hymen

---

steroids) or primary gonadal failure (high gonadotropins and low sex steroids). Differential diagnosis of the former includes benign variants of normal and many secondary causes of hypogonadism, whereas the latter always indicates gonadal pathology (Box 6-1). Normal endocrine function in conjunction with anatomic anomalies that hinder menstrual flow comprise the third category.

1. Hypogonadotropic hypogonadism (low luteinizing hormone [LH] and follicle-stimulating hormone [FSH]): hypothalamic-pituitary dysfunction or immature gonadal axis
2. Hypergonadotropic hypogonadism (high FSH and LH values): primary gonadal failure
3. Eugonadism (normal FSH and LH values): primary amenorrhea secondary to uterine, cervical, or vaginal structural defects

---

Hypogonadotropic Hypogonadism

Hypogonadotropic hypogonadism encompasses miscellaneous conditions ranging from a familial pattern of constitutional delay to central nervous system lesions impairing hypothalamic or pituitary function. This category includes genetic defects in gonadotroph differentiation or pituitary development and all secondary causes of central hypogonadism such as systemic illness, undernutrition, psychosocial stress, trauma, or infiltrative diseases. By far the most common diagnosis in this category is constitutional delay in growth and development.

Constitutional Delay in Growth and Development

An exaggerated delay of pubertal onset in an otherwise healthy child is a common variant of normal in which the physical and biochemical markers of puberty resemble those of a younger child. Puberty occurs spontaneously but at a later age with a concomitant delay in the pubertal growth spurt. A family history of delayed puberty is usually elicited. Many more males than females seek medical attention with this diagnosis in comparison with other causes of hypogonadism. Children with constitutional delay exhibit a decline in growth velocity at ages 2 to 3 years with crossing of height percentiles and delay in skeletal maturation. Growth subsequently proceeds at a low normal rate and bone age remains delayed for age until the pubertal growth spurt. Pubertal staging and stature are commensurate with bone age rather than chronological age. At the usual age of puberty, the short stature (often 2-3 SDs below the mean for age) of these children becomes more noticeable as they maintain a prepubertal growth rate while their peers enter puberty and have accelerated growth. Final height is achieved late and is often in the low-normal range but consistent with genetic potential. Although constitutional delay is considered a benign condition, decreased bone mineral density in young adult men with a history of constitutional delay has been reported.

Before making a diagnosis of constitutional delay, systemic illnesses and other causes of hypogonadism should be excluded with a comprehensive history and review of systems and a thorough physical examination. Constitutional delay in puberty can be difficult to distinguish from isolated hypogonadotropic hypogonadism, often requiring long-term monitoring to determine if puberty occurs spontaneously. Although not definitive, assessment of adrenarche can be helpful because children with constitutional delay generally have a later adrenarche and lower values of dehydroepiandrosterone sulfate (DHEAS) than do those with hypogonadotropic hypogonadism. Early morning testosterone values are an early marker of impending pubertal changes; 100% of boys with a value greater than 0.7 nmol/L (20 ng/dL) manifest signs of puberty within 15 months. Gonadotropin determination has been less useful. Neither basal nor gonadotropin-releasing hormone (GnRH)-stimulated FSH and LH values discriminate between these two conditions. Reports of differential responses to potent GnRH agonists or to successive doses of GnRH offer promise for development as diagnostic tests.

Idiopathic Hypogonadotropic Hypogonadism

Idiopathic hypogonadotropic hypogonadism (IHH) and Kallmann syndrome are isolated defects in GnRH secretion with no other hormonal deficits and no structural lesions of the hypothalamus or pituitary. Individuals with either of these conditions have complete or partial absence of LH pulses that can be restored with pulsatile administration of GnRH, indicating that the defect is at the hypothalamic level. Children with IHH have sexual infantilism and delayed skeletal maturation. Males have eunuchoid body proportions (upper-to-lower segment ratio of <1 and a >6-cm difference between arm span and standing height), a high pitched voice, and prepubertal testes. Females have no breast development and primary amenorrhea. Gonadotropin deficiency is occasionally diagnosed in newborn infants with cryptorchidism and microphallus because LH-stimulated testosterone secretion during late gestation is required for complete testicular descent and phallic growth. Hypogonadotropic hypogonadism can also present as slowly progressive or arrested puberty, decreased libido, impotence and oligospermia or azoospermia in men, and secondary amenorrhea and infertility in women.

The majority of patients with isolated gonadotropin deficiency and complete sexual infantilism lack LH pulses, a surrogate marker for GnRH pulse generator activity. A milder phenotype is observed with the *developmental arrest pattern* of gonadotropin secretion. These individuals have the sleep entrained pattern of early puberty, with predominantly nighttime pulses. Puberty can be stalled after onset or progress to spermatogenesis without full virilization, as seen with the *fertile eunuch syndrome.*

IHH can be sporadic (66%) or familial (34%), and several gene mutations have been identified in both forms (Table 6-1). Among a series of 106 patients seen at Massachusetts General Hospital, inheritance was X-linked in 11%, autosomal dominant in 64%, and autosomal recessive in 25%. The degree of hypogonadism and the LH pulse

profile can both vary within the same pedigree. GnRH receptor mutations can cause disordered LH pulse frequency or amplitude, or the LH can be bioinactive.

Kallmann Syndrome

Kallmann syndrome, IHH and anosmia or hyposmia, is the most common form of isolated gonadotropin deficiency (1 in 10,000 males and 1 in 50,000 females). Most cases are sporadic, and of these, less than 5% have mutations in the *KAL* gene (Xp22.3) encoding anosmin-1. Of the familial forms, X-linked recessive *(KAL-1)* is the most common, followed by autosomal dominant *(KAL-2)* and then autosomal recessive *(KAL-3).* Half of families with X-linked inheritance have deletions or point mutations of the *KAL* gene. Anosmin-1 is a neural cell adhesion protein that provides a scaffold for GnRH neurons and olfactory nerves during their embryonic migration from the olfactory placode to the medial basal hypothalamus and olfactory bulb, respectively. Consequently, olfactory bulbs are absent or structurally abnormal on magnetic resonance imaging in the majority of patients with Kallmann syndrome.

The embryonic expression of the *KAL* gene explains other associated clinical findings such as synkinesia (i.e., mirror movements of the hands; corticospinal tract involvement), abnormal eye movements (oculomotor nucleus), visual defects (retina), nystagmus and ataxia (cerebellum), midfacial clefts (midfacial mesenchyme), and renal agenesis (mesonephros and metanephros) (Figure 6-1). Unilateral renal agenesis has been described in 50% of boys with *KAL* gene mutations. Other manifestations include gynecomastia, short metacarpals, pes cavus, sensorineural defects, and epilepsy. As with other forms of hypogonadotropic hypogonadism, Kallmann syndrome can also present at birth with microphallus and cryptorchidism. Members of a family with the same *KAL* mutation have phenotypic variability suggesting some compensation by redundant proteins. Carrier females may have hyposmia, delayed menarche, or irregular menses but are usually fertile.

DAX-1 Gene Mutations

Mutations of the *DAX-1* gene located in the *DSS* (dosage-sensitive sex reversal) region at Xp21 cause hypogonadotropic hypogonadism at puberty in conjunction with early-onset adrenal insufficiency (X-linked adrenal hypoplasia congenita). *DAX-1* is an orphan nuclear receptor that is essential for development of the adrenal cortex and regulation of gonadotropin secretion at both the hypothalamic and pituitary levels. In most cases, the hypothalamic-pituitary dysfunction is not evident until puberty. Similar gonadotropin deficiencies have been described in a woman with homozygous *DAX-1* mutations, whereas female carriers are reported to have delayed puberty. A contiguous gene

Table 6-1   Gene Mutations Causing Hypogonadotropic Hypogonadism (HH)*

Gene	Gene Locus	Phenotype	Location of Central Nervous System Defect	LH	FSH	Inheritance
KAL	Xp22.3	HH, anosmia	Hypothalamus	↓	↓	X-linked recessive
DAX-1	Xp21	Congenital adrenal hypoplasia, HH	Hypothalamus, pituitary	N/↓	N/↓	X-linked recessive
SF1	9q33	XY sex reversal with müllerian structures, adrenal failure	Hypothalamus, pituitary	N/↓	N/↓	Autosomal recessive?
Leptin	7q31.3	Obesity, HH	Hypothalamus	N/↓	N/↓	Autosomal recessive
Leptin receptor	1p31	Obesity, HH	Hypothalamus	N/↓	N/↓	Autosomal recessive
HESX1	3p21.1-21.2	Septo-optic dysplasia, panhypopituitarism	Pituitary	→	→	Autosomal recessive
LHX3	9q34	Short stature, hypothyroidism, HH, hypoprolactinemia, cervical spine rigidity	Pituitary	↓	↓	Autosomal recessive
PROP1	5q	Short stature, hypothyroidism, HH, hypoprolactinemia	Pituitary	N/↓	N/↓	Autosomal recessive
GnRHR	4q21.2	HH	Pituitary	N/↓	N/↓	Autosomal recessive
LHβ	19q13.3	Isolated LH deficiency	Pituitary	→↑	N/↑	Autosomal recessive
FSHβ	11p13	Isolated FSH deficiency	Pituitary	↑	→	Autosomal recessive

CNS, central nervous system; GnRHR, gonadotropin-releasing hormone receptor; LH, luteinizing hormone; FSH, follicle-stimulating hormone.

*Adapted from Layman LC: Genetics of human hypogonadotropic hypogonadism, Am J Med Genet 1999;89:242; and Ackermann JC, Weiss J, Lee EJ, et al: Inherited disorders of the gonadotropin hormones, Mol Cell Endocrinol 2001;179:89, with permission.

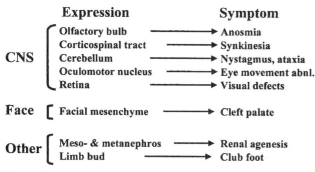

Figure 6-1   Correlation between the sites of *KAL* gene expression in human and chick with the observed clinical phenotype of Kallmann syndrome. (Reprinted from Layman LC. Genetics of human hypogonadotropic hypogonadism, Am J Med Genet 1999;89:242, with permission.)

deletion on Xp21 can lead to an association of this disorder with Duchenne muscular dystrophy and glycerol kinase deficiency. As with *KAL-1*, genotype-phenotype correlations have been poor even within families, suggesting compensation by modifier genes. *DAX-1* also plays a role in ovarian formation; thus, duplication of this gene causes sex reversal in genetic males.

Gonadotropin-Releasing Hormone Receptor Mutations

GnRH binds to a G protein–coupled receptor (4q13.1) that signals through the phosphoinositol pathway to increase intracellular calcium and stimulate gonadotropin synthesis and secretion. Mutations in the GnRH receptor gene have been identified in one third of familial cases of hypogonadotropic hypogonadism without anosmia and in 2% to 7% of patients with IHH (Figure 6-2). These mutations compromise GnRH action to varying extents by interfering with ligand binding or decreasing phospholipase C activation and phosphoinositol

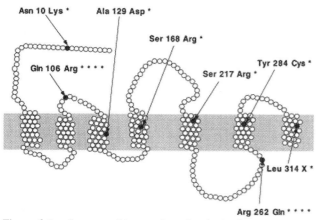

Figure 6-2   Structure of the gonadotropin-releasing receptor and location of inactivating mutations. Each star represents a mutation identified in an independent family (with one or more affected patients). (Reprinted from de Roux N, Milgrom E: Inherited disorders of GnRH and gonadotropin receptors, Mol Cell Endocrinol 2001;179:84, with permission.)

production. For example, Tyr284Cys and Ala129Asp cause complete hypogonadotropic hypogonadism, whereas Gln106Arg, Ser217Arg, and Arg262Gln are partial defects. Thus far, no mutations of the GnRH gene have been found in patients with hypogonadotropic hypogonadism.

Males with mutations of the GnRH receptor are hypogonadal with small, sometimes undescended testes. Females have poor breast development and amenorrhea. Gonadotropins and sex steroid levels are low. Despite the receptor defect, 75% exhibit a rise in LH and FSH with a single intravenous dose of GnRH (100 µg), whereas 50% require pulsatile administration of GnRH. Thus, a mutation in the GnRH receptor does not necessarily preclude therapy with pulsatile GnRH.

Miscellaneous Single-Gene Defects

Prohormone convertase (5q15-q21) mutations disrupt GnRH processing to cause hypogonadotropic hypogonadism and impair processing of insulin and pro-opiomelanocortin to cause obesity. Inheritance is autosomal recessive, and only a single case has been reported so far.

A defect in the *leptin* gene (Arg105Trp; 7q31.3) causes extreme obesity, hyperinsulinemia, and hypogonadotropic hypogonadism. The pubertal delay can be treated with exogenous GnRH, gonadotropins, or sex steroids. Unlike the leptin-deficient *ob/ob* mice, human leptin deficiency does not cause stunted growth, hyperglycemia, or hypercortisolemia. Defects in the *leptin receptor gene* (1p31) manifest a similar phenotype, but leptin is elevated.

Mutations in *PROP-1* (5q), a pituitary transcription factor, cause autosomal recessive deficiency of growth hormone, thyrotropin, prolactin, FSH, and LH. The pituitary fails to respond to growth hormone releasing hormone (GHRH), thyrotropin releasing hormone (TRH), or GnRH. Males have small genitalia, delayed or incomplete secondary sexual maturation with infertility, and growth failure. A 2-bp deletion (301-302delAG) accounts for 55% of familial and 12% of sporadic cases of combined pituitary hormone deficiency, but many other missense mutations and deletions have been identified. The onset and severity of pituitary dysfunction vary widely within the same genotype.

Midline defects such as septo-optic dysplasia or absence of the corpus callosum may be associated with pituitary gland hypoplasia. In septo-optic dysplasia, abnormal development of the prosencephalon leads to optic nerve involvement (pale optic discs with pendular nystagmus and even blindness) and hypothalamic defects, including growth hormone deficiency, diabetes insipidus, hypocortisolism, hypothyroidism, and hypogonadotropic hypogonadism. An Arg53Cys missense mutation in *HESX*, a homeobox gene that affects DNA binding, has been identified in a family of affected individuals with septo-optic dysplasia.

Hypothalamic and Pituitary Tumors

Craniopharyngiomas, the most common tumor causing hypopituitarism in childhood, account for 6% of all brain tumors in children and for 80% to 90% of tumors arising in the pituitary region. The peak incidence is between 5 and 14 years of age. Although the initial symptoms are usually neurological, namely headaches (13%) and visual disturbances (35%), endocrine dysfunction is already present in 70% to 80% of all patients at diagnosis. Up to 75% of patients have growth failure and growth hormone deficiency, 40% have gonadotropin deficiency, and 25% have ACTH and TSH deficiency. Postoperatively, panhypopituitarism, including diabetes insipidus, is common. Cushing disease and pituitary adenomas are rare causes of hypogonadism in children. Head trauma, central nervous system radiation, surgery, infections, and infiltrative disorders can disrupt hypothalamic or pituitary function and cause hypogonadotropic hypogonadism.

Genetic Syndromes

Hypogonadotropic hypogonadism is common in *Prader-Willi syndrome*. Other features include muscular hypotonia, mental retardation, short stature, obesity, and small hands and feet. Prader-Willi syndrome is caused by loss of function of the paternal allele for imprinted genes such as *SNRPN,* a spliceosomal protein, and *SNURF,* a gene that regulates imprinting because of deletions or maternal uniparental disomy of chromosome 15q11-q13.

Noonan syndrome is a relatively common disorder (1:1000-2500) characterized by delayed puberty, proportionate short stature, valvular pulmonic stenosis and/or hypertrophic cardiomyopathy (68%), cryptorchidism (60%), nuchal webbing with a low hairline, and chest deformities. The characteristic facial features include hypertelorism, down-slanting palpebral fissures, malrotated low-set ears, high arched palate, and micrognathia. The phenotype can include mild developmental delay and mental retardation, learning disabilities, language delay, and hearing loss. Puberty generally occurs spontaneously, although primary gonadal failure may also occur secondary to bilateral cryptorchidism. Noonan syndrome can be autosomal dominant or recessive in inheritance, or sporadic. Miscellaneous mutations in protein tyrosine phosphatase, nonreceptor type II, *PTPN11* (chromosome 12q24.1), have been identified in one third to one half of patients who have undergone molecular analysis.

Bardet-Biedl syndrome is characterized by mental retardation, pigmentary retinopathy, polydactyly, obesity, and hypogonadism. Females with this syndrome have both hypogonadotropic hypogonadism and primary gonadal failure. The genetic basis is unknown.

Autosomal recessive syndromes such as *multiple lentigines* and *Carpenter syndrome* are also associated with hypogonadotropic hypogonadism.

Lifestyle and Body Composition Changes

Intense Exercise (Female Athletic Triad)

The female athletic triad of primary or secondary amenorrhea, disordered eating, and osteoporosis illustrates the potential deleterious effects of intensive exercise training on the HPG axis. A progressive increase in the intensity of exercise leads to menstrual irregularity due to luteal-phase defects, then oligomenorrhea and anovulation, and finally amenorrhea. The hormonal correlates of this are an initial decrease in frequency of LH pulses followed by more severe disorders of pulsatility, and then complete functional arrest of the HPG axis. The incidence of hypogonadism and menstrual dysfunction depends on nutritional status and the type, intensity, and duration of exercise. Up to 50% of ballet dancers and high-intensity runners, as opposed to 12% of swimmers, become amenorrheic. The body fat hypothesis of Frisch and McArthur attributes this difference to the lower percentage of body fat in runners and ballet dancers ($\cong15\%$) compared with that in swimmers ($\cong15\%$). On the other hand, when ballet dancers interrupt their training, menses often return without altering the lean body–to–fat mass ratio, suggesting that exercise may have an independent role. Currently, low energy availability rather than change in body fat composition or the stress of exercise is believed to be the critical factor. When the availability of metabolic fuel falls below a critical level due to decreased intake and/or increased energy expenditure, the HPG axis is downregulated, a mechanism similar to that caused by eating disorders. This can be avoided by increasing intake to compensate for the increased energy expenditure.

The second component of the female athletic triad, disordered eating, has been reported in up to 32% of college age athletes and begins at an average age of 14 years. Disordered eating habits, such as binging, self-induced vomiting, and laxative and diuretic abuse, are regarded by many athletes as harmless. The prevalence is highest among gymnasts ($\cong15\%$) and long distance runners and field hockey players ($\cong15\%$). Despite comparable total caloric intake, athletes with this syndrome consume 50% less fat and more carbohydrate and fiber than their menstruating counterparts.

Osteoporosis, the third component of the triad, is a serious complication of exercise-induced hypogonadism and amenorrhea. Although weight-bearing exercise can improve bone mineral density, exercise that is intense enough to cause amenorrhea leads to bone loss, even at weight-bearing sites, and increased risk of stress- and running-related fractures. Consequently, amenorrheic athletes have a lower lumbar bone mineral density than do eumenorrheic athletes matched for sport, age, weight, height, and training schedule.

In boys and men undergoing endurance exercise training, the hypothalamic-pituitary-testicular axis is perturbed to the extent of reducing testosterone concentrations, but puberty is rarely delayed or arrested. Although the long-term consequences of reduced testosterone concentrations in athletes are unknown, its effects in other androgen-deficient states indicate that spermatogenesis and bone mineralization may be compromised.

Undernutrition and Anorexia Nervosa

Food restriction and weight loss are well-known causes of menstrual disorders. Reduced energy availability from caloric restriction alters LH pulsatility to a greater extent than that seen with the female athletic triad. In healthy cycling women, moderate degrees of food restriction lead to low estradiol levels and anovulation despite normal LH levels. After 2.5 weeks of severe starvation, LH pulsations revert to a prepubertal pattern. A 10% to 15% loss of body weight (corresponding to a 30% loss in body fat) can delay puberty or cause menstrual irregularities and amenorrhea. The hypogonadism leads to a 20% to 68% prevalence of osteoporosis in different studies. Decreased insulin-like growth factor-I levels, GH resistance, and hypercortisolism potentiate the effect of hypogonadism and nutritional deficiencies on bone loss. Moreover, osteopenia due to anorexia nervosa is more severe in adolescents than in adults, even when the duration of amenorrhea is comparable. Adolescence is a period of rapid bone mass accumulation, with 90% of peak bone mass achieved by the age of 18 years. This active bone mass accrual is significantly reduced with adolescent anorexia nervosa and cannot fully "catch up" with weight recovery.

Systemic Illnesses

Any major systemic illness, particularly inflammatory bowel disease, malignancies, and chronic infections, can cause pubertal delay and poor growth. Poor nutrition, chronic illness, pain, and psychosocial factors can all disrupt the HPG axis.

Chronic iron overload secondary to multiple transfusions in children with severe thalassemia or hemochromatosis causes pituitary damage and hypogonadotropic hypogonadism. Anterior pituitary involvement is selective, with gonadotropes and lactotropes being affected earlier than other pituitary cells. Boys with thalassemia have low nocturnal gonadotropins and a poor LH response to GnRH. Their testosterone response to human chorionic gonadotropin (hCG) is lower than that of boys with constitutional delay, implying that there is also damage to the testes.

Hypogonadism associated with human immunodeficiency virus infections can cause both primary and secondary hypogonadism. Weight loss and severe illness lead to hypogonadotropic hypogonadism, whereas direct involvement of the gonads by the virus, opportunistic infections, or associated malignancy causes primary gonadal failure. Severe immune dysfunction is also associated with significant delays in pubertal development.

Hypergonadotropic Hypogonadism

Males

Klinefelter Syndrome

Klinefelter syndrome, a common cause of primary hypogonadism (1 in 600 males), is characterized by testicular failure, androgen deficiency, and impaired spermatogenesis. The karyotype is 47,XXY in two thirds of patients and mosaic (46,XY/47,XXY) or a variant (48,XXXY, 49,XXXXY) in the remaining third. The extra X chromosome is acquired through nondysjunction during parental gametogenesis or a mitotic error in the zygote. Paternal nondysjunction accounts for 53% cases of Klinefelter syndrome, maternal meiotic errors for 43%, and postzygotic errors for 3%. The incidence of maternal meiotic I errors increases with increasing maternal age.

Pathogenesis

Testosterone values in cord blood of neonates with Klinefelter syndrome are usually lower than those of non-affected infants, and germ cells are already reduced in number during infancy. During childhood, LH, FSH, testosterone, and the testosterone response to GnRH are all in the normal prepubertal range. At puberty, however, LH, FSH, and sex hormone–binding globulin (SHBG) become elevated, whereas testosterone is low or low-normal and free testosterone and inhibin are low. The testes become small and firm and develop the classic features of hyalinization and fibrosis of the seminiferous tubules and oligospermia with eventual azoospermia. Spontaneous fertility, however, has been reported in men with 46,XY/47,XXY mosaicism.

Clinical Features

Although testicular atrophy and hyalinization of the seminiferous tubules appear to be invariant features of Klinefelter syndrome in adults, the timing of testicular failure and the variability of associated features are related to the degree of mosaicism. Prepubertal testicular failure is rare but causes pubertal delay and results in eunuchoid body proportions, with arm span greater than height by 2 cm or more, long legs, and tall stature. The genitalia are usually normally formed, but the phallus may be small in size. Facial, axillary, and pubic hair are sparse and body habitus is more feminine with decreased muscle mass and a feminine fat distribution. Gynecomastia is common and differs from that of most high-estrogen states in having interductal rather than ductal hyperplasia.

Leydig cell failure after the onset of puberty has milder manifestations, with more extensive pubic and facial hair and varying degrees of gynecomastia. Despite a normal onset of puberty, an eunuchoid habitus with long lower extremities causing disproportionate tall stature is common and postulated to be caused by duplication of genes modulating growth on the extra X chromosome. The phallus is normally virilized, although the testes are small, often less than 4 mL in volume. Infertility, small testes, and elevated gonadotropin levels are common (90-100% of patients). Other findings include low testosterone values (65-85% of patients), decreased facial and pubic hair (30-80%), gynecomastia (50-75%), and a small phallus (10-25%). The hypogonadism can lead to significant osteopenia and osteoporosis, which are alleviated by timely implementation of testosterone replacement.

Delayed puberty is the more common manifestation of Klinefelter syndrome, but precocious puberty has been reported and occurs 5.5 times more frequently than expected. Precocious puberty may be idiopathic or secondary to hypothalamic hamartomas and gonadal or extragonadal germ cell tumors.

Associated Disorders

Men with Klinefelter syndrome have an increased incidence of mild adult-onset diabetes mellitus, autoimmune disorders such as Hashimoto thyroiditis, systemic lupus erythematosus, rheumatoid arthritis, Sjögren syndrome, deep venous thrombosis, pulmonary embolism, and venous ulcers. Thinning of the dental enamel from enlargement of the pulp cavity causes problems with dental decay. The low testosterone levels and reduced numbers of lymphocytes and suppressor T cells may contribute to the propensity for autoimmune disease. Testosterone replacement has been reported to ameliorate clinical symptoms and improve immune function.

Breast cancer is increased by 20-fold in men with Klinefelter syndrome with estimated incidences of 0.9% to 3%. Gynecomastia is a predisposing factor, although the increased risk is not considered high enough to support prophylactic mastectomy. Extragonadal germ cell tumors are also more common in Klinefelter syndrome, possibly due to persistently elevated gonadotropin levels. The possibility of an underlying increased risk for malignancy is supported by the report of an abnormally high transformation frequency by simian virus 40 (SV40) of fibroblasts from 47,XXY patients.

Individuals with Klinefelter syndrome may have neuropsychological impairment and behavioral problems. During childhood, speech and language development and the acquisition of motor milestones, strength, and coordination can be delayed. Although full-scale IQs are similar to controls and siblings, academic difficulties are common due to verbal processing deficits, diminished short-term memory, poor data retrieval skills, and an increased incidence of attention deficit disorder. Emotional immaturity, poor self-esteem, social stress and anxiety, apathy, and poor impulse control lead to underachievement at school. Individuals with more than one extra X chromosome have greater intellectual impairment. Anxiety, neuroses, psychoses, and depression are not unusual in such adults. Testosterone replacement is reported to improve psychological well-being and social functioning.

Management

Klinefelter syndrome is usually diagnosed at puberty when pubertal delay, eunuchoid proportions, and small testes lead to evaluation and subsequent diagnosis. Occasionally, the diagnosis is made by prenatal amniocentesis or because of behavioral or school performance problems. Testosterone treatment is started at the time of diagnosis or at puberty if the diagnosis is recognized early, and treatment should be continued throughout life. Replacement of testosterone allows normal development of pubertal characteristics and a masculine body habitus, prevents osteopenia and osteoporosis, increases the numbers of lymphocytes (specifically suppressor T cells), and improves self-esteem and behavior.

Individuals with Klinefelter syndrome can produce sperm with no cytogenetic abnormalities and have fathered children with normal sex chromosomes. In 20% of men with Klinefelter syndrome, primarily those with a mosaic karyotype, germ cells can be recovered from testicular biopsy samples for selection of viable spermatogonia and cryopreservation. Some spermatozoa carry an extra X chromosome, suggesting the need for further selection of sperm from biopsy specimens to avoid transmission of this syndrome by assisted reproduction techniques. In vitro fertilization by intracytoplasmic injection of sperm has successfully produced nonaffected infants.

Mutations in Gonadotropin Genes and Receptors

An *LHβ* gene mutation has been identified in a 17-year-old boy with pubertal delay, small testes, and normal male genitalia. LH was elevated, whereas FSH and testosterone were low and testicular biopsy revealed spermatogenic arrest with complete absence of Leydig cells. Molecular analysis identified a homozygous Gln54Arg point mutation in exon 3 that impaired binding to the LH receptor, making the LH biologically inactive. Although postnatal Leydig cells were absent, the external genitalia were virilized, confirming that *fetal* Leydig cell development and testosterone synthesis are not dependent on fetal LH secretion.

The LH receptor (chromosome 2p21) is a G protein–coupled receptor with seven transmembrane domains. LH binding activates adenylate cyclase and, at high concentrations, phospholipase C to stimulate Leydig cell development and regulate testosterone synthesis. The phenotype of 46,XY individuals with LH receptor mutations varies according to the severity of the mutation. Milder defects cause a reduction in Leydig cell number and present as delayed puberty with normal or undervirilized genitalia. The wölffian ducts may be incompletely developed and testes may or may not be descended. Absence of the receptor with complete unresponsiveness to either LH or hCG causes XY sex reversal. The external genitalia are female, both müllerian and wölffian structures are absent, and intra-abdominal testes are present but lack Leydig cells.

Males with mutations of the genes for *FSHβ* or its receptor do not have delayed puberty. Spermatogenesis may be impaired, but the development of secondary sexual characteristics proceeds normally because LH signaling is unaffected.

Miscellaneous Causes of Testicular Dysfunction

Testicular injury from *irradiation* or *gonadotoxic chemotherapy* causes gonadal dysfunction in cancer patients and those undergoing radiation for bone marrow transplantation. Radiotherapy-induced testicular damage from direct or scatter irradiation is dose dependent. Germinal epithelium is more susceptible in the sexually mature testes, whereas Leydig cells are more radiosensitive in the prepubertal testes. The stage of germ cell differentiation also affects radiosensitivity; hence, spermatogonia are damaged by doses as low as 0.1 Gy, whereas spermatids are affected at doses of 4 to 6 Gy. The recovery of spermatogenesis occurs as early as 9 to 18 months after irradiation when the dose is less than 1 Gy but can take more than 5 years with doses above 4 Gy. Chemotherapy-induced testicular damage and recovery are likewise dependent on the specific cytotoxic drug and the dose administered. Alkylating agents such as melphalan, cyclophosphamide, chlorambucil, and busulfan; antimetabolites such as cytarabine and vinca alkaloids; and other cytotoxic agents such as cisplatin and procarbazine are all gonadotoxic. The germinal epithelium is more sensitive than Leydig cells; thus, azoospermia or oligospermia may be present despite normal or low-normal testosterone secretion.

In animals, suppression of testicular function with GnRH analogues alone or with testosterone or flutamide, and with testosterone alone or with estradiol reduces the extent of testicular damage from chemotherapy or radiation. Similar clinical trials in humans have been less efficacious. Other experimental techniques in animals include testicular biopsy to collect and cryopreserve stem cells before starting therapy for later implantation. In humans, semen collection and cryopreservation is possible in older adolescents and adults but not feasible in prepubertal boys.

Mumps orchitis is rare since the institution of routine measles, mumps, and rubella (MMR) vaccination. Moreover, prepubertal children with mumps are rarely affected and, if so, usually have unilateral involvement (80%) rather than the bilateral orchitis that occurs in adults. Treatment with interferon-α2B can prevent the testicular atrophy and fibrosis that occurs in 30% to 50% of affected individuals. Other viral infections, such as coxsackievirus infection and dengue, also cause orchitis with residual testicular damage, whereas the orchitis caused by Epstein-Barr virus, adenovirus, echovirus, varicella, and influenza usually resolve without significant sequelae.

Prenatal testicular torsion causes irreversible testicular injury, often resulting in complete testicular loss with only fibrotic tissue remaining. Testicular torsion after birth is an emergency mandating immediate surgical intervention to preserve testicular blood flow and function. Occasionally testes are damaged during surgical repair of cryptorchid testes, particularly high positioned abdominal testes. Some cryptorchid testes, however, are intrinsically malformed with impaired androgen secretion and spermatogenesis. Traumatic insults to the testes may also damage the testes and cause testicular failure.

Liver cirrhosis is an uncommon etiology of hypogonadism in prepubertal boys. Chronic liver disease inhibits testosterone synthesis and increases SHBG levels, resulting in reduced free testosterone levels. Gonadotropins are initially high but become suppressed with liver failure. *Chronic renal failure* is also associated with primary testicular failure and elevated gonadotropins. Sickling of red cells within the testicular blood vessels damages the testes in patients with *sickle cell anemia*.

Many intersex disorders are associated with primary gonadal failure due to defective testis formation, the inability to synthesize or respond to androgens, or prophylactic gonadectomy because of increased risk for malignancy (discussed in Intersex Disorders).

Females (Primary Ovarian Failure)

Turner Syndrome

Turner syndrome due to haploinsufficiency of X chromosome genes is the most common sex chromosome anomaly and the major cause of primary hypogonadism in females. The presence of normal cell lines in fetal membranes is believed to be essential for placental function and fetal survival; thus, up to 15% of 45,X conceptuses are spontaneously aborted. Consequently, although 3 of 100 female conceptuses have a 45,X karyotype, only 1 in 2000 to 5000 liveborn females have this karyotype. If Turner syndrome is diagnosed prenatally, fetal echocardiography and ultrasonography are recommended to identify cardiac and renal structural anomalies and cystic hygromas, which increase the risk for fetal demise. In the absence of nuchal lymphedema, physical signs of Turner syndrome are usually minimal. During counseling, the wide variability in presentation of somatic features and the high probability of short stature and ovarian failure should be discussed.

Clinical Features

At birth, the diagnosis of Turner syndrome is suggested by swelling of the hands or feet from congenital lymphedema, a low hairline with excess nuchal skin and webbing (pterygium coli), ear deformities, dysplastic nails, a broad chest with hypoplastic nipples, and cardiac or renal malformations. Bicuspid aortic valves and aortic coarctation are the most common cardiac anomalies. After the newborn period, growth failure and lack of pubertal development or amenorrhea are the most common symptoms bringing this disorder to medical attention. Other associated features include cubitus valgus, multiple pigmented nevi, a high arched palate, short fourth metacarpals, defective dentition, scoliosis, idiopathic hypertension, and recurrent otitis media. Cognitive function is usually normal, although visuospatial organization may be affected and attention deficit is not uncommon. In addition to short stature and gonadal failure, endocrine manifestations include autoimmune thyroiditis, glucose intolerance, insulin resistance, and osteoporosis.

Short stature and gonadal dysgenesis are the most consistent findings in Turner syndrome; associated somatic features may be minimal. Even when other features are absent, unexplained growth failure in girls should prompt cytogenetic studies to rule out this disorder. The short stature has been linked to haploinsufficiency of the *SHOX* (short stature homeobox–containing gene on the X chromosome) gene in the pseudoautosomal region at distal Xp. Growth velocity decelerates to subnormal rates by 2 to 4 years of age, although growth failure may first manifest during infancy. A pubertal growth spurt is absent. Ten percent of girls with Turner syndrome have scoliosis, which contributes to the short stature. Mean adult height of women with Turner syndrome is almost 20 cm below the population mean but correlates strongly with mid-parental height.

Management

At diagnosis, echocardiography or magnetic resonance imaging is recommended to assess cardiac status. Fifty percent of affected children have bicuspid aortic valves, and up to 20% have coarctation of the aorta. Echocardiograms should be repeated every 5 years to monitor the diameter of the aortic root, as dilatation can occur even without structural abnormalities. Renal ultrasonography is recommended to identify aberrant vasculature and abnormalities in the collecting system or in the structure and position of the kidneys (e.g., horseshoe kidney).

Despite normal growth hormone responses to provocative testing, growth hormone therapy has improved growth rates and adult height in girls with Turner syndrome and is the standard of care in the United States. Provocative growth hormone testing is not indicated before starting therapy. The suggested dose of recombinant human growth hormone is 0.35 to 0.375 mg/kg/week given as daily subcutaneous injections, but lower doses also substantially improve growth velocity. Prompt initiation of growth hormone therapy at the onset of growth failure is likely to offer the best outcome for improving final height. The use of growth hormone in girls with Turner syndrome has been associated with disproportionate growth of the hands and feet, more episodes of otitis media, and an increase in size and number of pigmented nevi.

Most girls with Turner syndrome have primary gonadal failure and require exogenous estrogen for sexual maturation. The duration of growth hormone therapy before initiating estrogen replacement is a positive predictor of final adult height. This beneficial aspect of postponing estrogen therapy must be weighed against its deleterious effects on bone mineralization and the psychosocial stress of delayed sexual maturation. We advocate starting low-dose estrogen at 12 to 14 years of age and slowly increasing the dose over 2 to 3 years to achieve pubertal maturation at a normal pace. Conjugated estrogens (Premarin) 0.3 mg every other day or 5 μg ethinyl estradiol daily for 12 months is followed by 0.3 mg of Premarin or 10 μg ethinyl estradiol daily for the next 12 months. The estrogen dose is increased to Premarin 0.625 mg or 20 μg ethinyl estradiol before adding 5 mg medroxyprogesterone acetate (Provera) for 12 days each month to initiate cyclical uterine bleeding. Transdermal estrogen patches are now available in sufficiently low doses to allow gradual induction of puberty. One study has shown improved uterine development with transdermal estrogen therapy compared with oral estrogen. With timely initiation of GH and estrogen therapy, an adult height of 150 cm is a reasonable goal in most girls with Turner syndrome.

Approximately 5% of girls with Turner syndrome have Y chromosomal material; this possibility needs to be considered in all virilized girls. The risk of gonadoblastoma is increased in patients with an intact Y chromosome or with pericentromeric fragments or markers for the Y chromosome; these patients should have prophylactic removal of the gonads.

Girls with Turner syndrome have viable oocytes in fetal life and infancy but undergo accelerated oocyte loss. Residual ovarian function is sufficient in 15% to 25% of girls to initiate breast development, but only 5% to 10% progress to spontaneous menarche, and pregnancies are reported in only 1% to 3%. Elevated and/or rising gonadotropin levels are associated with progressive ovarian failure. Contraceptive and genetic counseling should be offered to individuals with residual ovarian function. Pregnancies are associated with a high risk of spontaneous miscarriages (26%) and stillbirths (6%). Thirty percent of live-born infants have various congenital anomalies, including Down syndrome, spina bifida, and congenital heart disease, and 35% have Turner syndrome; therefore, amniocentesis is recommended for all pregnant women with this syndrome. In vitro fertilization techniques using donated oocytes have reported success rates as high as 50% to 60%. Children born after oocyte donation have no additional risks. Cryopreservation of oocytes harvested early in life for later implantation is an area of ongoing research interest.

Osteopenia is common in women with Turner syndrome. During childhood, cortical sites are affected to a greater extent than trabecular sites, and the defect is one of impaired bone formation. During adolescent and adult years, trabecular sites are more affected due to increased bone turnover. Long-term treatment with growth hormone in the prepubertal and early to midpubertal years optimizes bone mineral density and may potentiate attainment of peak bone mass when estrogen is provided. Estrogen replacement, adequate calcium intake ($\geq$1.2 g/day), and weight-bearing activities all help promote bone mineralization.

Autoimmune thyroiditis occurs in 10% to 30% of girls with Turner syndrome; thus, annual screening for elevations in thyroid stimulating hormone is recommended. Glucose intolerance and insulin resistance are common, but the incidence of diabetes mellitus is not increased and screening for glucose tolerance is not routinely recommended. Both growth hormone treatment and obesity exacerbate insulin resistance; hence, weight control is helpful.

Recurrent otitis media resulting from anatomical malformations of the eustachian tubes should be treated aggressively to avoid the frequent development of conductive hearing loss. Continued screening for auditory deficits is recommended as progressive sensorineural hearing loss in the 1500- to 2000-Hz range may develop as the patient becomes older.

Autoimmune Ovarian Failure

Autoimmune ovarian failure is a component of the autoimmune polyglandular syndromes (APGS) and has been reported in both types I and II. Sixty percent of girls older than 13 years of age with the type I syndrome (Addison disease, hypoparathyroidism, and candidiasis) develop ovarian failure, which may precede the onset of Addison disease by 8 to 14 years. Ten percent of individuals with type II APGS develop premature ovarian failure. Steroid cell antibodies (St-C-Ab) are detectable in 78% of women with premature ovarian failure who also have Addison disease. A lymphoplasmacellular infiltrate is evident around steroid-producing cells, and the ovaries may appear cystic, possibly due to the high levels of gonadotropins.

Associated autoimmune disorders are present in more than one third of girls and women with autoimmune ovarian failure. Autoimmune thyroid disease is the second most prevalent endocrinopathy, followed by Addison disease. Other associated conditions are pernicious anemia, diabetes mellitus, and myasthenia gravis. No antibody markers are available to diagnose autoimmune ovarian failure in humans, although a gene encoding an ooplasm-specific antigen has been isolated in mice with autoimmune oophoritis. It has been designated MATER (Maternal Antigen That Embryos Require) based on its role in preimplantation development. Immunization of rabbits with heterologous zona pellucida antigens also causes immune destruction of ovarian follicles. Short courses of high-dose glucocorticoids, cyclosporin A and plasmapheresis have resulted in temporary improvement of the autoimmune ovarian failure.

Mutations in the Luteinizing Hormone and Follicle-Stimulating Hormone Genes and Receptors

In females, isolated FSH deficiency (elevated FSH, low LH and estradiol) presents as delayed puberty and/or infertility with impaired follicular development. Although GnRH stimulates a rise in LH but not FSH, exogenous FSH has successfully induced fertility in at least one woman with this defect. Homozygous mutations in the *FSHβ* gene have been identified; the most common is a 2-bp deletion (Val61X) in exon 3, a frameshift mutation that causes premature termination. The truncated FSH is unable to dimerize or bind to the FSH receptor and has decreased immunoactivity and bioactivity. Missense mutations have also been identified.

Two main phenotypes have been reported in individuals carrying an inactivating mutation of the *FSH receptor gene*. The first is the Finnish phenotype associated with a homozygous Ala189Val mutation, which affects receptor trafficking to the cell surface. Females with this mutation have absent or poorly developed secondary sexual characteristics, primary amenorrhea, and high gonadotropins. Ovaries are small and have only primordial and primary follicles. In the other phenotype, a partial defect exists in FSH receptor signaling. Women with this defect have primary amenorrhea with low estrogen and high FSH. The ovaries are of normal size with antral follicles that develop to varying extents depending on the severity of the functional defect in the receptor.

The 46,XX individuals with mutations in the LH receptor present with amenorrhea but develop secondary sexual characteristics. Gonadotropins are elevated, whereas estradiol and progesterone are low. Follicles develop only to the antral stage, suggesting a role for LH in late follicular maturation.

Miscellaneous Causes of Ovarian Dysfunction

Premature ovarian failure occurs in 50% of individuals exposed to pelvic irradiation for malignant disease. The severity and duration of ovarian dysfunction depend on the radiation dose and fractionation and on age at time of treatment. The LD_{50} for oocytes is about 4 Gy; exposure to more than 8 Gy causes permanent ovarian failure. Radiation damage causes interstitial fibrosis, hyalinization of blood vessels, and developmental arrest and reduced numbers of primary follicles. Surgical repositioning of the ovaries behind the uterus or laterally to the paracolic gutters to reduce radiation exposure has successfully preserved ovarian function.

Cytotoxic chemotherapy causes less impairment of gonadal function in females than in males; however, premature ovarian failure still occurs in more than 60% of treated women. Gonadotoxic agents include cyclophosphamide, busulfan, procarbazine, and etoposide. The actively proliferating cells in the mature ovary are more sensitive to cytotoxic chemotherapy than the nondividing cells in the prepubertal ovary. GnRH analogues have been used successfully to induce a prepubertal milieu during chemotherapy with alkylating agents, with spontaneous resumption of ovulation and menses in most long-term survivors. Antiestrogens and oral contraceptives have also been used before chemotherapy for the same purpose. Gonadal suppression thus merits consideration in all reproductive-age females undergoing chemotherapy. Egg retrieval for in vitro fertilization and embryo cryopreservation are viable methods of preserving fertility for married couples but are not feasible in young girls. As an alternative, cryopreservation of ovarian sections for autotransplantation is under clinical investigation, although the theoretical risk of reintroducing malignant stem cells raises concerns.

Certain chemicals and environmental toxins may cause ovarian damage, such as 2-bromopropane, a cleaning solvent, which caused ovarian failure in 16 Korean laborers.

With the implementation of routine MMR vaccination, mumps oophoritis has become an extremely uncommon cause of hypergonadotropic ovarian failure. Ovarian failure has also been associated with *Shigella* infections, malaria, and varicella.

In the classic form of *galactosemia,* a deficiency in uridine diphosphate galactose causes ovarian damage starting during intrauterine life.

Steroidogenic defects in estradiol synthesis such as mutations of the genes for steroidogenic acute regulatory protein (StAR), 17α-hydroxylase, 17,20-lyase, 17β-hydroxysteroid dehydrogenase, and aromatase are discussed in Chapter 7.

Eugonadal Primary Amenorrhea (With Normal Breast and Pubic Hair Development)

Partial or Complete Noncanalization of the Vagina; Imperforate Hymen

Girls with vaginal agenesis or an imperforate hymen often have cyclical endometrial shedding that accumulates in the uterus and fallopian tubes due to outflow obstruction (cryptomenorrhea). Secondary sexual characteristics are generally well developed, but menarche fails to occur. A history of cyclical lower abdominal pain is often elicited. The müllerian structures become distended and painful from accumulated menstrual blood and may be palpable on abdominal examination. A vaginal examination and ultrasonogram are diagnostic. Surgery is necessary to correct the anatomical obstruction to menstrual flow.

Evaluation

Evaluation of pubertal delay should include a careful history of general health and nutrition, growth pattern, neurological symptoms, anosmia, past history of radiation, chemotherapy or surgery, exercise intensity, and family history of the onset and pattern of pubertal development (absent, delayed onset, "stalled puberty"). On physical examination, a careful standing height with upper-to-lower segment ratio and arm span (for early detection of an eunuchoid habitus), assessment of subcutaneous fat, pubertal staging including testicular size and position in boys, a test for anosmia, and a complete neurological assessment are particularly important. The growth pattern should be assessed with serial heights plotted on a growth chart and compared with standard curves for "late maturers."

A complete blood count, sedimentation rate, and biochemical profile help exclude chronic diseases. Simultaneous slowing of growth should prompt measurement of thyroid function and insulin-like growth factor-I to identify associated endocrine dysfunction. Prolactinomas sometimes present as stalled puberty; thus, a prolactin level should be included in the evaluation. DHEAS, sex steroids (testosterone or estradiol using ultrasensitive assays), FSH, and LH provide an assessment of the HPG axis. A karyotype should be obtained in children with hypergonadotropic hypogonadism to rule out Klinefelter or Turner syndrome.

If gonadotropins are low without an obvious cause of hypogonadotropic hypogonadism such as unequivocal anorexia nervosa or a systemic illness, cranial magnetic resonance imaging with gadolinium for pituitary imaging is essential to identify intracranial pathology. A pelvic sonogram may be able to delineate müllerian structures and define the nature of the gonads. A bone age is helpful for determination of skeletal maturation in relation to growth and pubertal development.

GnRH stimulation testing does not differentiate between constitutional delay in puberty and IHH: a family history of constitutional delay and a growth pattern suggestive of a "late bloomer" usually point to the former condition. Although routine GnRH testing is not diagnostic, clinical studies suggest that the gonadotropin response to potent GnRH agonists or to GnRH after priming with GnRH for 36 hours may differentiate between the two conditions.

MANAGEMENT OF AND TREATMENT OPTIONS FOR DELAYED PUBERTY

Delayed puberty secondary to systemic illness, excessive exercise, or weight loss can be corrected with treatment or resolution of the primary disorder. If puberty does not resume in a timely fashion, sex steroid therapy can be initiated to induce puberty. The therapeutic goals are to induce age- and gender-appropriate secondary sexual characteristics and improve psychosocial health. Estrogen or testosterone therapy also induces a pubertal growth spurt and improves bone mineralization. To avoid rapid epiphyseal closure, initial therapy is begun at doses that are well below adult replacement doses and then gradually increased to achieve pubertal maturation at a normal pace. Long-term sex steroid therapy in individuals with persistent hypogonadism helps maintain an eugonadal state and optimize bone mineralization.

Hormone Replacement Therapy in Males

Puberty Induction and Maintenance

In boys, treatment is started at 12 to 14 years of age or, in older individuals, at the time of diagnosis. Testosterone enanthate or cypionate is started at a dose of 50 mg intramuscular every 4 weeks and increased by 25 to 50 mg every 6 to 12 months to a maximum of 200 mg every 2 to 3 weeks. Accelerated bone age advancement and growth rate are indications for decreasing the dose. Severe acne, fluid retention, and prolonged painful erections also mandate dose reduction. Local side effects include tenderness at the injection site and allergic reactions to the vehicle (sesame or cottonseed oil). Another option is the use of a daily trans-

dermal gel or patch that avoids the high peaks and troughs observed with depot testosterone injections. The transdermal formulations, however, are designed to provide adult androgen replacement; therefore, the lower doses needed for induction of puberty have not been established. Androgel 1% (Unimed Pharmaceuticals, Inc., Deerfield, IL) is dispensed in packets of 2.5 or 5 g that deliver 25 or 50 mg of testosterone when applied to the shoulders, upper arms, or abdomen. Androderm (Watson Pharmaceuticals, Inc., Corona, CA) patches for nonscrotal areas deliver 2.5 or 5 mg of testosterone daily. Testoderm (Alza Pharmaceuticals, Palo Alto, CA) is available for scrotal skin as either Testoderm (4- or 6-mg delivery system) or Testoderm with adhesive (6 mg) and, for nonscrotal areas, as Testoderm TTS (5 mg). Doses are adjusted on the basis of testosterone levels obtained after 2 to 3 weeks of use. Recommended sampling times are the morning after applying Androgel or the Androderm patch and 2 to 4 hours after applying any of the Testoderm patches. Local skin irritation can be minimized with topical steroids. Disadvantages of the transdermal patches include difficulty with adhesion in individuals involved in strenuous physical activity and cross-transfer of testosterone to other individuals from skin contact.

In boys with hypogonadotropic hypogonadism and functional testes, low-dose hCG can be used as an alternative to testosterone in a dosage of 200 to 500 units administered every other day. Although this regimen has the advantage of increasing testicular size, thus providing cosmetic benefits, the obvious disadvantage is the frequency of administration. Moreover, excessive stimulation of Leydig cells also increases estrogen production, which causes gynecomastia. This is avoided by using the lowest effective dose of hCG.

In patients with constitutional delay of growth and puberty, a short course of low-dose testosterone is often sufficient to initiate pubertal maturation, improve growth rate, and alleviate psychosocial distress. Spontaneous progression of puberty often ensues when therapy is discontinued after 6 months. The experimental addition of letrozole, an aromatase inhibitor, to monthly testosterone enanthate injections has been demonstrated to improve adult predicted height in boys with constitutional delay of growth and puberty.

Induction of Fertility

Fertility in patients with hypogonadotropic hypogonadism requires treatment with gonadotropins or pulsatile GnRH therapy. Pulsatile GnRH (pulse frequency every 2 hours) is effective in inducing testicular growth and spermatogenesis in individuals with hypothalamic defects, but gonadotropins are the treatment of choice if the pituitary is dysplastic or has sustained extensive damage. hCG and recombinant FSH/human menopausal gonadotropins with hCG have all been used successfully.

Hormone Replacement Therapy in Females

Puberty Induction and Maintenance

Low-dose estrogen therapy is initiated at 10 to 12 years of age to induce breast budding without advancing bone age. Initiation of estrogen therapy is delayed in girls with Turner syndrome to 12 to 14 years to optimize the effects of growth hormone therapy. The initial dosage of estrogen is either 0.3 mg conjugated estrogens every other day or 5 μg of ethinyl estradiol daily. Transdermal estrogen patches (delivering 0.025 mg/day) applied twice weekly are also available for induction of breast development. Transdermal estrogen is useful in children with poor compliance and in those with a family history of thromboembolism. The dose of estrogen is increased gradually every 6 to 12 months to achieve full replacement doses within 2 to 3 years. Full estrogen replacement at a dose of 0.625 mg conjugated estrogens or 20 μg ethinyl estradiol ensures maintenance of feminization and protection against osteoporosis. Cyclical progesterone (5-10 mg daily of medroxyprogesterone acetate or 200-400 mg micronized progesterone [Prometrium, Solvay Pharmaceuticals, Inc., Marietta, GA]) is added for 12 days every month after full estrogen replacement to ensure cyclical endometrial shedding and decrease the risk of endometrial dysplasia.

If pubertal delay results from chronic illnesses, undernutrition, or excessive exercise, treatment is directed at the primary condition. When hyperprolactenemia is the cause of pubertal delay, hypothyroidism should be excluded, and a cranial imaging study is necessary to identify prolactinomas. Therapy is then initiated with the dopamine agonists bromocryptine mesylate or cabergoline. Starting bromocryptine at a low dose of 1.25 mg at bedtime minimizes the major side effect of nausea. The dose is then increased gradually to 2.5 mg BID or TID to normalize the prolactin levels. Cabergoline has the advantage of biweekly administration and fewer side effects. It is begun at a dosage of 0.25 mg twice weekly and may be gradually increased to 1 mg twice weekly, if required.

Androgens may be helpful for inducing hair growth in girls lacking pubic hair, but male pattern baldness, clitoral enlargement, and voice changes are possible side effects.

Induction of Fertility

Pulsatile GnRH therapy using a pulse frequency that mimics that seen across a menstrual cycle is effective in inducing ovulation in women with hypothalamic hypogonadism. When hypogonadism is due to pituitary dysfunction, either hCG or human menopausal gonadotropin (hMG)/recombinant FSH with hCG is used. GnRH therapy has the advantage of higher conception rates with fewer multiple pregnancies.

MAJOR POINTS

In girls, puberty is considered delayed if breast development has not started by age 13, or with failure to attain menarche and immature breast development at age 15. *Primary amenorrhea* is defined as failure to attain menarche by age 16 in the presence of normal breast development.

In boys, puberty is considered delayed in the absence of testicular enlargement (>4 mL) or pubic hair at age 14.

In addition to delay in the onset of puberty, an unusually slow pace of puberty or arrested pubertal development warrants further evaluation to exclude pathology.

Pubertal delay can result from hypogonadotropic hypogonadism (hypothalamic or pituitary dysfunction or immaturity), hypergonadotropic hypogonadism (low sex steroids with a normal compensatory rise in gonadotropins), or eugonadotropic hypogonadism (structural defects in the development of the uterus, cervix, and vagina).

Hypogonadotropic hypogonadism encompasses the most frequent cause of pubertal delay in boys—constitutional delay of growth and development—but also includes a number of pathological etiologies. The diagnosis of constitutional delay is a diagnosis of exclusion.

The association of anosmia with pubertal delay (hypogonadotropic hypogonadism) is highly suggestive of Kallmann syndrome.

Hypergonadotropic hypogonadism (low sex steroids and elevated follicle-stimulating hormone and luteinizing hormone) is diagnostic of a pathological cause of delayed puberty.

Turner syndrome needs to be considered in a short girl with pubertal delay (hypergonadotropic hypogonadism), especially in the absence of a family history of delayed puberty.

An enuchoid habitus, slow or delayed puberty (with normal or elevated follicle-stimulating hormone), and relatively small testes for the degree of pubertal maturation are suggestive of Klinefelter syndrome.

The optimal timing for gonadal steroid replacement to induce puberty is dependent on the growth and skeletal maturation of the adolescent. Ideally, testosterone or estrogen is started at a low dose and gradually increased at a pace similar to endogenous puberty until adult replacement doses are achieved.

SUGGESTED READINGS

Ackermann JC, Weiss J, Lee EJ, et al: Inherited disorders of gonadotropin hormones, Mol Cell Endocrinol 2001;179:89.

American Academy of Pediatrics, Committee on Genetics: Health supervision for children with Turner syndrome, Pediatrics 1995;96:1166.

Amory JK, Anawalt BD, Paulsen CA, et al: Klinefelter syndrome, Lancet 2000;356:333.

Argente J: Diagnosis of late puberty, Horm Res 1999;51(suppl 3):95.

Blumenfeld Z, Haim N: Prevention of gonadal damage during cytotoxic therapy, Ann Med 1997;29:199.

Brook CGD: Treatment of late puberty, Horm Res 1999;51(suppl 3):101.

de Roux N, Milgrom E: Inherited disorders of GnRH and gonadotropin receptors, Mol Cell Endocrinol 2001;179:83.

DiMeglio LA, Pescovitz OH: Disorders of puberty: inactivating and activating mutations, J Pediatr 1997;131:S8.

Hayes FJ, Seminara SB, Crowley WF Jr: Hypogonadotropic hypogonadism, Endocrinol Metab Clin North Am 1998;27:739.

Howell S, Shalet S: Gonadal damage from chemotherapy and radiotherapy, Endocrinol Metab Clin North Am 1998;27:927.

Kulin H: Delayed puberty, J Clin Endocrinol Metab 1996;81:3460.

Layman LC: Genetics of human hypogonadotropic hypogonadism, Am J Med Genet 1999;89:240.

Palmert MR, Boepple PA: Variation in the timing of puberty: clinical spectrum and genetic investigation, J Clin Endocrinol Metab 2001;86:2364.

Saenger P: Growth promoting strategies in Turner syndrome, J Clin Endocrinol Metab 1999;84:4345.

Seminara SB, Oliveira LMB, Beranova M, et al: Genetics of hypogonadotropic hypogonadism, J Endocrinol Invest 2000;23:560.

Smyth CM, Brenner WJ: Klinefelter syndrome, Arch Intern Med 1998;158:1309.

Styne DM: New aspects in the diagnosis and treatment of pubertal disorders, Pediatr Endocrinol 1997;44:505.

Wickman S, Sipila I, Ankarberg-Lindgren C, et al: A specific aromatase inhibitor and potential increase in adult height in boys with delayed puberty: a randomized controlled trial, Lancet 2001;357:1743.

Wu FCW, Brown DC, Cutler GE, et al: Early morning plasma testosterone is an accurate predictor of imminent pubertal development in prepubertal boys, J Clin Endocrinol Metab 1992;76:26.

Yen SSC: Effects of lifestyle and body composition on the ovary, Endocrinol Metab Clin North Am 1998;27:915.

CHAPTER 7

Intersex Disorders

MADHUSMITA MISRA

MARY M. LEE

INTRODUCTION

The designation of a newborn infant as a boy or girl is usually evident from the appearance of the external genitalia at delivery. Parents and medical personnel seldom anticipate that the process of sex differentiation may go awry, making gender indeterminate at birth. When the phenotype of the external genitalia is ambiguous or discordant with fetal ultrasonogram or prenatal karyotype, concerns arise about a potential intersex condition. In these children, clinical decisions regarding sex assignment and long-term management of gender role remain challenging, despite tremendous advances during the past decade in understanding the basic biology of gonadal determination and sex differentiation.

GONADAL DETERMINATION AND SEX DIFFERENTIATION

The progression of molecular events in gonadal determination and sex differentiation is being defined more precisely as an increasing number of genes in these developmental pathways are identified (Figure 7-1). Chromosomal (46,XX or 46,XY) or genetic sex is established at fertilization with the Y chromosome carrying the primary determinant of the male-specific pathway, the testis-determining gene *(SRY)*. Before induction of *SRY* expression, however, XX and XY embryos are morphologically undifferentiated and have common embryological precursors of the gonads and external genitalia and both sets of internal genital ducts.

Primitive Undifferentiated Gonad

Primitive germ cells are first recognizable in the dorsal endoderm of the yolk sac at 3 to 4 weeks' gestational age.

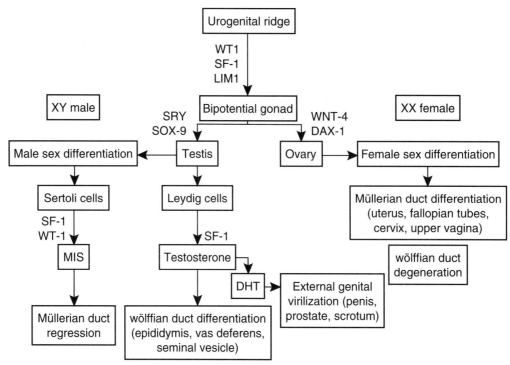

Figure 7-1   Pathways of Gonadal Determination and Sex Differentiation. Sequential events leading from the undifferentiated urogenital ridge to a fully differentiated male or female are depicted on this flow diagram. Some of the genes involved in gonadal formation and testicular and ovarian differentiation are shown.

During the next 2 weeks, these cells migrate to the hindgut and then through the dorsal mesentery to populate the primitive gonad that has arisen from the mesoderm of the urogenital ridge. A number of genes have been revealed as key players in formation of the undifferentiated gonad through finding the phenotype of gonadal agenesis in genetically engineered mice with null mutations of these genes. Of these, two transcription factors, *WT1* (the product of the Wilms' tumor suppressor gene) and steroidogenic factor-1 (*SF-1*), are the best characterized. *WT1* is essential for kidney and gonad morphogenesis, whereas *SF-1* plays a critical role in development of the adrenal gland, pituitary, and gonad. After initial gonadogenesis, *WT1* and *SF-1* are postulated to activate other downstream genes that regulate sex-specific gonadal determination, such as *DAX-1* and *SRY*.

A heterozygous loss of function mutation of *WT1* (11p13) in humans causes the WAGR contiguous gene syndrome (Wilms' tumor, aniridia, mental retardation, and minor genitourinary abnormalities). A less common but more severely affected phenotype is associated with dominant negative point mutations in the zinc finger region of *WT1* that abrogate DNA binding to the wild-type allele. The phenotype associated with these dominant negative mutations is the Denys-Drash syndrome, characterized by Wilms' tumor, diffuse mesangial sclerosis leading to end-stage renal failure in the first few years of life, and genital ambiguity. The gonadal phenotype varies from complete sex reversal in 46,XY individuals (streak gonads and female genitalia) to genital ambiguity with dysgenetic gonads and undervirilization. A similar gonadal phenotype of gonadal dysgenesis and genital ambiguity is present in Frasier syndrome, which is caused by mutations within intron 9 of the *WT1* gene. In this related syndrome, Wilms' tumor does not develop and patients develop focal glomerular sclerosis with a less severe renal impairment that is of later onset.

SF-1 is initially expressed in the undifferentiated urogenital ridge, where it acts in concert with *WT1* to induce gonadal and adrenal formation. At later developmental stages, *SF-1* is upregulated in the differentiating testis and repressed in the ovary to regulate somatic cell differentiation and induce steroidogenic enzyme expression in both adrenals and gonads. The phenotype of gonadal agenesis and male-to-female sex reversal with an *Sf-1* mutation is similar to that of *Wt1*. In contrast to the renal abnormalities found with a deletion of *Wt1*, however, *Sf-1* knock-out mice have defective hypothalamic and pituitary function and adrenal agenesis. In humans, the majority of *SF-1* mutations may be lethal because of its essential role in the formation of the adrenal gland and production of all steroid hormones. The rare patients reported with *SF-1* mutations manifest adrenal failure in infancy and 46,XY sex reversal.

Testicular Differentiation

The embryonic gonad remains indifferent until *SRY* is activated at day 42 to initiate the male developmental pathway (Figure 7-2; see Figure 7-1) During the next few days, testicular organization occurs as the primordial germ cells are incorporated into testicular cords. Within these primitive seminiferous cords, the primordial germ cells start to differentiate and proliferate in response to *SRY*. The somatic cells within the cords differentiate into Sertoli cells, whereas the interstitial mesenchymal cells differentiate into Leydig cells, the two major hormone-producing cell types of the testis (see Figure 7-2).

The identification of *SRY* as the primary testis-determining gene was accomplished by positional cloning in patients with XX sex reversal. Its role in testis determination was subsequently confirmed by the generation of sex-reversed XX mice transgenic for *Sry*, a Sox family transcription factor with a high mobility group (HMG) DNA-binding motif. The HMG box is the site of numerous *SRY* (Yp11.3) mutations causing human 46,XY sex reversal, verifying the importance of this region for *SRY* action. Although specific gene targets of *SRY* have not been identified, experimental data support several possibilities for its mechanism of action: *SRY* may be a classic transcriptional activator, it may repress genes that inhibit testicular devel-

opment, or it may alter gene expression by bending DNA. The phenotype of patients with *SRY* loss of function mutations ranges from complete gonadal dysgenesis (46,XY sex reversal) to true hermaphroditism or partial gonadal dysgenesis with genital ambiguity and testicular dysgenesis. Conversely, a gain of function mutation resulting from a Y-to-X translocation bearing the *SRY* gene is responsible for some cases of 46,XX male sex reversal.

SOX9 (17q24.3-25.1) is an *SRY*-related HMG box transcription factor that is critical for testicular determination. *SOX9* is initially expressed at low levels in both male and female urogenital ridges in the bipotential embryo. As the gonads start to differentiate, the expression of *SOX9* is induced in males and repressed in females, similar to that of *SF-1*. Its function in testicular determination is confirmed by the development of testes and sex reversal in XX mice transgenic for *SOX9*. Heterozygous *SOX9* dominant negative mutations cause testicular dysgenesis and 46,XY sex reversal in humans. This gonadal phenotype is an inconsistent feature of campomelic dysplasia, a syndrome attributed to *SOX9* mutations that is characterized by congenital bowing of long bones, brachydactyly, micrognathia, and congenital cardiac and renal anomalies.

The inability to demonstrate translocation of the *SRY* gene in all patients with 46,XX sex reversal and the finding of intact *SRY* and *SOX9* genes in some women with 46,XY

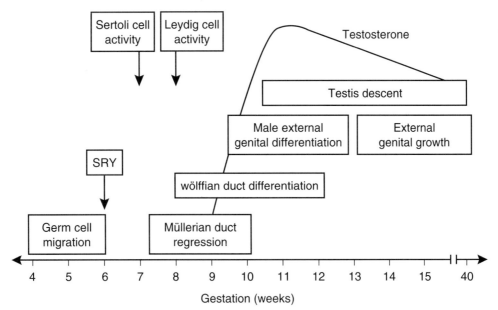

Figure 7-2   Temporal Pattern of Events in Male Sex Differentiation. During the period of germ cell migration, undifferentiated wölffian and müllerian ducts are formed in all embryos. The onset of *SRY* expression at 6 weeks stimulates organization of the testes and differentiation of the Sertoli and Leydig cells. *Sertoli cell activity* refers to the secretion of müllerian inhibiting substance to induce müllerian duct regression, and *Leydig cell activity* refers to the secretion of testosterone to promote male sex differentiation, with the increase in fetal serum testosterone concentrations represented by the dark line. (Adapted with permission from Hughes LA: Minireview: sex differentiation, Endocrinology 2001;142:3281.)

sex reversal reinforce the role of other genes in the testicular determination pathway. Such genes are likely to be found within small chromosomal deletions such as 9p24, 10q, and 12q13 that are present in patients with *SRY*-independent 46,XY sex reversal or gonadal dysgenesis. Candidate genes include *DMRT* (9p23.3-24.1), a testicular gene essential for Sertoli cell development, and *Dhh* (Desert hedgehog, 12q13.1), a gene critical for Sertoli cell–germ cell interactions and germ cell maintenance.

Ovarian Differentiation

In female embryos, the primitive gonad remains undifferentiated until the ninth week of gestation when ovarian determining factors such as *Wnt-4* and *DAX-1* initiate ovarian differentiation. The dividing germ cells are loosely organized into irregular cords. The oocytes commence meiotic prophase but become arrested at the diplotene stage of prophase and are surrounded by somatic cells to form primordial follicles. Follicular development is maximal at 20 to 25 weeks' gestation and occurs in parallel with differentiation of the somatic cells to granulosa or theca cells. Germ cells that are not incorporated into follicles undergo attrition to cause the decrease in number from 6 or 7 million to 2 million at term.

Ovarian development requires the interactions of two genes, *WNT-4,* a secreted growth factor, and *DAX-1,* a nuclear hormone receptor in the DSS region (dosage-sensitive sex reversal, adrenal hypoplasia congenita, X-linked) of the X chromosome (Xp21). *WNT-4* and *DAX-1* are both expressed in the undifferentiated gonad and then repressed in the developing testis and upregulated in the ovary. *WNT-4* may act in concert with *DAX-1* to antagonize *SRY* action and promote ovarian differentiation. Although *WNT-4* knock-out mice have XX sex reversal, this association has not been reported in humans. Mutations or deletions of *DAX-1* cause congenital adrenal hypoplasia and hypogonadotropic hypogonadism, while gonadal development is unaffected. However, a duplication of either *WNT-4* or *DAX-1* can interfere with normal testicular development to cause gonadal dysgenesis as a dosage-dependent form of 46,XY sex reversal.

Differentiation of the Genital Ducts

Sex differentiation of the wölffian (male) and müllerian (female) internal genital ducts depends on the local hormonal milieu (Figure 7-3; see Figure 7-2). As testicular cords organize in the differentiating testis, *SF-1* and *WT1* act cooperatively to activate the expression of müllerian inhibiting substance (MIS) in the Sertoli cells. MIS signals through the mesenchymal cells to indirectly stimulate apoptotic cell death of the müllerian duct epithelial cells in males. MIS-induced regression of the müllerian ducts starts by 8 weeks and is complete by the third month, leaving a vestigial remnant as the prostatic utricle. Shortly after the onset of MIS expression, *SF-1* induces the expression of the cytochrome P450 steroid hydroxylases and 3β-hydroxysteroid dehydrogenase to initiate testosterone synthesis by Leydig cells. During this stage of gonadal development, testosterone production is gonadotropin independent. Testosterone has no direct action on the müllerian ducts but potentiates MIS actions to facilitate complete regression of the müllerian ducts. The high local concentrations of

Figure 7-3   Differentiation of the Male and Female Genital Ducts. Both sets of genital ducts are present in the indifferent stage and differentiate according to the local hormonal milieu from 7 to 12 weeks. Female development occurs in the absence of male hormones. Male development proceeds in response to the actions of testosterone on the wölffian ducts and müllerian inhibiting substance on the müllerian duct. (Reprinted with permission from Grumbach MM, Conte FA: Disorders of sexual differentiation. In Larsen PR, Kronenberg HM, Melmed S, et al, editors: Williams' Textbook of Endocrinology, 10th ed, Philadelphia, 2003, WB Saunders.)

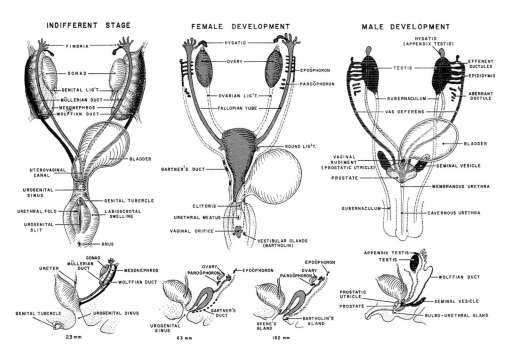

testosterone stimulate differentiation and growth of the wölffian structures (epididymis, vas deferens, seminal vesicles) between 9 and 14 weeks of embryonic life.

In females, differentiation of the genital ducts occurs without a need for active production of hormones. Müllerian ducts differentiate into the Fallopian tubes, uterus, cervix, and upper vagina in the absence of MIS, whereas the wölffian ducts degenerate in the absence of testosterone (see Figure 7-3).

Differentiation of the External Genitalia

In parallel with internal genital duct development, differentiation of the genital tubercle, urethral folds, and labioscrotal swellings takes place (Figure 7-4). In males, although testosterone is able to promote wölffian duct development, virilization of the external genital requires reduction of testosterone to its more active metabolite, dihydrotestosterone (DHT) by 5α-reductase-2. The expression of this enzyme at the undifferentiated genital tubercle and urogenital sinus enables testosterone to be converted to DHT at its site of action. DHT stimulates fusion of the urethral folds to form the corpora spongiosa enclosing the cavernous urethra and the labioscrotal swellings to form the scrotum. DHT also mediates prostate differentiation and growth of the genital tubercle into the glans penis. The critical window for genital virilization is before 12 weeks; androgen exposure after this time can cause hypertrophy of the phallus but not midline fusion (see Figure 7-2). Much of phallic growth occurs between 20 to 40 weeks, when testosterone production becomes dependent on pituitary luteinizing hormone (LH) stimulation. Descent of the testes into the scrotal sac is also a late event mediated in part by androgens.

In the absence of androgens and MIS, differentiation of the genitalia proceeds independently of ovarian function and inherently follows the female pathway (see Figure 7-4). The fused müllerian ducts contact the urogenital sinus to

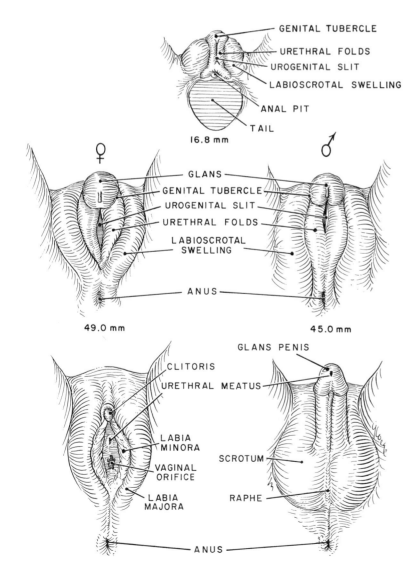

Figure 7-4 Differentiation of Male and Female External Genitalia. The external genitalia are initially identical in male and female embryos. Sexually dimorphic differentiation proceeds after gonadal determination and the secretion of testosterone by the fetal testis. Male development requires local conversion of testosterone to its more biologically active reduced product, dihydrotestosterone. Female development occurs in the absence of androgenic stimulation. Differentiation of the external genitalia is complete by 12 to 14 weeks. Exposure to androgen after this period manifests primarily as phallic enlargement (Reprinted with permission from Grumbach MM, Conte FA: Disorders of sexual differentiation. In Larsen PR, Kronenberg HM, Melmed S, et al, editors: Williams' Textbook of Endocrinology, 10th ed, Philadelphia, 2003, WB Saunders.)

form the müllerian tubercle. This stimulates endodermal proliferation and extension of the uterovaginal plate to the perineum to form a separate vaginal orifice. The plate canalizes to form the vagina at 20 weeks. The urogenital tubercle becomes the clitoris and the urethral and labioscrotal folds remain unfused and form the labia minora and majora.

Müllerian Inhibiting Substance and Testosterone

To achieve normal differentiation of the internal and external genital structures in males, MIS and testosterone and their receptors, and downstream signaling pathways must be intact. MIS, or anti-müllerian hormone (AMH), is a 140-kDa glycoprotein in the transforming growth factor (TGF)-β family of growth and transcription factors. MIS is produced as a prohormone that undergoes proteolytic cleavage to generate a bioactive C terminus that binds to cell surface serine-threonine kinase receptors. Mutations in the MIS gene (19p) or its receptor (12q) result in the persistent müllerian duct syndrome. In affected males, the absence of normal MIS action enables the müllerian ducts to differentiate and persist as rudimentary or incompletely developed müllerian structures. The retained müllerian

structures interfere with testicular descent and often manifest as unilateral testicular ectopia with both testes descended through the same inguinal canal. Androgen synthesis is essentially unaffected; therefore, the wölffian ducts and external genitalia virilize normally.

Male sex differentiation requires sufficient synthesis of testosterone at the appropriate time. Initial testosterone synthesis during the period of genital differentiation is gonadotropin independent, but continued production of testosterone in later pregnancy is dependent on human chorionic gonadotropin (hCG) or LH. Genetic mutations of any of the testosterone biosynthetic enzymes or the cholesterol transporter can diminish androgen production and disrupt masculinization of the internal and external genitalia. Inability to convert testosterone to DHT (5α-reductase-2 gene defect) causes undervirilization of the external genitalia, but wölffian duct development remains normal. DHT and testosterone bind to the androgen receptor, a steroid hormone nuclear receptor. The androgen receptor is bound to chaperone (heat shock) proteins in the absence of ligand (Figure 7-5). Androgen binding produces a conformational change that releases the heat shock protein and activates the receptor. The activated steroid recep-

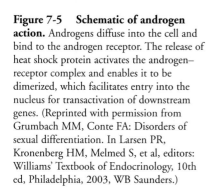

Figure 7-5 Schematic of androgen action. Androgens diffuse into the cell and bind to the androgen receptor. The release of heat shock protein activates the androgen–receptor complex and enables it to be dimerized, which facilitates entry into the nucleus for transactivation of downstream genes. (Reprinted with permission from Grumbach MM, Conte FA: Disorders of sexual differentiation. In Larsen PR, Kronenberg HM, Melmed S, et al, editors: Williams' Textbook of Endocrinology, 10th ed, Philadelphia, 2003, WB Saunders.)

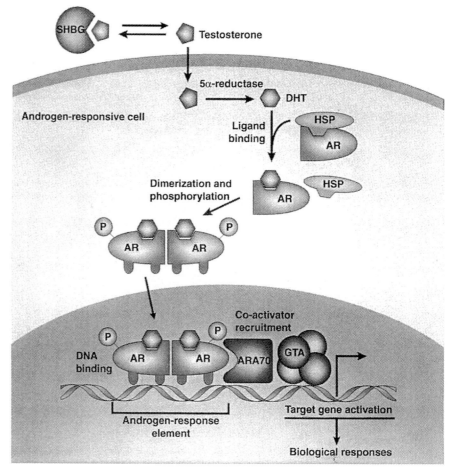

tor complex dimerizes, enters the nucleus, and binds to steroid-responsive elements to elicit androgen-mediated transcriptional events. Androgen resistance due to a defect in the androgen receptor or signaling pathway causes varying degrees of undervirilization of both internal and external genitalia. All of these conditions affecting androgen synthesis or action are characterized by undervirilization of the genitalia with complete or nearly complete müllerian duct regression because MIS action is only minimally affected.

DIFFERENTIAL DIAGNOSIS OF INTERSEX CONDITIONS

Classification of intersex conditions into four pathophysiological categories provides an organized framework for the evaluation of children with genital ambiguity (Table 7-1). These categories are as follows:

1. Abnormality in the primary process of gonadal morphogenesis
2. Virilized genetic female with ovaries (female pseudohermaphroditism)
3. Undervirilized genetic male with testes (male pseudohermaphroditism)
4. Congenital embryopathy independent of hormone production

Disorders of Gonadal Morphogenesis

Primary defects in gonadal morphogenesis are often associated with a chromosomal anomaly or a mutation or deletion of one of the genes critical for gonadal formation and testicular differentiation. In general, the aberrant

Table 7-1   Differential Diagnosis of Intersex Conditions

Disorders of Gonadal Morphogenesis	Gene Map Symbol (Locus)
Gonadal dysgenesis (partial and complete)	*SRY* (Yp11.3)
Campomelic dysplasia	*SOX1* (17q24.3-q25.1)
Associated with primary adrenal failure	*SF1* (9q33)
Denys-Drash and Frasier syndromes	*WT1* (11p13)
Dosage-sensitive sex reversal	*DAX-1* (Xp21.3-p21.2)
Associated with polyneuropathy	*Dhh* (12q13.1)
Mixed gonadal dysgenesis	
True hermaphroditism	
Congenital anorchia/vanishing testis syndrome	
Virilized female	
Congenital adrenal hyperplasia	
21α-Hydroxylase deficiency	*CYP 21* (6p21.3)
11β-Hydroxylase deficiency	*CYP 11B1* (8q24.3)
3β-Hydroxysteroid dehydrogenase deficiency	*HSD3B2* (1p13.1)
Defect in 17β-hydroxysteroid dehydrogenase	*17β-HSD3* (9q22)
Aromatase deficiency *CYP 19* (15q21.1)	
In utero exposure to androgens or progestational agents	
Undervirilized male	
Androgen insensitivity (complete, partial, mild)	*AR* (Xq11-12)
Disorders of testosterone biosynthesis	
Lipoid adrenal hyperplasia	*StAR* (8p11.2), *CYP 11A* (P450scc)
Defect in 17α-hydroxylase/lyase	*CYP 17* (10q24.3)
Defect in 17β-hydroxysteroid dehydrogenase	*17β-HSD3* (9q22)
5α-Reductase 2 deficiency	*SRD5A2* (2p33)
Leydig cell hypoplasia	*LCGR* (2p21)
Smith-Lemli-Opitz syndrome	*DHCR7* (11q12-q13)
Persistent müllerian duct syndrome	
Type 1	*MIS/AMH* (19p12.3-p13.2)
Type 2	*MIS/AMHR2* (12q13)
Embryopathy	
Penoscrotal transposition	
Penile agenesis	
Hypospadias	
Bladder and cloacal exstrophy	
Rokitansky-Kuster-Hauser syndrome	
Müllerian aplasia	
Miscellaneous syndromes associated with genital ambiguity	

formation or impaired differentiation of an undifferentiated gonad to a testis imparts an increased risk for malignant transformation. Therefore, management usually includes gonadectomy and replacement of estrogens or androgens at the time of puberty to induce secondary sexual maturation (details provided in Chapter 6). Ovarian dysgenesis from haploinsufficiency of the X chromosomes, however, is not associated with an increased risk for malignancy; thus, gonadal exploration is usually unnecessary. The extent of genital virilization generally correlates with gonadal histology and is useful as a parameter of androgen exposure in the decision regarding gender assignment. More so than for the other intersex categories, sex assignment also considers the appearance and function of the external genitalia.

Complete or Partial Gonadal Dysgenesis

In children with complete gonadal dysgenesis, the gonads never differentiate and regress to form streaks (46,XY sex reversal). The somatic cells in the streak gonads remain undifferentiated and are unable to produce testosterone or MIS; thus, the internal and external genitalia develop along the inherently female pathway, sometimes with subtle evidence of minor virilization. If the genitalia are female in appearance, a discrepancy between the prenatal cytogenetic analysis and phenotype may lead to early diagnosis; otherwise, the condition may remain unrecognized until the failure of puberty occurs. At that time, primary gonadal failure (elevated FSH and LH) in a patient with eunuchoid body proportions, normal stature, a small uterus with nonvisualized ovaries, and a 46,XY karyotype suggest the diagnosis. If the karyotype is 46,XX or unknown, the differential diagnosis of primary gonadal failure at puberty also includes autoimmune ovarian failure, Turner syndrome, or, rarely, an FSH receptor gene defect. In patients with gonadal dysgenesis, the elevated gonadotropins at puberty occasionally stimulate the residual nests of hilar cells sufficiently to produce testosterone and cause clitoromegaly and hirsutism.

In the partial or incomplete form, the gonads are dysgenetic rather than streaks. The phenotype can range from mild clitoromegaly and posterior labial fusion to more obvious genital ambiguity. Development of the müllerian structures is variable and can be discordant between the two sides, depending on the extent of Sertoli cell function in each gonad. Gender assignment is usually female. Virilization may occur at puberty if the gonads are not removed. The risk for gonadoblastomas (seminomas and dysgerminomas) in individuals with gonadal dysgenesis is 10% to 30%. Spontaneous estrogen effects such as breast development or virilization may be the initial manifestation.

Gonadal mosaicism is the most frequently identified cause of gonadal dysgenesis. Defects in genes that are essential for gonadal differentiation and testis determination, such as *SRY*, *SOX9*, and *WT1* (the Wilms' tumor suppressor gene), and gene duplications of *DAX-1* or *WNT4* have also been implicated in gonadal dysgenesis. In the majority of patients with gonadal dysgenesis, however, no genetic defects have been found, suggesting the possibility of mutations in unidentified genes in the testicular determination pathway.

Mixed Gonadal Dysgenesis

Children with mixed gonadal dysgenesis have asymmetrical gonadal histology, typically with a streak gonad and a contralateral dysgenetic or normal testis. In the dysgenetic gonad, Sertoli cell secretion of MIS is usually better preserved than Leydig cell production of testosterone. The phenotype can be male, ambiguous, or female in appearance with variable and often asymmetrical rudimentary müllerian structures. A hemiuterus and fallopian tube are often present on the side of the streak gonad. If one gonad is a normal testis, testosterone secretion may be adequate for full virilization of the external genitalia and secondary sexual maturation, in which case the diagnosis may be difficult to detect.

The incidence of gonadoblastoma in dysgenetic testes is 20%, of which one third are germ cell tumors. Carcinoma in situ is even more common. When gender assignment is male, early gonadal biopsy is necessary to determine the nature of the testicular tissue and direct further management. If the biopsy reveals normal testicular histology and endocrine function is intact with normal androgens and gonadotropins, the testis can be left in place. Close monitoring with annual imaging studies (sonography, computed tomography, or magnetic resonance imaging) and a repeat biopsy at the onset of puberty and then again at 20 years of age are recommended. If carcinoma in situ is absent at these time points, malignant transformation of a histologically normal testis is less likely. Dysgenetic testes and streak gonads are removed early because of their increased malignant potential.

The karyotype associated with this condition is 45,X/46,XY. Prenatal cytogenetics has revealed a higher than expected incidence (1.7:10,000) of this karyotype. The majority (90%-95%) were associated with normal male external genitalia, although an autopsy series found ovotestes in 2 of 11 cases with normal male genitalia. This karyotype can also be associated with a Turner syndrome phenotype.

True Hermaphroditism

True hermaphroditism is a rare intersex condition in which an individual has both testicular and ovarian tissue.

The largest numbers of cases have been reported from Africa and Europe. Children with this disorder have ambiguous genitalia ranging from a female phenotype with slight clitoromegaly to a minimally undervirilized male phenotype. More commonly, the genitalia are clearly ambiguous with microphallus (with or without chordae), hypospadias (commonly penoscrotal or perineoscrotal), fused labioscrotal folds, and cryptorchidism. Müllerian structures develop on the side with an ovary, whereas müllerian structures are absent and a vas deferens and an epididymis may be present on the side with a testis. When the gonad is an ovotestis, there is partial müllerian regression and wölffian duct differentiation. Some cases are diagnosed at puberty with the development of discordant secondary sexual characteristics. Males may present with prominent gynecomastia or cyclical penile bleeding and females may present with virilization and amenorrhea.

Possible gonadal combinations include an ovotestis with an ovary (50%), bilateral ovotestes (30%), and an ovary and a testis (20%). The most frequent gonad is an ovotestis, followed by an ovary, then a testis. Ovaries are more likely to be located on the left side (76.5%), whereas ovotestes or testes are more common on the right (60.3%). This distribution may be due to the effect of asymmetric gonadal growth on gonadal differentiation. Ovaries remain intraabdominal, whereas gonads containing testicular tissue may lie within the abdomen or undergo varying degrees of descent, depending on the extent of testicular tissue in the gonad. Thus, an ovotestis may be abdominal (50%), inguinal (26%), or labioscrotal (24%) in position. In an ovotestis, the firm, pale, convoluted appearing ovarian tissue can be clearly demarcated from the smooth yellow testicular tissue. On ultrasonography, testicular tissue appears fine and granular with a homogeneous echogenicity, whereas an ovary is hypoechoic with identifiable follicles.

The diagnosis of true hermaphroditism requires the presence of functional ovarian and testicular tissue containing ovarian follicles and distinct seminiferous tubules, respectively. The testicular tissue is often immature and dysgenetic, however, the estimated risk for malignant transformation is 5%, less than that observed with complete or partial gonadal dysgenesis. Interstitial and peritubular fibrosis, hyalinization of the basement membranes of tubules, tubular atrophy, and hyperplastic Sertoli cells have been described. Complete spermatogenesis producing functional sperm is rare. Ovarian tissue, on the other hand, is generally normal, even in an ovotestis. Primordial follicles are present before puberty and follicles develop to various stages in the mature ovary. Ovulation and pregnancy are possible.

When the gender assignment is female, an ovary is left in place, but testes and ovotestes are resected to avoid virilization at puberty. Occasionally only the testicular part of an ovotestis is excised, while the ovarian tissue is retained in situ to preserve ovarian function and fertility. When the gender assignment is male, a histologically normal testes can be left in place but the contralateral ovary or ovotestes is usually resected.

The karyotype can be 46,XX (70%), mosaic (20%), or 46,XY (10%). If dysgenetic gonads are present, a Y chromosome complement is likely to be found. Almost all (99%) of patients of African or mixed African origin have a 46,XX karyotype, whereas 40% of European patients have sex chromosome mosaicism. True hermaphroditism and gonadal dysgenesis have been found within the same pedigree. Postulated causes of true hermaphroditism include germline *SRY* mutations, selective activation of testicular differentiation in part of the gonad, asymmetrical gonadal growth and differentiation, and chimerism of 46,XX and 46,XY embryos.

Congenital Anorchia or the Vanishing Testes Syndrome

Congenital anorchia overlaps the spectrum of gonadal dysgenesis but is attributed to loss of the testes or gonads secondary to vascular insult rather than a molecular defect in gonadal formation. The karyotype is therefore 46,XY and the extent of virilization depends on the developmental stage at which testicular function is lost (see Figure 7-2). Deficient androgen secretion before 8 weeks' gestation leads to a female internal and external phenotype that includes differentiated müllerian structures. If the loss of function occurs during the critical period for male differentiation from 8 to 10 weeks' gestation, the genitalia are ambiguous, with variable development of the wölffian and müllerian ducts. If the vascular insult and testicular loss occur after 12 to 14 weeks' gestational age, although the internal and external genitalia are male in appearance and the müllerian structures are absent, virilization is incomplete. The deficiency of androgens during the second and third semesters may lead to hypospadias and failure of the phallus to increase in size.

Virilization in a Genetic Female (Female Pseudohermaphroditism)

Virilization of the genitalia in a child with a 46,XX karyotype and normally differentiated ovaries is typically due to nongonadal androgens, most commonly from the fetal adrenal (see Table 7-1). Rarely, the androgens are of placental or maternal origin. The excess androgens do not disrupt müllerian duct development; therefore, the uterus and fallopian tubes are normally formed. The timing and extent of androgen exposure during the critical stages of sex differentiation dictate the magnitude of the masculinizing effects. Early exposure to androgens can fully virilize the external genitalia, whereas late exposure may cause only clitoromegaly. Management involves treatment of the primary condition to avoid ongoing androgen exposure. Because the ovaries are usually functional, hormonal therapy is seldom needed for secondary sexual maturation at puberty unless the gender of rearing is male. Severe virilization may require urogenital reconstruction.

Congenital Adrenal Hyperplasia

Congenital adrenal hyperplasia (CAH), a condition caused by autosomal recessive enzymatic defects in cortisol biosynthesis, is by far the most common cause of virilization in genetic females (Figure 7-6). In the predominant virilizing forms of CAH, 21α-hydroxylase and 11β-hydroxylase deficiencies, the affected enzyme is necessary for synthesis of cortisol and aldosterone but not for androgens. The compensatory rise in corticotropin releasing hormone (CRH) and corticotropin (ACTH) in response to inadequate serum cortisol stimulates adrenal steroidogenesis and causes adrenal hyperplasia. Consequently, adrenal androgens and the steroid precursors proximal to the enzymatic defect accumulate, contributing to the clinical manifestations of this condition. The management of virilization secondary to cortisol biosynthetic defects consists of providing sufficient glucocorticoids to suppress the ACTH drive to prevent stimulation of adrenal steroidogenesis.

21α-Hydroxylase Deficiency (P450c21)

Mutations or deletions of the *CYP21* gene (6p21.3) account for over 90% of cases of CAH, with an incidence of 1 in 14,000 live births and a carrier frequency of 1 in 60. Both male and female infants have hyperpigmentation due to high ACTH levels, and subtle symptoms of adrenal insufficiency such as feeding intolerance and irritability are present early. The extent of virilization of female infants depends on the severity of the enzymatic defect (Figure 7-7). Although adrenal androgens are already elevated during the initial stages of sex differentiation at 8 to 10 weeks, complete masculinization of the external genitalia is rare. An enlarged phallus with the urethral opening on the shaft or at the base of the phallus and fused well-rugated labioscrotal folds are more common. The genitalia of affected males are imperceptibly affected; therefore, if newborn screening is unavailable, males present at 1 to 2 weeks of age in an acute adrenal crisis with emesis, hyponatremic dehydration, and hyperkalemia. Milder cases of CAH are sometimes missed at birth and present in early childhood with pubic hair, clitoromegaly or phallic growth, and accelerated linear growth. About 70% of infants with 21α-hydroxylase deficiency have significant salt wasting, which can cause rapid metabolic decompensation, lending urgency to the rapid diagnosis of infants with intersex conditions. Marked elevations of

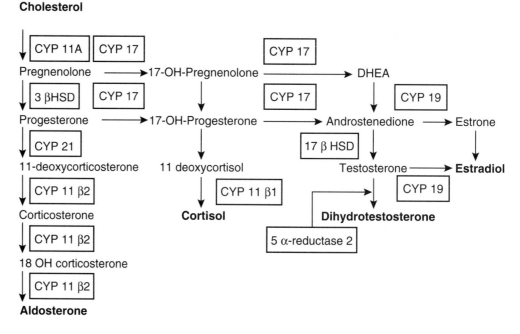

Figure 7-6 Sex Steroid Biosynthetic Pathway. The enzymatic steps necessary for the biosynthesis of aldosterone, cortisol, testosterone, and estradiol. Mutations in enzymes that impair cortisol synthesis lead to compensatory adrenal hyperplasia and signs of glucocorticoid deficiency, whereas mutations affecting only sex steroid production have minimal systemic symptoms.

CYP 11 β2 (11β hydroxylase, 18 hydroxylase, 18 oxidase)
CYP 17 (17α hydroxylase, 17,20 lyase)
CYP 19 (aromatase)

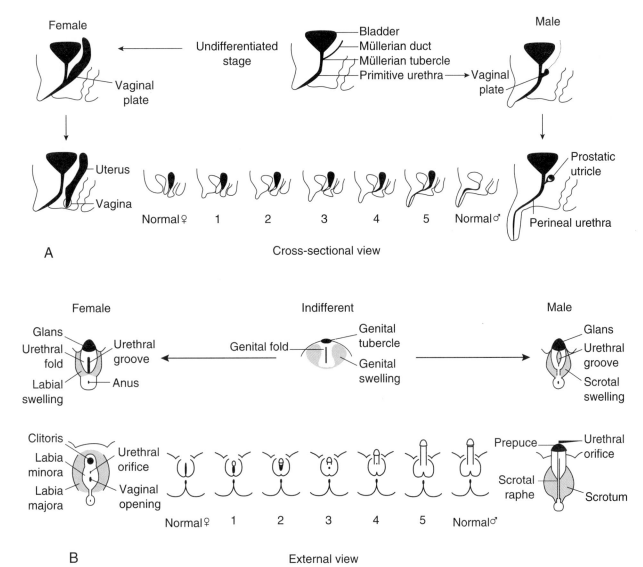

Figure 7-7   Virilization of the Urogenital Sinus and Genitalia in 46,XX Patients with Congenital Adrenal Hyperplasia. The varying degrees of virilization of the urogenital sinus and genitalia are depicted in the cross-sectional *(A)* and external *(B)* views and staged as proposed by Andrea Prader. Normal female and male sex differentiation are shown for comparison. (Redrawn with permission from White PC, Speiser PW: Congenital adrenal hyperplasia due to 21-hydroxylase deficiency, Endocr Rev 2000;21:245.)

17-hydroxyprogesterone, androstenedione, and testosterone are pathognomonic.

In infants with adrenal crisis, vigorous volume expansion with isotonic saline, followed by rehydration with 5% to 10% dextrose and 0.45% normal saline, and stress doses of intravenous steroids, rapidly stabilizes the clinical status. Glucocorticoid and mineralocorticoid replacement decreases androgen production by suppressing ACTH secretion and halts further virilization in infants and children. Clitoromegaly becomes less obvious over time as the labia majora and minora grow in size. Steroids are gradually tapered to physiological replacement doses of oral hydrocortisone (10-15 mg/m^2/day) in two or three divided doses. Fludrocortisone at a dosage of 0.05 to 0.2 mg/day is necessary in all children with salt-wasting forms of CAH (low sodium, high potassium, and high renin levels). Aldosterone deficiency can be subclinical in children with a diagnosis of simple virilizing CAH; thus, the addition of fludrocortisone may improve metabolic control and permit lower doses of hydrocortisone.

Other Virilizing Forms of Congenital Adrenal Hyperplasia

11β-Hydroxylase Deficiency

11β-hydroxylase deficiency, the second most common cause of CAH, has an incidence of 1 in 100,000. The clinical features of infants with defects in the *CYP11B1* gene (8q24.3) are similar to those with 21α-hydroxylase deficiency except for the development of low renin hypertension at older ages. The biochemical findings of elevated ACTH, 17-hydroxyprogesterone, androstenedione, and testosterone also overlap, but 11-deoxycortisol and 11-deoxycorticosterone are disproportionately elevated in this disorder. At high concentrations, 11-deoxycorticosterone binds to the mineralocorticoid receptor and causes hypertension.

3β-Hydroxysteroid Dehydrogenase Deficiency

Defects in the *HSD3B2* gene (1p13.1) result in deficiency of 3β-hydroxysteroid dehydrogenase (3β-HSD), an enzyme necessary for synthesis of cortisol, aldosterone, and sex steroids. This disorder is associated with mild virilization in affected females due to peripheral conversion of the elevated dehydroepiandrosterone (DHEA) to androgens. In contrast to 21-hydroxylase and 11-hydroxylase deficiencies, 3β-HSD deficiency affects testosterone synthesis; therefore, males are undervirilized. Elevated DHEA, dehydroepiandrosterone sulfate (DHEAS), and 17-hydroxypregnenolone and a markedly increased ratio of 17-hydroxypregnenolone to 17-hydroxyprogesterone are diagnostic.

Aromatase Deficiency

Aromatase deficiency (*CYP19* gene, 15q21.1) is a rare autosomal recessive cause of virilization in 46,XX individuals. Aromatase converts in utero fetal and maternal adrenal androgens to estrogens; a deficiency of either placental or fetal aromatase activity causes elevated circulating androgens and severe virilization of the fetal genitalia. With placental aromatase deficiency, the mother also becomes progressively virilized during the pregnancy.

In Utero Exposure to Androgens or Progestational Agents

A less common cause of virilization in a 46,XX infant is in utero exposure to androgens of nonfetal origin. No medical therapy is necessary for the infant, as removal from the intrauterine milieu eliminates the source of the androgens. Maternal use of androgens or drugs with androgenic potency such as progestational agents or some anticonvulsants has been implicated in fetal virilization. Maternal and fetal virilization can also be caused by arrhenoblastomas and other rare androgen-secreting ovarian and adrenal tumors. The minor elevations in testosterone associated with hyperthecosis or polycystic ovarian syndrome seldom cause fetal virilization because of efficient placental aromatization of androgens to estrogens.

Undervirilization in a Genetic Male (Male Pseudohermaphroditism)

Male sex differentiation is a complex process that depends on the active secretion and interaction of two testicular hormones and the responsiveness of their target tissues; consequently, the differential diagnosis of undervirilization in genetic males encompasses a heterogeneous group of disorders. Any perturbation in androgen action during the period of sex differentiation or phallic enlargement can impair genital virilization in a child with a 46,XY karyotype and normally formed testes. The timing and extent of androgen exposure and action are both critical for complete masculinization of the internal and external genitalia. In most cases of genital ambiguity due to inadequate virilization in genetic males, only the androgen pathway is affected; MIS expression and induction of müllerian duct regression is intact. Müllerian remnants may persist, however, because androgens are needed to potentiate MIS action for complete involution of the müllerian ducts. In evaluating an undervirilized genetic male, several clinical points are important to keep in mind: (1) the severity of the genital ambiguity can vary within a single diagnosis, (2) the clinical phenotype is often indistinguishable among different etiologies for the genital ambiguity, and (3) the diagnostic evaluation is frequently inconclusive without identification of a specific etiological condition (Table 7-1).

Defects in Testosterone Biosynthesis

An enzymatic defect in any of the enzymes required for testosterone biosynthesis can attenuate testosterone production and compromise full virilization of the genitalia. Some of these enzymatic defects also disrupt cortisol synthesis and cause CAH, whereas others are specific to the testosterone pathway (see Figure 7-6). The disorders associated with a defect in the cortisol biosynthetic pathway are treated by replacement of glucocorticoids and mineralocorticoids (discussed earlier). Among the conditions that cause inadequate virilization, sex steroids are necessary at puberty for secondary sexual maturation in all cases.

Congenital lipoid adrenal hyperplasia is a rare disorder that results from a mutation in the gene coding for steroidogenic acute regulatory protein (*StAR*) (8p11.2). Formerly attributed to a deficiency of the side chain cleavage enzyme (P450scc), only one family has been identified with a mutation in this gene; most patients who have been studied have loss of function mutations or deletions of *StAR*. The loss of *StAR* activity results in the inability of cholesterol to be transported from the outer to the inner mitochondrial membrane, an essential step for the acute, stimulated synthesis of all gonadal and adrenal steroids.

Consequently, cholesterol lipids accumulate in steroidogenic cells of the adrenal cortex and the gonads and further damage these cells, hindering basal synthesis of steroids as well. Affected males are severely undervirilized to the extent that the external genitalia may appear female or only minimally ambiguous, the wölffian structures are hypoplastic, and the testes are undescended. The vagina ends in a blind pouch because the müllerian ducts regress normally. Affected females have normal genitalia so the condition may not be recognized at birth. If undiagnosed, severe acute adrenal insufficiency causes rapid metabolic decompensation, and early death is not uncommon. ACTH is elevated, but all steroids and steroid precursors are low. Full steroid replacement with both glucocorticoids and mineralocorticoids is necessary for this and the following two disorders. Because of the female-appearing genitalia, 46,XY males with this condition usually undergo orchiectomy and are reared as females. At puberty, estrogen is given for breast development and low-dose testosterone can be used to promote growth of pubic and axillary hair.

3β-Hydroxysteroid dehydrogenase deficiency (HSD3B2) is associated with male undervirilization; the phallus is typically small with incomplete scrotal fusion and hypospadias. Affected 46,XX females are partially virilized. The defect in this enzyme compromises testosterone production with resultant low serum testosterone. DHEA is elevated and can be converted peripherally to androgens to cause virilization of affected patients. 17-hydroxypregnenolone is elevated, thereby increasing the ratio of 17-hydroxypregnenolone to 17-hydroxyprogesterone.

17α-Hydroxylase/lyase deficiency due to a mutation in the *CYP17* gene (10q24.3) affects conversion of 17-hydroxypregnenolone to DHEA, a precursor in the sex steroid pathway. The decreased production of testosterone causes genital ambiguity in genetic males. Although 17α-hydroxylase/lyase is also necessary for cortisol and aldosterone production, adrenal insufficiency is often subclinical due to elevated precursor steroids. At high concentrations, corticosterone has glucocorticoid activity and 11-deoxycorticosterone has mineralocorticoid activity. Moreover, the enzymatic properties of this bifunctional enzyme can be differentially affected and are modulated by cofactors.

17β-Hydroxysteroid dehydrogenase deficiency is an autosomal recessive condition caused by mutations in the *17β-HSD3* gene (9q22). The conversion of androstenedione to testosterone is impaired, leading to ambiguous or female genitalia. Considerable virilization may occur at puberty from peripheral conversion of androstenedione to testosterone. A milder late-onset form presents with pubertal gynecomastia in an adolescent with a normal male phe-notype. An abnormally high ratio of androstenedione to testosterone in response to hCG stimulation is diagnostic. In an affected female, the elevated DHEA and androstenedione can be metabolized to an active androgen to cause significant virilization.

5α-Reductase-2 deficiency, also referred to as pseudovaginal perineal-scrotal hypospadias, is an autosomal recessive disorder caused by mutations of the *SRD5A2* gene (2p23). This enzyme reduces testosterone to its more active metabolite, dihydrotestosterone (DHT), at target tissues. DHT is required for male sex differentiation of the external genitalia and for growth of facial hair. In this disorder, the external genitalia are ambiguous (perineoscrotal hypospadias and microphallus), a urogenital sinus and pseudovagina are generally present, and spermatogenesis is impaired in the cryptorchid testes. Development of the internal structures is unaffected because DHT is not required: the wölffian ducts differentiate fully in response to testosterone and the müllerian ducts undergo normal regression. The external genitalia become virilized during puberty and fertility is possible. An elevated ratio of testosterone to DHT (T/DHT) is diagnostic. In prepubertal children, the basal ratio may be normal, but the hCG-stimulated ratio should increase. DHT values are between 5 and 60 ng/dL at birth in males and then decrease rapidly in the first week of life. From 30 to 60 days, DHT increases transiently to 12 to 85 ng/dL and then decreases a few months later to the prepubertal range (<3 ng/dL). Values in females are up to 15 ng/dL at birth and decrease rapidly to less than 3 ng/dL. The normal T/DHT ratio is less than 12 at birth and then decreases to 5 until 6 months of age. During childhood, a higher ratio of 11 is observed. In adults, the normal T/DHT ratio is 8 to 16, and affected males usually have a ratio greater than 36.

Sex assignment is a challenge in children diagnosed with this disorder. The extent of in utero masculinization and the T/DHT ratio in early infancy are useful indicators of enzymatic activity, but significant virilization can occur at puberty. At that time, a number of 46,XY individuals raised as female are reported to have successfully switched to a male gender role in the Dominican Republic. Hence, male gender assignment may be preferable even when the genitalia are ambiguous. Topical administration of DHT (25 mg/day, 2% by weight in a cold cream base) increases phallic length, but the product is not easily available. Pharmacological doses of testosterone can be converted by the type 1 nongenital 5α-reductase isozyme to normalize DHT levels and induce further virilization. Males may require extensive surgical repair; however, postponing surgery until the effects of pubertal androgens are known and the individual can participate in the decision-making process may be prudent.

Leydig Cell Hypoplasia (Inactivating Mutations of the Luteinizing Hormone Receptor)

Leydig cell hypoplasia is a rare autosomal recessive disorder caused by an inactivating mutation of the lutropin-chorionic gonadotropin receptor (LCGR). The phenotype is similar to that of a severe testosterone biosynthetic defect. The external genitalia are female or ambiguous and gonads are undescended. Müllerian regression is complete but wölffian structures are hypoplastic or absent. Leydig cells are absent in prepubertal patients and either absent or reduced in number at puberty. The serum testosterone is low and fails to rise with hCG stimulation. In contrast to testosterone biosynthetic defects, no precursor steroids are elevated.

In severe forms, sex assignment is usually female. Gonadectomy is performed and estrogen replacement begun at puberty. The extent of masculinization of the genitalia can be used as a parameter of central nervous system exposure to androgens and capacity for testosterone production. In those individuals who are raised as males, testosterone therapy is started at puberty to increase phallic size and induce secondary sexual maturation.

Androgen-Insensitivity Syndromes

Androgen-insensitivity syndrome (AIS), the most frequently identified cause of undervirilization in a genetic male, has an incidence of 1 in 20,000 live male births. AIS is caused by loss of function mutations or deletions of the androgen receptor (Xq11-12) (see Figure 7-5). The phenotype varies from normal female genitalia due to total unresponsiveness to androgens to subfertility in a fully virilized adult man with a mild defect. There may be a family history of female relatives with delayed menarche, primary amenorrhea, and/or sparse sexual hair or of male relatives with gynecomastia, hypospadias, or infertility.

Complete Androgen-Insensitivity Syndrome

The 46,XY individuals with complete androgen-insensitivity syndrome (CAIS) manifest as phenotypic females with female external genitalia, sometimes with an underdeveloped clitoris or labia minora, a short blind-ending vagina that is generally sufficient for coitus, and no uterus. Symmetrical inguinal (60%) gonads are often palpated, although gonads may also be labial (7%) or intra-abdominal (15%). Müllerian structures are absent, although in up to one third of cases a rudimentary uterus or other anlagen persists. Wölffian derivatives are poorly differentiated.

CAIS is diagnosed in the newborn period only when bilateral masses are palpated in the labia or inguinal canals of an infant with female genitalia or if the phenotype at birth is discordant with a prenatal karyotype of 46,XY. Many cases are diagnosed in an adolescent girl who presents with primary amenorrhea, absent or sparse pubic and axillary hair, and normal breast development. The breasts are often well developed, whereas the nipples may be juvenile. During infancy, the hormonal profile is similar to that of male infants. At puberty, FSH is normal or slightly elevated, and LH is elevated. Testosterone is in the high-normal male range and estrogen is intermediate between normal male and female ranges. Peripheral aromatization of testosterone to estrogen is responsible for the breast development. Androgen receptor binding activity, assessed in cultured genital skin fibroblasts, is usually absent in CAIS. Western blot analysis can confirm the absence of androgen receptor protein, and mutational analysis of the androgen receptor gene is definitive but not readily available.

Bilateral orchiectomy is recommended because the overall incidence of gonadal malignancy is about 9%. Some prefer leaving the testes intact during pubertal maturation to allow spontaneous feminization from peripheral conversion of testosterone to estrogen. Orchiectomy is then performed and estrogen replacement started. However, malignant transformation of the gonads during childhood has been reported, so we support early orchiectomy. Moreover, if inguinal hernia repair is necessary, removal of the testes at that time avoids a second surgical procedure.

Partial Androgen-Insensitivity Syndrome

Partial androgen-insensitivity syndrome (PAIS) results in a spectrum of disorders that ranges from a female phenotype with clitoromegaly and/or minimal posterior labial fusion (Lub syndrome) to genital ambiguity with an intermediate-sized phallus, urogenital sinus, labioscrotal folds with or without rugation, and posterior fusion (Gilbert-Dreyfus syndrome) to a male phenotype with microphallus, perineal hypospadias, cryptorchidism, and/or bifid scrotum (Reifenstein syndrome) to an unequivocally male phenotype with a minor defect such as isolated hypospadias or azoospermia. Wölffian structures are not fully differentiated, whereas müllerian structures are absent. Puberty is characterized by virilization of the external genitalia, growth of sexual hair, and significant gynecomastia. The clinical phenotype varies considerably even within families bearing the same genetic mutation.

The phenotype resembles that of 17β-hydroxysteroid dehydrogenase deficiency, but the ratio of androstenedione to testosterone is normal. Testosterone, estradiol, and LH are normal or high; FSH is usually normal. Less than half of patients with suspected PAIS have abnormal androgen binding. Those with normal receptor binding activity may have a defect in DNA binding or transcriptional activation. Identification of a mutation in the coding region of the androgen receptor gene is diagnostic, but mutational analysis is not available commercially. Moreover, mutations have been identified in only two thirds of patients with suspected PAIS. Thus, PAIS is often a presumptive diagnosis when other etiologies have been excluded.

In PAIS, the severity of the phenotype is often the basis for gender assignment because it reflects the degree of androgen resistance and may provide an estimate of central nervous system androgenization. Assessment of phallic growth in response to a short course of testosterone is often useful when a male sex of rearing is contemplated. If virilization occurs, the testes can be left in place, and reconstructive surgery such as hypospadias repair or orchidopexy performed as appropriate. When there is no response to testosterone, a female gender assignment should be considered.

Mild Androgen-Insensitivity Syndrome

Mild androgen-insensitivity syndrome (MAIS) manifests as impaired spermatogenesis and infertility or subfertility in conjunction with gynecomastia, sparse pubic hair, and minimally reduced testicular volume. The same mutation can cause PAIS or MAIS. Kennedy syndrome is a form of MAIS associated with spinobulbar motor neuropathy in which pubertal gynecomastia is followed by decreased libido and impotence and later, in the 40s and 50s, by testicular atrophy, impaired spermatogenesis, oligospermia, and infertility. However, because the testicular atrophy is a late occurrence, many males with this syndrome father children.

Genetics of Androgen-Insensitivity Syndrome

Mutations in the androgen receptor gene can be identified by standard DNA sequencing techniques and by single-strand conformational polymorphism/polymerase chain reaction, but the genotype–phenotype correlation is poor except for gene deletions associated with CAIS, and mutations in the coding region are not found in 25% to 30% of patients with suspected AIS. Complete deletion of the gene accounts for 1%, and partial deletions account for 4% of identified genetic defects. The majority (>90%) are point mutations. The same point mutation may have variable expression within a family pedigree. This has been attributed to genetic background factors such as coregulatory proteins or to somatic mosaicism.

The effect of mutations in different domains of the androgen receptor on androgen binding and signaling, however, has been well characterized. The first of the eight exons encodes the N-terminal fragment and has a role in transcriptional activation. Nearly all mutations in exon 1 cause premature termination of translation and CAIS. This region has two homopolymeric amino acid repeats that are polymorphic in size: polyglutamine (9-36 repeats) and polyglycine (10-31 repeats). Kennedy syndrome, a motor neuropathy associated with MAIS, results from expansion of the polyglutamine tract beyond 38 repeats. Mutations of exons 2 and 3, the receptor DNA binding domain (composed of two zinc-containing fingers), interfere with DNA binding but androgen binding is preserved. Exons 5 to 8, the most frequent site for missense mutations, encode the ligand binding domain. These mutations either completely disrupt androgen binding or alter binding affinity such that higher concentrations of androgens are necessary for receptor activation. A small hinge region between the DNA and ligand binding domains may be important for receptor activation.

Persistent Müllerian Duct Syndrome

The persistent müllerian duct syndrome (PMDS) is an autosomal recessive disorder characterized by well-developed müllerian duct derivatives in 46,XY males with cryptorchid testes and otherwise normal male internal and external genitalia. Because the external genitalia are fully virilized, this condition is a variant of normal development and not usually considered an intersex condition. Transverse testicular ectopia in a child with unilateral cryptorchidism and an inguinal hernia is a common presentation of PMDS (80%). The uterus, fallopian tubes, and both testes are found in a hernial sac. Alternatively, PMDS can present as bilateral cryptorchidism with the uterus and tubes in the abdomen and intra-abdominal testes in the round or broad ligaments. The testes are hypermobile and have an increased risk of torsion and malignant changes. Fertility appears to be reduced because of inadequate communication of the testes with male excretory ducts, complications of orchiopexy, or the cryptorchid state.

The diagnosis generally arises during an evaluation for cryptorchidism or when müllerian structures are observed during abdominal or pelvic surgery. Serum MIS is undetectable or low in cases caused by gene defects but normal with receptor defects. However, an undetectable MIS in a child with bilateral cryptorchidism is also consistent with anorchia or vanishing testes. The diagnosis of PMDS can be made by performing an hCG stimulation test. A normal rise in testosterone is consistent with PMDS, and an absent response is predictive of anorchia. A sonogram of the pelvis to identify müllerian structures is also helpful. Early orchidopexy should be performed to optimize testicular function. The fallopian tubes and uterus are excised carefully to avoid compromising blood supply to the testes and damaging the vas deferens, which is usually embedded in the lateral uterine wall and cervix.

Almost 50% of patients with PMDS have mutations in the MIS gene (19p), most commonly in exons 1 and 5. Another 40% have mutations in the gene for the MIS receptor; 50% of these have a common 27-bp deletion in exon 10. Up to 15% of patients with PMDS have no discernible mutations in the coding sequences for either the MIS gene or receptor.

Gonadotropin, Growth Hormone, or Human Chorionic Gonadotropin Deficiency

Gonadotropin deficiency and placental insufficiency have both been associated with cryptorchidism and microphallus. During sex differentiation, testosterone synthesis is initially gonadotropin independent; thus, midline fusion and differentiation of the genitalia proceed normally. By the second trimester, testosterone secretion by the Leydig cells is probably regulated by LH or hCG. A deficiency in either hormone leads to inadequate production of androgens during the period of penile growth and may manifest as microphallus. A similar phenotype is seen with GH deficiency as GH potentiates the effects of androgens on phallic growth.

Miscellaneous Causes of Undervirilization

The Smith-Lemli-Opitz syndrome due to a mutation of the sterol-Δ7-reductase gene (11q12-q13) leads to failure to thrive, genital ambiguity, and congenital abnormalities in brain, heart, lung, and kidney development. The genital ambiguity may be severe or present as isolated hypospadias. This enzyme is necessary for the synthesis of cholesterol, a precursor for all steroid hormone production, including androgens. A deficiency of this enzyme leads to low steroids and increased 7-dehydro-cholesterol, the immediate precursor to cholesterol.

Congenital Embryopathy

Anomalies of urogenital development that are independent of the karyotype and gonadal hormone action may occur during embryogenesis, frequently in association with other congenital anomalies. In these cases, the gonads are concordant with the karyotype. Examples are penoscrotal transposition, penile agenesis with imperforate anus, bifid phallus with bladder extrophy, and vaginal anomalies. The 46,XX infants are typically raised as females, whereas sex assignment in 46,XY infants traditionally depended on genital anatomy and the potential for function after corrective surgery. However, an equally important consideration in this decision may be the influence of fetal androgens on gender identity, as demonstrated by recent case reports of 46,XY infants with cloacal extrophy who were raised as girls but desired sex reassignment at adolescence. The appropriate sex assignment of infants in this category is being readdressed and is an area of much controversy and debate.

Hypospadias occurs if fusion of the penile urethra is incomplete. This is one of the most common congenital anomalies, occurring in 4 to 8 of 1000 liveborn male infants. First-degree hypospadias with the urethral opening on the glans penis is not usually associated with other urogenital anomalies and seldom requires extensive evaluation or correction. More severe forms with the urethral opening along the shaft or the base of the penis or on the perineum warrant investigation for underlying intersex conditions, particularly if associated anomalies are present. Although most cases are multifactorial in origin, mild PAIS and sex chromosome abnormalities can present as isolated hypospadias. Maternal intake of progestational agents, maternal cocaine use, and exposure to environmental estrogens and antiandrogens have all been implicated.

Both vaginal atresia and müllerian aplasia (Rokitansky-Kuster-Hauser syndrome) present as primary amenorrhea in adolescents with normal breast and pubic hair development. The karyotype is 46,XX, and hormonal profiles are normal with intact ovaries. These developmental defects may be familial. Specific gene defects are starting to be identified, such as one family with müllerian aplasia due to a defect in the gene for hepatic transcription factor 2.

EVALUATION

Any divergence in development of the external genitalia from the norm may indicate an intersex condition. The diagnosis of an intersex condition is unequivocal in an infant with a phallus intermediate in length between normal standards for a clitoris and penis (6.4 mm to 2.2 cm at birth), incomplete fusion of the labioscrotal folds, an aberrantly located urethral opening, and nonpalpable gonads. The finding of an abnormal phallic size or labioscrotal fusion alone is considered a genital anomaly associated with an underlying intersex condition, but cryptorchidism or hypospadias may be isolated findings without such association. On the other hand, intersex conditions may also present without any genital ambiguity as exemplified by children with CAIS or pure gonadal dysgenesis.

The finding of ambiguous genitalia in a newborn is psychologically stressful for the family and requires prompt attention by an experienced team that includes an endocrinologist, an urologist or a pediatric surgeon, a child psychiatrist or psychologist, and the family's pediatrician. Involvement of clergy and introduction to support groups or other families with similar issues are helpful for emotional support. Parents should be shown the genitalia of their baby and reassured that although the genitalia are incompletely formed or overly developed, the condition occurs as part of a developmental process, similar to other more common congenital anomalies. Parents should be made aware of the difficulty in determining the appropriate sex assignment for their infant until the evaluation is complete and kept fully informed of the progress of the diagnostic work-up. A systematic and thorough evaluation using a multidisciplinary approach to diagnosis and management is essential. Although most conditions are not medically urgent, timely recognition of a common cause of genital ambiguity, salt-wasting CAH, circumvents life-threatening decompensation.

History and Examination

The evaluation starts with a detailed history that should include exposure to androgenic and progestational agents in intrauterine life, maternal virilizing symptoms, and family history of ambiguous genitalia, unexplained infant deaths, primary amenorrhea, infertility, and inguinal hernias with prolapsed gonads. The physical examination should focus on identifying syndromic features, determining the position of the gonads, and establishing the genital anatomy. Asymmetrical positioning of the gonads is suggestive of asymmetrical development of the gonads as seen with disorders in gonadal morphogenesis. Any gonad palpated below the external inguinal ring is presumed to contain testicular tissue; ovarian tissue without any testicular components rarely descends below the inguinal ring. For example, infants with true hermaphroditism may have an abdominal ovary and a testis or an ovotestis in the scrotum or labial folds. The size of the phallus, position of the urethral opening, extent of chordae, and development of the labioscrotal folds are noted. The uterus, when present, is sometimes palpable on gentle rectal examination as a firm, midline, pencil-sized structure. Genital pigmentation may be due to hypersecretion of ACTH associated with CAH.

Laboratory Studies

Cytogenetic analysis with high-resolution banding should be performed in all infants and children with ambiguous genitalia. The sex chromosomes can be specifically examined by fluorescent in situ hybridization (FISH) using centromeric probes for the X chromosome and centromeric or long arm probes for the Y chromosome. FISH for *SRY* may be helpful in patients with sex reversal. Molecular studies are also available in research laboratories to identify genetic mutations in many of the genes involved in sex differentiation. This includes, but is not limited to, *SOX 9, DAX-1,* and *SF-1* genes in the steroidogenic pathway for cortisol and testosterone biosynthesis, MIS and its receptor, 5α-reductase, and the receptors for androgens and LH (see Table 7-1).

If CAH is a possibility, electrolytes should be followed closely, and 17-hydoxyprogesterone and other adrenal precursors are measured to delineate specific enzymatic deficiencies. If the enzymatic defect is severe enough to cause genital abnormality, basal steroid values and ratios should be abnormal. Occasionally, measurement of adrenal steroid precursors after stimulation with 125 to 250 µg of ACTH is needed to confirm a diagnosis. The inclusion of 17-OH-progesterone in the newborn screen in most states allows early diagnosis of virilizing CAH infants who are not recognized clinically.

The sexually dimorphic expression of MIS in prepubertal children makes it useful for identifying testicular tissue in children with intersex conditions. Unlike testosterone, MIS is produced only in the gonads. Serum MIS concentrations are high in prepubertal males and low in females, with no overlap in values before the age of 6 years (Figure 7-8). Although the range of values starts to overlap at this time, mean values in older children are still clearly distinguishable (43 ng/mL in boys and 2.7 ng/mL in girls). Consequently, in young boys, an MIS value within the male range is predictive of testicular tissue. Conversely, except for rare cases of PMDS, an undetectable MIS value is highly predictive for absent testicular tissue. Moreover, MIS values

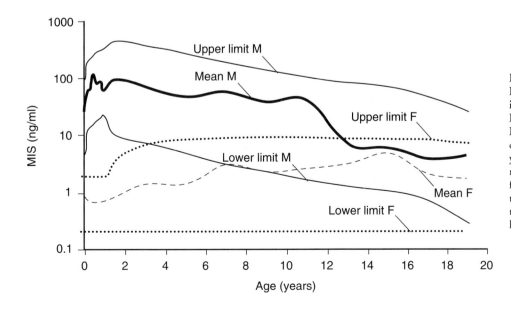

Figure 7-8   Serum Müllerian Inhibiting Substance (MIS) Values in Males and Females (Solid Black Line) and Girls (Broken Black Line). Serum MIS values are easily distinguishable in the prepubertal years between males and females with no overlap in values within the first few years of life. In contrast to testosterone, which is also secreted by the adrenal, MIS is a gonad-specific hormone.

correlate with the extent of parenchymal tissue and may be helpful for distinguishing among different intersex diagnoses. A low MIS value is suggestive of a dysgenetic or hypoplastic testicular tissue associated with a disorder of morphogenesis. An MIS value in the normal or elevated male range is consistent with a structurally intact testis as seen in disorders of testosterone biosynthesis or androgen insensitivity.

Assessment of testosterone is valuable for determining the etiology of an undervirilized genetic male but may not help with initial differential diagnosis. Serum testosterone concentrations in 46,XX girls with CAH can be elevated to a range that is indistinguishable from that of newborn males. In infants with disorders of morphogenesis, serum testosterone is quite variable: low with dysgenetic gonads and low or normal with ovotestes. In virilized genetic males, measurement of testosterone, DHT, and testosterone precursors helps identify testicular enzymatic defects or androgen insensitivity.

Basal testosterone values adequately reflect androgen production only during early infancy when testosterone production transiently increases. At birth, testosterone values in males are elevated (75-400 ng/dL) but decrease within a few days to 20 to 50 ng/dL. From 4 to 12 weeks of life, testosterone levels rise to 100 to 400 ng/dL. By 6 months, testosterone declines to the prepubertal values of less than 10 ng/dL. In females, serum testosterone is lower at birth (20-65 ng/dL) than that of males and then decreases further during the first month to comparable prepubertal values of less than 10 ng/dL. During much of childhood, serum testosterone values are low and indistinguishable between males and females. With puberty, testosterone values gradually increase in males to the normal adult range of 300 to 1000 ng/dL and remain in the much lower range of 10 to 50 ng/dL in females.

The low testosterone values during late infancy and childhood make it difficult to assess androgen biosynthetic capacity to differentiate between an ovary and testis. Stimulation with hCG is required for an adequate estimate of testicular function in the prepubertal testis. We administer hCG at a dosage of 1500 unit/m² on days 1 and 3 and measure testosterone levels at baseline and on days 3 and 6. A doubling of testosterone values from baseline to day 3 and again from day 3 to day 6, with a peak testosterone greater than 50 ng/dL, is indicative of functional testicular tissue. A number of other protocols for hCG stimulation have been proposed, including a single dose of hCG, daily hCG administration for 5 days, or every other day for 1 week to 3 weeks; all serve to increase testosterone production. In prepubertal children, the Leydig cells are relatively refractory; thus, two injections of hCG may not sufficiently stimulate androgen production. A prolonged stimulation test with administration of hCG every other day for 2 to 6 weeks may be needed to adequately assess the capacity for androgen synthesis.

A robust rise in testosterone is observed with AIS and 5α-reductase deficiency and a minimal increment is noted in testosterone biosynthetic defects or disorders of morphogenesis. No rise is observed with LH receptor defects or gonadal agenesis or in virilized genetic females. Androstenedione, DHEA, and DHT are also measured to assess sequential steps in the androgen pathway.

The addition of gonadotropin measurements provides an index of the hypothalamic-pituitary-gonadal axis. Both LH and FSH are secreted in a pulsatile pattern; thus, basal values are usually of limited use unless elevated. At birth, LH abruptly rises almost 10-fold in male infants, stimulating a rise in testosterone in the first 3 hours of life. Within the first 24 hours, LH decreases to low values until 2 weeks of age, when it starts to rise transiently and peaks at 2 months. By 6 months, LH again declines to low prepubertal values. In male infants, the pulse amplitude of LH is much higher than that of FSH, resulting in stimulation of testosterone synthesis in the first few months. In female infants, the greater FSH pulse amplitude stimulates increased estrogen secretion during the first 2 to 3 years of age.

During infancy and puberty, when the hypothalamic-pituitary-gonadal axis is active, gonadotropins are responsive to negative feedback by sex steroids. As a result, FSH and LH increase when testosterone is deficient, whether due to an enzymatic defect or to absent or dysgenetic gonads. Elevated gonadotropins at these periods are therefore indicative of either absent gonads or deficient androgen action. During the remainder of childhood, however, gonadotropins are in a low prepubertal range and remain low even in children with gonadal dysgenesis or anorchia. Consequently, gonadotropins are helpful diagnostically when elevated but less useful if in the normal prepubertal range.

The diagnostic work-up sometimes includes a short trial of depot testosterone to assess the response of the phallus to testosterone; this is particularly useful in infants with PAIS. Genital tissue biopsy for androgen receptor binding studies is helpful if AIS is suspected. In some cases, gonadal biopsy is necessary for diagnosis or to detect gonadoblastoma or carcinoma in situ. Laparoscopy may be needed to identify and remove dysgenetic testes.

Imaging Studies

Imaging studies to define the internal genitalia are an essential aspect of the evaluation for an intersex condition. A pelvic ultrasound may be able to identify abdominal gonads and müllerian structures, especially in the hands of an experienced operator. Transrectal sonography is being used in some centers to improve resolution. Magnetic resonance imaging may better define the anatomy of the vagina, cervix, and müllerian structures and is more sensitive for localizing the gonads. However, both sonography and magnetic resonance imaging can miss small ectopic gonads. A retrograde genitogram helps delineate the anatomy of the urogenital sinus and the entry of the vagina and urethra. This is sometimes performed in conjunction with a cystoscopic examination.

MANAGEMENT OF AND TREATMENT OPTIONS FOR INTERSEX DISORDERS

Classically, rapid sex assignment and early surgical correction to match the gender of rearing have been advocated. A key consideration in sex assignment was the potential for future sexual and reproductive function, keeping in mind the etiology, the anatomy of the genitalia, and the limitations of reconstructive surgery. This emphasis on genital anatomy and function was based on a fundamental assumption of gender neutrality in infancy, which has been questioned. The appearance of the external genitalia was also believed to affect the establishment of gender identity. Recent reports suggest that in utero androgen imprinting of the fetal brain may also be critical for establishing gender identity. Moreover, genetic and hormonal events during childhood and puberty may affect gender identity and adult sexuality. Therefore, fetal and postnatal virilization of the central nervous system has become an important additional consideration for sex assignment.

Diamond and Sigmundson have recommended male sex assignment for 46,XY infants with mild PAIS, isolated hypospadias or microphallus, 5α-reductase or 17β-reductase deficiency, and severely virilized 46,XX infants with CAH. Female sex assignment is recommended for 46,XY infants with CAIS, severe PAIS, pure gonadal dysgenesis and less-virilized 46,XX infants with CAH. Sex assignment in conditions such as mixed gonadal dysgenesis and true hermaphroditism depends on the size of the phallus and the extent of labioscrotal fusion. The mean and the −2 SDs for stretched penile length are 3.8 and 3.0 cm for a male term infant and 3.0 and 2.3 cm for an infant born at 34 weeks, respectively. Standards are also available for very low birth weight (VLBW) and extremely low birth weight (ELBW) infants. An extremely small phallus with minimal corporal tissue raises concerns about the phallic response to androgens and a comparable lack of fetal central nervous system virilization. Although these recommendations provide useful guidelines, many cases do not fit neatly into one of these categories, and each infant must be evaluated individually.

After the diagnostic evaluation is complete, sex assignment should be made thoughtfully by consensus decision of the team, and discussed in depth with the family.

When a child presents with ambiguous genitalia after early infancy, the previously assigned sex is usually supported. Sex reassignment is considered only when the gender identity of the child is discordant with the assigned sex.

The timing of urogenital reconstructive surgery is highly controversial. The traditional approach advocates early surgical repair to enable concordance of the external genitalia with the gender of rearing. Clitoral recession, labioscrotal reduction, and vaginal exteriorization performed as a one-step procedure during infancy eliminates the trauma of repeated surgical procedures. In recent years, however, there has been a move toward delaying surgery because of limited long-term data on the psychological outcome of early versus late surgery and concerns regarding impairment of genital sensation. Proponents of this approach argue that urogenital reconstructive surgery is a cosmetic procedure that should be postponed until the child is able to provide informed consent. Moreover, some individuals with intersex conditions request sex reassignment as young adults, lending further credence to the need to reevaluate traditional approaches regarding urogenital reconstructive surgery. A compromise solution until long-term data is available is to assign sex early but to postpone surgery until a consensus is reached among the family members and medical care providers regarding the ultimate gender identity and role of the individual patient.

If the assigned sex is male, a short course of testosterone can be given to promote phallic growth. Orchiopexy should be performed by 12 months of age to optimize testicular function and to facilitate monitoring for malignancies. Dysgenetic testes and ovotestes at increased risk of malignancy should be removed. Corrective surgery for hypospadias, chordae, or genital anomalies can be undertaken as a one-step procedure at 6 to 18 months of age but is not essential unless urinary function is compromised. Supplemental sex steroids are often necessary to induce puberty. Testosterone cypionate or enanthate at a dosage of 50 mg intramuscular monthly is begun at 12 to 14 years of age. The dose is increased by 25- to 50-mg increments every 6 to 12 months to achieve full masculinization over 3 years. Full replacement dose in adult males is 200 mg every 2 to 3 weeks. Testosterone can also be given via patch or cream (discussed in Chapter 6). Fertility is possible in men with secondary or tertiary gonadal insufficiency by treatment with pulsatile gonadotropin-releasing hormone or gonadotropins.

When the assigned sex is female, removal of testicular tissue or dysgenetic gonads at risk for malignancy is recommended and urogenital reconstructive surgery may be needed. Hormone replacement is necessary to induce pubertal maturation. Low-dose estrogen replacement is initiated in girls at 11 to 12 years of age as 0.3 mg conjugated estrogens every other day or 50 to 100 ng ethinyl estradiol/kg/day. The dose of estrogen is increased gradually every 6 to 12 months to achieve complete pubertal maturation in 2 to 3 years, when cyclical progesterone is added. Estrogen can also be delivered via transdermal patches (discussed in Chapter 6). A regimen of 20 μg ethinyl estradiol or 0.625 mg conjugated estrogens daily, with 5 to 10 mg medroxyprogesterone acetate added on days 15 to 28, or a low-dose contraceptive with comparable hormone doses maintains feminization and should protect against osteoporosis and cardiovascular disease. Progesterone decreases the risk of endometrial dysplasia in those with an uterus but is unnecessary in individuals without a uterus.

CONCLUSION

Despite major advances in the understanding of the pathophysiology of intersex conditions, the clinical management and long-term outcome of these complex conditions remain controversial and a focus of ongoing studies. Nevertheless, a comprehensive diagnostic evaluation and the involvement of an experienced multidisciplinary team are of utmost importance in the care of an infant or a child with an intersex condition. Although general principles and recommendations provide useful guidelines for the clinician, individual attention to the specific considerations for each child with one of these rare conditions facilitates his or her optimal management and helps ensure improved outcomes.

MAJOR POINTS

The embryo and gonad are initially undifferentiated. In male embryos, the induction of *SRY* initiates a transcriptional cascade of events that results in testis determination and consequent differentiation of the genitalia. In the absence of *SRY* expression, the gonad differentiates as an ovary and the genitalia are female in appearance.

Specific molecular defects of genes in the sex determination pathway cause abnormalities in sexual differentiation, primarily by disrupting formation of the bipotential gonad or complete testis determination, and can be associated with syndromic conditions.

In genetic males, the secretion of two hormones by the fetal testis is essential for normal male sexual differentiation of the internal and external genitalia. Müllerian inhibiting substance secreted by Sertoli cells induces regression of the müllerian ducts, the precursor of the female internal reproductive tract. Testosterone secreted by Leydig cells stimulates wölffian duct differentiation to form the male

MAJOR POINTS—Cont'd

reproductive tract. The testosterone is then converted to dihydrotestosterone to virilize the external genitalia.

In a genetic female, the müllerian ducts differentiate into the fallopian tubes, uterus, cervix, and upper vagina in the absence of müllerian inhibiting substance, and the wölffian ducts regress in the absence of testosterone. Endogenous or exogenous androgen exposure can virilize a genetic female to varying extents depending on the timing and extent of androgen exposure.

The most common cause of virilization in a genetic female is congenital adrenal hyperplasia caused by molecular defects in the gene for 21α-hydroxylase.

The most common cause of undervirilization in a genetic male is androgen insensitivity caused by molecular defects in the androgen receptor gene.

Asymmetry of gonadal position is often associated with a disorder of gonadal formation.

Ovarian tissue generally does not descend below the external inguinal ring. Therefore, a gonad palpable below the external inguinal ring implies that testicular tissue is present and excludes the diagnostic category of "a virilized genetic female."

If müllerian structures are present, the differential diagnosis would include a disorder of gonadal morphogenesis, a virilized genetic female, or the persistent müllerian duct syndrome. If müllerian structures are absent, implying normal Sertoli cell function, undervirilization of a genetic male due to a disorder restricted to the androgen pathway is likely. This includes conditions such as androgen insensitivity, testosterone biosynthetic defects, and inactivating mutations of the luteinizing hormone receptor.

Gender assignment and management can be a challenge and must be individualized for each patient. Management decisions should consider the etiology of the condition, appearance of the genitalia, potential androgen imprinting of the developing brain, ongoing effects of postnatal exposure to androgens, and psychosocial factors.

SUGGESTED READINGS

Achermann JC, Meeks JJ, Jameson JL: Phenotypic spectrum of mutations in DAX-1 and SF-1, Mol Cell Endocrinol 2001; 185:17.

Ahmed SF, Hughes IA: The genetics of male undermasculinization, Clin Endocrinol (Oxf) 2002;56:1.

Clarkson MJ, Harley VR: Sex with two SOX on: SRY and SOX9 in testis development, Trends Endocrinol Metab 2002;13:106.

Diamond M, Sigmundson HK: Management of intersexuality: guidelines for dealing with persons with ambiguous genitalia, Arch Pediatr Adolesc Med 1997;151:1046.

Grumbach MM, Conte FA: Disorders of sexual differentiation. In Larsen PR, Kronenberg HM, Melmed S, et al, editors: Williams' Textbook of Endocrinology, 10th ed, Philadelphia, 2003, WB Saunders.

Hughes IA: Mini-review: sex differentiation, Endocrinology 2001;142:3281.

Kaye CI, Cunniff C, Frias JL, et al: Evaluation of the newborn with developmental anomalies of the external genitalia, Pediatrics 2000;106:138.

Koopman P: Sry, Sox9 and mammalian sex determination. In Scherer G, Schmid M, editors: Genes and Mechanism in Vertebrate Sex Determination, Basel, Switzerland, 2001, Birkhauser Verlag.

Krob G, Braun A, Kuhnle U: True hermaphroditism: geographical distribution, clinical findings, chromosomes and gonadal histology, Eur J Pediatr 1994;153:2.

Lane AH, Lee MM: Mullerian inhibiting substance: a nontraditional marker of gonadal function, Curr Opin Endocrinol Diabetes 2001;8:296.

Lerman SE, McAleer IM, Kaplan GW: Sex assignment in cases of ambiguous genitalia and its outcome, Urology 2000;55:8.

McPhaul MJ: Molecular defects of the androgen receptor, Recent Prog Horm Res 2002;57:181.

Meyer-Bahlburg HFL: Gender and sexuality in classic congenital adrenal hyperplasia, Endocrinol Metab Clin North Am 2001;30:155.

Miller WL: Disorders of androgen biosynthesis, Semin Reprod Med 2002;20:205.

Muller J, Ritzen EM, Ivarsson SA, et al: Management of males with 45,X/46,XY gonadal dysgenesis, Horm Res 1999;52:11.

Quigley CA, De Bellis A, Marschke KB, et al: Androgen receptor defects: historical, clinical, and molecular perspectives, Endocr Rev 1995;16:271.

Sarafoglou KS, Ostrer H: Familial sex reversal: a review, J Clin Endocrinol Metab 2000;85:483.

Tilmann C, Capel B: Cellular and molecular pathways regulating mammalian sex determination, Recent Prog Horm Res 2002;57:1.

Tuladhar R, Davis PG, Batch J, et al: Establishment of a normal range of penile length in preterm infants, J Paediatr Child Health 1998;34:471.

Warne GL, Zajac JD: Disorders of sexual differentiation, Endocrinol Metab Clin North Am 1998;27:945.

White PC, Speiser WP: Congenital adrenal hyperplasia due to 21-hydroxylase deficiency, Endocr Rev 2000;21:245.

Wilson JD: Androgens, androgen receptors, and male gender role behavior, Horm Behav 2001;40:358.

GROWTH

Disorders of Growth

ADDA GRIMBERG

DIVA D. De LEÓN

INTRODUCTION

The scientific study of children's growth and development began with the publication of the first textbook on growth, *Wachstum der Menschen in die Lange* by Johann Augustin Stoeller, more than 270 years ago (1729). This textbook did not contain any record of actual measurements; the first real growth study was reported a few years later in a doctoral thesis by Christian Friedrich Jampert. Jampert measured and recorded the height, weight, and other dimensions of a series of boys and girls at the Royal Orphanage of Berlin, completing the first cross-sectional growth study (1754). Count Philibert Guéneau de Montebeillard established the first longitudinal study of height when he recorded the heights of his son from birth to 18 years (1759-1777). This record has been extensively used and cited throughout the years. Until the end of the 19th century, pediatric textbooks included little on the subject of growth. It was the introduction of pediatric endocrinology as a specialty, and especially the recognition of growth hormone (GH) deficiency (GHD), that gave more impetus to the clinical study of growth.

NORMAL PHYSIOLOGY

The Growth Hormone Axis

GH (somatotropin), the principal mediator of somatic growth in childhood, acts within an axis of both positive stimuli and negative feedback loops (Figure 8-1). GH is synthesized and secreted by the somatotrophs, which comprise about half the cells of the anterior pituitary gland. The anterior pituitary communicates directly with the hypothalamus through a special fenestrated portal circulation, the exception to the blood-brain barrier. The hypothalamic-pituitary unit is located at the base of the third ventricle,

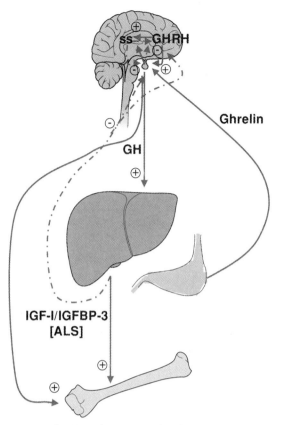

Figure 8-1   The Growth Hormone (GH) Axis. GH release by the pituitary gland is controlled by the hypothalamic factors somatostatin (ss) and growth hormone–releasing hormone (GHRH). It is also stimulated by ghrelin, which is produced in the stomach. GH stimulates hepatic production of the circulating 150-kDa complex, composed of insulin-like growth factor I (IGF-I), IGF binding protein-3 (IGFBP-3), and the acid-labile subunit (ALS). IGF-I provides negative feedback control to both the pituitary and hypothalamus. Stimulatory signals are presented by *solid arrows*; inhibitory, by *dashed arrows*.

The GH pulses reach their greatest amplitude during puberty, a central effect of estrogen in both genders. Similarly, circulating levels of GH in females peak at the time of ovulation due to the estrogen-stimulated increase in frequency of the GH pulses.

GH synthesis is itself highly regulated. Expression of the pituitary GH gene, one of five closely related genes on chromosome 17q22-24, requires the pituitary transcriptional factor, Pit1. It is also stimulated by GHRH and thyroid hormone (T_3) and repressed by cortisol. Somatostatin does not affect GH synthesis, only its secretion. During transcription, alternative mRNA splicing results in 22- and 20-kDa GH isoforms, both of which circulate and stimulate linear growth.

GH circulates bound to serum binding proteins, especially the GH-binding protein (GHBP), which is the extracellular domain of the GH receptor (GHR). GH is released from the circulation to bind to its receptor, GHR, located in multiple target tissues and primarily the liver. A member of the cytokine receptor superfamily, GHR is a single-chain glycoprotein with a single transmembrane domain that activates the intracellular JAK/STAT signaling pathway. The number of hepatic GHRs increases postnatally, during puberty, and during pregnancy, another effect of estrogen. In addition to modulation of the number of GHRs, GH sensitivity can be regulated by an intracellular negative feedback loop; GH induces suppressors of cytokine signaling (SOCs) that inhibit GH-induced activation of the GHR/JAK2 complex.

According to the somatomedin hypothesis, GH actions are mediated by its stimulation of hepatic insulin-like growth factor (IGF)-I synthesis and release. It is now understood that GH has direct effects on target tissues independent of IGF-I and that IGF-I release can be both endocrine (hepatic) and autocrine/paracrine (locally within the target tissues). GH stimulates not only IGF-I production by the hepatocytes but also production of the acid-labile subunit (ALS) by hepatocytes and the IGF-binding protein (IGFBP)-3 by hepatic endothelia and Kupffer cells. All three proteins are released into the circulation as a 150-kDa complex. This complex is believed to prolong the half-life of circulating IGF-I and to control its delivery to the target tissues where it binds and activates the IGF receptor (IGF-1R). IGF-1R is a tyrosine kinase receptor, similar to the insulin receptor, that promotes cellular survival and mitogenesis. IGF-I provides additional negative feedback loops decreasing GH secretion, both directly at the somatotrophs and indirectly at the hypothalamus through stimulation of somatostatin.

A new GH-releasing factor, Ghrelin, was identified and cloned. Ghrelin is an octanoylated 28–amino acid peptide synthesized primarily by the X/A-like cells of the stomach. Ghrelin was discovered to be the endogenous ligand for the GH secretagogue receptor (GHS-R), a seven-transmembrane

allowing regulation by higher brain centers both through multiple afferent neural connections and through chemical agents from the cerebrospinal fluid.

Afferent signals from the brain and hypothalamus regulate the pulsatile GH secretion, which achieves its characteristic sleep entrainment by the age of 3 months. The arcuate nucleus of the hypothalamus contains neurons that secrete GH-releasing hormone (GHRH) when stimulated by norepinephrine and serotonin. In contrast, somatostatin (GH release–inhibiting hormone [abbreviated ss]) is synthesized by neurons in the hypothalamic paraventricular nucleus and other brain centers. Somatostatin inhibits GH secretion both directly at the somatotrope level and indirectly by suppressing GHRH release. In turn, both GHRH and GH stimulate somatostatin release, thereby turning off the GH secretion. GH also inhibits GHRH release in a short negative feedback loop. Pulses of GH occur when the brain enters stage IV sleep, a time of GHRH release and somatostatin withdrawal.

domain, G protein–coupled receptor that is expressed in the hypothalamus, pituitary, and other brain centers. In a study of seven healthy men, aged 24 to 32 years, stimulation of GH release was significantly greater by Ghrelin than GHRH, and synergistic when both agents were administered. Ghrelin has also been shown to potently induce feeding behavior, through the *c-fos*, neuropeptide Y, and agouti-related peptide pathways.

It is not surprising that a stomach product should stimulate GH secretion, as there are numerous connections between the GH axis and the metabolic status of the body. GH secretion is often blunted by obesity, glucose, and free fatty acids, whereas hypoglycemia and certain amino acids stimulate GH release. The number of hepatic GHRs decreases with fasting but increases with refeeding; their number is quickly modulated through internalization and microaggregation into coated pits. IGF-I production is very sensitive to nutritional status, especially protein and, to a limited extent, total caloric intake. The amount of circulating free IGF-I is further influenced by metabolic effects on IGFBP production, most notably suppression of hepatic IGFBP-1 by insulin. Conversely, GH exerts multiple metabolic effects apart from its stimulation of somatic growth. GH is an anabolic, insulin counterregulatory hormone, that stimulates lipolysis, promotes protein anabolism, lowers circulating total and LDL cholesterol levels, increases cardiac output, and improves bone mineralization. For these metabolic reasons, the Food and Drug Administration has approved GH replacement therapy for GH-deficient adults, even though they can no longer grow.

The Growth Plate

The growth of long bones occurs at the growth plate through a highly regulated sequence of chondroplasia and osteogenesis (Figure 8-2). Grossly, bone growth occurs in the direction toward the epiphysis, whereas the process at the cellular level proceeds in the opposite direction. Chondroplasia occurs in the reserve, proliferative, and upper hypertrophic zones of the growth plate. Prechondrocytes, the cartilage precursor cells, in the reserve zone differentiate into chondrocytes in a GH-dependent manner. Young chondrocytes then undergo clonal expansion (four cell divisions each) in the proliferative zone under IGF-I stimulation. In fact, part of the GH-induced differentiation of prechondrocytes into chondrocytes involves the expression of new genes like IGF-I, IGF-1R, and the estrogen receptor. After proliferation, the chondrocytes elongate in the upper hypertrophic zone under both GH and IGF-I influences. This elongation contributes about 60% of total growth, versus only 15% from the preceding cellular proliferation.

In the lower hypertrophic zone, the chondrocytes begin to produce a calcified matrix. The cells become entrapped and die by apoptosis within 4 days. They leave behind lacunae, which are penetrated by bone marrow in the resorption front. Ultimately, the lacunae are inhabited by osteoblasts and osteoclasts. The bone marrow is very rich in GHR. GH recruits osteoclasts from bone marrow monocytes and stimulates paracrine IGF-I production, which then leads to white blood cell proliferation. In addition to its central involvement in GH secretion, thyroid hormone is required at the growth plate for osteogenesis to occur. The mechanism whereby estrogen fuses the growth plate is still unknown.

Bone growth is also highly sensitive to biomechanical forces. For example, the strength of healthy load-bearing bones correlates with muscle strength, and the length of congenitally paralyzed limbs grows less than their nonparalyzed counterparts through postnatal mechanical effects on chondral modeling. The Utah paradigm of skeletal physiology examines the impact of biomechanical forces, especially muscular factors, on cartilage physiology and skeletal development.

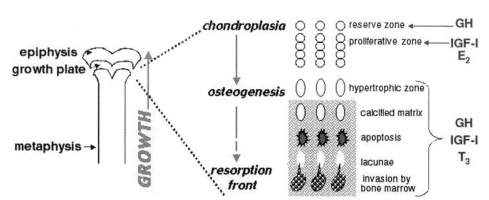

Figure 8-2   Growth at the Growth Plate. Growth of long bones occurs at the growth plate, seen grossly as bone elongation toward the epiphysis. The cellular events progress in the opposite direction, from chondroplasia through osteogenesis, under coordinated regulation by several hormones. GH, growth hormone; IGF-I, insulin-like growth factor I; E_2, estrogen; T_3, thyroid hormone. (Based on Hochberg Z: Clinical physiology and pathology of the growth plate. Best Pract Res Clin Endocrinol Metab 2002;16:399 with permission.)

GROWTH EVALUATION

The study of growth can be seen from three different perspectives. The first is the basic scientific study of growth per se. The second perspective is the use of growth as an index of the health and condition of society. This perspective is embodied in population surveys such as those of the U.S. National Center for Health Statistics (NCHS). The third perspective involves the study by the clinician of the growth of an individual patient. The routine measurements of weight and length at birth were first introduced in a Paris hospital in 1800, but it was not until 80 years later when the systematic following of infants in their first and second years was established.

Growth is a sensitive indicator of a child's health. Therefore, frequent and accurate assessment of growth as part of routine health maintenance is of primary importance in children.

Understanding the normal patterns of growth is a prerequisite to the diagnosis of growth disorders. Growth is a complex process and involves the interaction of multiple factors previously described in this chapter. Despite this complexity, children normally grow in a remarkably predictable manner. Deviation from the normal pattern of growth is frequently the first manifestation of a wide variety of disorders that is discussed later in this chapter.

Phases of Normal Growth

At each stage of life, from intrauterine development to the cessation of growth in adulthood, growth occurs at different rates. To better understand the process of growth, it is important to distinguish the different and partially superimposable phases of growth (Box 8-1).

Prenatal Growth

The most dramatic events in growth occur before birth, the transformation of a single cell into an infant. Prenatal growth varies dramatically, averaging 1.2 to 1.5 cm/wk. The velocity of linear growth reaches a peak at about 18 weeks of gestation, when the fetus is growing at a velocity of 2.5 cm/wk, and falls to almost 0.5 cm/wk immediately before birth. Growth in weight follows the same pattern, except that the peak is reached later. There is a difference in average length between boys and girls of around 0.8 cm by 30 weeks of gestation and 1 cm by 40 weeks. This difference is due to a slightly faster growth in boys since early in fetal life. Growth during the last few weeks of gestation slows down significantly due to the influence of uterine size, so that size at birth reflects the maternal environment more than genetic influences. After birth the growth rate increases again, and genetically large children catch up to their programmed curves in the 6 to 12 months after birth. In the same way, genetically small children slow down to follow their curves.

Intrauterine growth retardation, which can result from many different causes, can have a lasting effect on a child's growth throughout life. Regardless of the etiology, retardation in fetal growth when fetal growth is very rapid during early pregnancy may result in persistent postnatal growth impairment.

Growth During Infancy

After birth, the infant shifts from a growth rate that is predominantly determined by maternal factors to one that is increasingly related to his or her own genetic background, as reflected by midparental size (Box 8-2). Consequently, for about two thirds of normal infants, the linear growth rate shifts during the first 12 to 18 months. Thus, during the first year of life, growth velocity is rapid and highly variable, averaging 23 to 28 cm/yr. During this period, growth velocity is independent of endogenous GH. Prenatal influences on growth may continue, so the small-for-gestational age (SGA) neonate who has the genetic capacity to catch up to the normal range generally shows accelerated growth within the first 6 months after birth. In contrast, most SGA babies who do not show catch-up growth during the first 6 months continue to grow at a slow rate into childhood and are generally destined to be of small stature. Those who are relatively large at birth but whose genetic background is for smaller size tend to grow more slowly, as a physiological effort to balance the genetic and environmental components of growth.

Box 8-1	Average Growth Velocity at Different Phases	
1.	Prenatal growth	1.2 to 1.5 cm/wk
2.	Infancy	23 to 28 cm/yr
3.	Childhood	5 to 6.5 cm/yr
4.	Puberty	8.3 cm/yr (girls)
		9.5 cm/yr (boys)

Box 8-2	Calculating Mid-Parental Height
For boys: Father's height + (mother's height + 13 cm)/2	
For girls: Mother's height + (father's height − 13 cm)/2	

Growth During Childhood

During the second and third years of life, growth velocity declines rapidly, averaging 7.5 to 13 cm/yr. Longitudinal studies of the first 2 years after birth show that the differential between boys' and girls' growth velocities diminishes during the first year, until during the second year when the girls' velocity is actually greater.

By the end of the third year, growth rate has settled into a steady, consistent pattern that persists throughout the childhood years until puberty. On average, a healthy child grows at a velocity of approximately 5 to 6.5 cm/yr during the childhood years and usually does not deviate significantly from this pattern until the onset of puberty. Growth chart maintenance at regular intervals helps to establish the individual growth pattern relative to normative data and facilitates assessment when a meaningful change in growth pattern occurs.

Growth During Puberty

Puberty plays a dual role in growth: height velocity is markedly accelerated; the rate of skeletal maturation is also increased with resultant fusion of epiphyseal cartilage. Thus puberty can be considered as a growth-promoting event as well as the final height-limiting process. Several hormonal factors may interact to determine the pubertal growth spurt: GH, IGF-I, and sex steroids of gonadal and adrenal origins. In both sexes, the role of gonadal steroids is obvious from the remarkable acceleration of linear growth that occurs at the time of sexual maturation, whether that event is early, normal, or delayed. In the absence of normal GH and IGF-I secretion, gonadal steroids have limited growth-promoting effects. This is suggested by the subnormal increase of the growth rate in hypopituitary boys treated with testosterone before GH therapy was available. Additional evidence for the effects of sex steroids in the absence of GH action is obtained from patients with Laron dwarfism. Among eight of these patients followed throughout puberty, three girls did not show any significant growth spurts. In contrast, in three boys and two girls who grew at a mean rate of 2.9 cm/yr before puberty, height velocity increased to 6.5 cm/yr during sexual maturation. These observations suggest that sex steroids may have a direct growth effect independent of GH and IGF-I. Nonetheless, the acceleration of growth caused by sex steroids in the absence of normal GH and IGF-I is minimal compared with the normal pubertal spurt. In patients with sex steroid deficiency and normal GH secretion, no pubertal growth spurt occurs. Patients with congenital hypogonadism have a normal pattern of prepubertal growth. However, no obvious pubertal growth spurt occurs in GH-treated boys with gonadotropin deficiency unless sex steroids are also administered. Numerous researchers have shown that sex steroids, especially estrogens, modulate GH secretion, in particular, increasing the amplitude of GH secretory episodes. GH in turn stimulates IGF-I production, accounting for or reflecting the increased growth velocity.

The onset of puberty brings a rapid growth velocity, but frequently, this acceleration in growth may be preceded by an apparent slowing down or falling off of the individual growth curve. Pubertal growth begins earlier in girls than in boys but is 3 to 5 cm greater in magnitude in boys than in girls. The adult sex difference, averaging 13 cm, is due mainly to the earlier termination of growth in girls. Boys have 2 years more in which to grow before entering puberty. Thus boys, when their puberty starts, are about 8 to 10 cm taller than girls when their puberty started 2 years earlier. The boys' larger pubertal spurts add the remaining differences.

The peak height velocity during the pubertal growth spurt is comparable with the rate of growth during the second year of life. The average peak height velocity is 8.3 cm/yr in girls and 9.5 cm/yr in boys. The time of onset of the pubertal growth spurt varies in normal children, reflecting the concept of a "tempo of growth" or rate of maturation, as emphasized by Tanner. The physiological basis for differences in tempo among individuals is unknown but it appears to have genetic influences. Tempo and final height are practically unrelated in normal children. Whether the pubertal growth spurt occurs early or late exerts little influence on final height in most normal boys and girls. This statement does not necessarily hold for children with true precocious puberty. In both sexes, sexual precocity increases the immediate growth rate and the total pubertal height gain, compared with average maturers. There is increased duration of puberty, which increases the total pubertal height gain, but the increased rate of bone maturation markedly reduces the period of prepubertal growth so that the net effect is final height loss. In both sexes, delayed puberty reduces the immediate growth rate and the total pubertal height gain, compared with average maturers. Also, there is, at least in boys, a reduced duration of puberty. However, the reduced rate of bone maturation increases the prepubertal height gain so the final height is not affected.

Growth ceases when the skeleton achieves adult maturity. The vertebral column continues to grow for a while after the limbs have stopped, as do shoulder and chest widths. Whether growth has finished cannot be judged from chronological age. Often auxologists take an increment of less than 1 cm over one full year as an indicator of the end of growth, but some data indicate that after this there is an average further gain of 1 cm.

Measurement

Accurate and reproducible measurements of height are essential for monitoring growth. Individual measurements at a single point in time detect absolute short or tall stature, but two or more measurements over a period of time are needed to detect a change in growth velocity, regardless of the starting height. The guidelines of the American Academy of Pediatrics state that children should be measured every 2 months until age 6 months, every 3 months from age 6 to 18 months, and then yearly until age 18 years. Effective growth monitoring needs precise measurement, accurate plotting on appropriate charts, and correct interpretation.

Although measuring techniques have improved during the past two decades, recent studies of routine child measurement techniques in pediatric practices throughout the United States have shown severe deficiencies. Measuring height is subject to error as a result of poor technique, variations between instruments and observers, movement of the child, diurnal variations, and plotting mistakes. Incorrect measurements may result in failure to identify growth pathology or in apparent deviations for a child who is actually growing normally.

Supine length is routinely measured during the first 24 months, whereas erect height is assessed in older children. Between 24 and 36 months, measurements can be made on children in either a recumbent or standing position. It is important to plot the child using the appropriate growth chart depending on whether a supine or an erect height was obtained; a child's standing height is less than his or her length, and plotting height on a length chart will give the false perception that growth has decelerated. For measurement of supine length, it is best to use a firm box with an inflexible board against which the head lies, with a movable footboard on which the feet are placed perpendicular to the plane of the supine length of the infant. The use of cloth or plastic measuring tapes should be avoided. Correctly measuring a neonate or infant is a two-person job. Optimally, the child should be relaxed, the legs should be fully extended, and the head should be positioned in the "Frankfurt plane" with the line connecting the outer canthus of the eyes and the external auditory meatus perpendicular to the long axis of the trunk. The infant should be gently stretched. The footplate should be placed against the feet, making sure the toes are vertical to the heels.

When children are old enough to stand erect, it is best to use a stadiometer to determine height. Swinging or floppy arm devices can result in grossly inaccurate readings due to the angle of the arm to the measuring device, in addition to the positioning and posturing of the child. A stadiometer consists of a moving headplate (placed at a precise 90-degree angle to the wall) and a metal measuring tape. There are different models of stadiometers, but essentially any device that meets the requirement of a completely flat wall, precise 90-degree angles at both feet and head, and an accurate metal measuring tape can provide accurate, reproducible measurements of growth, provided appropriate measuring techniques are used. To appropriately measure a standing child, the child should stand up straight, heels together, toes comfortably apart, and the head aligned in the Frankfurt plane. The heels, back of legs, buttocks, shoulders, and occiput should touch the vertical surface of the stadiometer or the wall. The lordotic curve in the lumbar region can be minimized by having the child relax the shoulders. Additionally, the measurer can gently press the abdomen toward the wall to reduce the space between the lower back and the wall. The head should be level, with the child looking straight ahead stretched upward to compensate for diurnal height variations. The individual doing the measuring can accomplish this by placing his or her hand beneath the angle of the child's jaw and lifting gently. To eliminate the effect of diurnal variation, measurements should be taken at or near the same time of the day. A reduction in stature averaging about 8 mm has been found during the first hour after rising from bed. During the next hours, the shrinkage is less, around 6 or 7 mm during the rest of the day. Virtually all the decrease is accounted for by sitting height, and it is primarily due to fatigue of the muscles of the spine. Taking three consecutive measurements and recording the mean value is one method of increasing the accuracy of growth measurements.

Other measurements that are important in the evaluation of a child with short stature but not necessarily for routine growth follow-up include sitting height and limb measurements. Sitting height is important in the differential diagnosis of short stature, particularly in relation to chondrodystrophies, and is also important in the follow-up of children treated with spinal irradiation. Limb segment measurements are also useful in the differential diagnosis of chondrodystrophies. The measurement of knee height (the distance from the upper surface of the knee to the lower surface of the heel) is useful when growth velocity is determined during a short period of time and in the study of fluctuations in growth rate, as it is more sensitive to short-term changes than statural height.

Growth Charts

A long list of heights and weights is very difficult to interpret, so numerical values should always be plotted on a growth chart. The original measurements should also be recorded because it is easy to make plotting errors. When plotting a child's height, it is important to use the appropriate growth chart (according to gender) and to adequately plot the age of the patient. It is not a good practice to round off the age of the patient to the closest year; the age should be plotted as accurately as possible. Growth charts allow us to compare the growth of an individual child with the growth of a standardized group of children who are believed to be healthy. Thus growth charts are very useful tools in child health surveillance, and their proper use and understanding are essential.

Growth charts fall into several categories, which include distance charts, velocity charts, cross-sectional charts, and longitudinal charts. In *distance charts,* stature is plotted against age, and they can be of the cross-sectional or longitudinal type. The second category of charts, *velocity charts,* plot annual increments. These charts are tempo conditioned, in that they allow for the variations in timing and intensity of the adolescent growth spurt. The velocity in many ways reflects the child's state at any particular time better than the distance, which represents the accumulation of events in all of the preceding years. For *cross-sectional charts,* the data are collected from the entire age range and a large sample of different children is used in each age band. In the *longitudinal (individual) charts,* the shape of the curve is derived from data collected from a relatively small sample of children followed over several years. Most of the charts used currently are based on cross-sectional population studies. The data on which the charts are based should relate to the population under consideration and should be updated at regular intervals.

Distance and Velocity Standards

Evaluation of a child's height must be performed in the context of normal standards. The NCHS publishes several growth charts, with separate charts for boys and girls appropriate for ages birth to 36 months and 2 to 20 years (Figures 8-3 through 8-6). During the transition from one growth chart to another, which usually occurs between 2 to 3 years of age, there may be an apparent discontinuity in the percentile of the child's growth. This is caused by the shift in measurements taken standing versus lying down. These charts compare individual children with the 5th, 10th, 25th, 50th, 75th, 90th, and 95th percentiles of normal American children but do not satisfactorily define children below the 5th or above the 95th percentile. NCHS released new growth charts in 2000 that are not only updated but also more representative of the American population, more accurately reflecting the nation's cultural and racial diversities. The charts are based on data gathered through the National Health and Nutrition Examination Survey (NHANES), the only survey that includes data from actual physical examinations on a cross section of Americans from all over the country. Charts based on cross-sectional data do

not take into account that time of puberty and therefore acceleration of linear growth varies from child to child. Some charts have been developed by Tanner and colleagues to address this issue (Figures 8-7 and 8-8). Such charts are of particular value in assessing growth during adolescence and puberty and for plotting sequential growth data on any given child.

Properly used, velocity standards are far superior to distance standards for rapidly picking up abnormalities. Velocity measures what has happened during the past year or 6 months, whereas distance measures the whole accumulated experience of childhood. Although there is considerable variability in the normal height velocity in children of different ages, between the age of 2 years and the onset of puberty children normally grow with remarkable fidelity relative to the normal growth curves. Any "crossing" of height percentiles during this age period should be noted and investigated, and abnormal height velocity always warrants further evaluation. Growth velocity is calculated using a minimum of two measurements, obtained across time, with the plotted data point representing the mean growth velocity achieved during the interval, as opposed to the measurable increment between the two time points. Growth velocity charts are useful in identifying a growth pattern reflecting the individual's achieved growth velocities over time compared with normal standards (Figures 8-9 and 8-10).

Charts for Children With Growth Pathology

There are charts available for certain genetic syndromes, including Turner syndrome (Figure 8-11), achondroplasia, and Down syndrome (Figures 8-12 through 8-15). Such growth profiles are invaluable for tracking the growth of children with these clinical conditions. The charts are used in essentially the same way as the charts for normal children. Deviation of growth from the appropriate disease-related growth curve suggests the possibility of a second underlying problem. For example, children with Down syndrome have a higher incidence of hypothyroidism (congenital and autoimmune), which can further impair their growth; thus, a deviation from their pattern of growth may be the first diagnostic clue.

Parental Target Height

Because genetic factors are important determinants of growth and height potential, it is useful to assess a patient's stature relative to that of siblings and parents. Although during the first 18 months to 2 years, the height of a child is not closely related to parental heights, by age 2 the correlation becomes sufficiently high for knowledge of parental height to lend a considerable increase in precision

Text continued on page 147

Birth to 36 months: Boys
Length-for-age and Weight-for-age percentiles

NAME _____

RECORD # _____

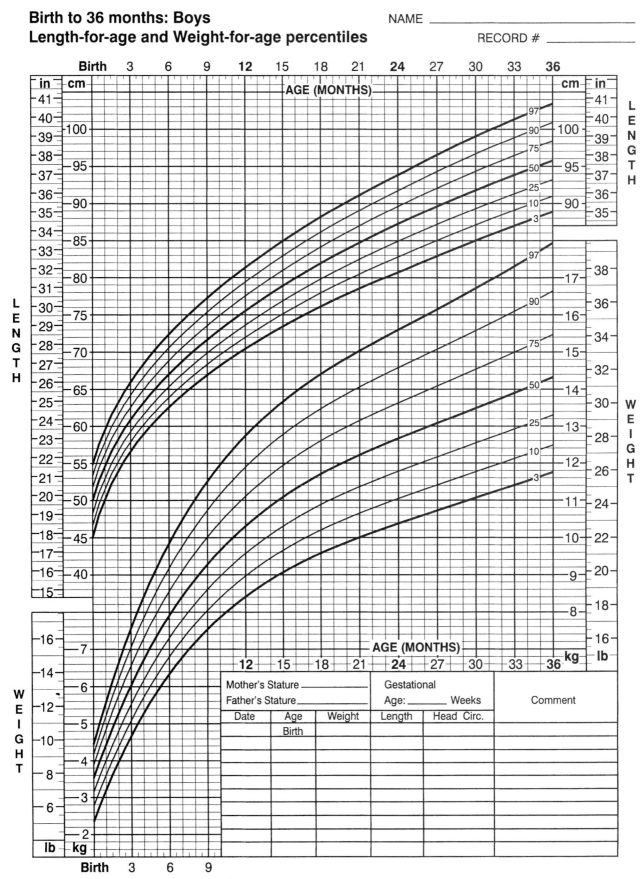

Figure 8-3   Growth Chart for Boys from Birth to 36 Months. Published May 30, 2000 (modified 4/20/01). Source: Developed by the National Center for Health Statistics in collaboration with the National Center for Chronic Disease Prevention and Health Promotion (2000). http://www.cdc.gov/growthcharts

Birth to 36 months: Girls
Length-for-age and Weight-for-age percentiles

NAME _____

RECORD # _____

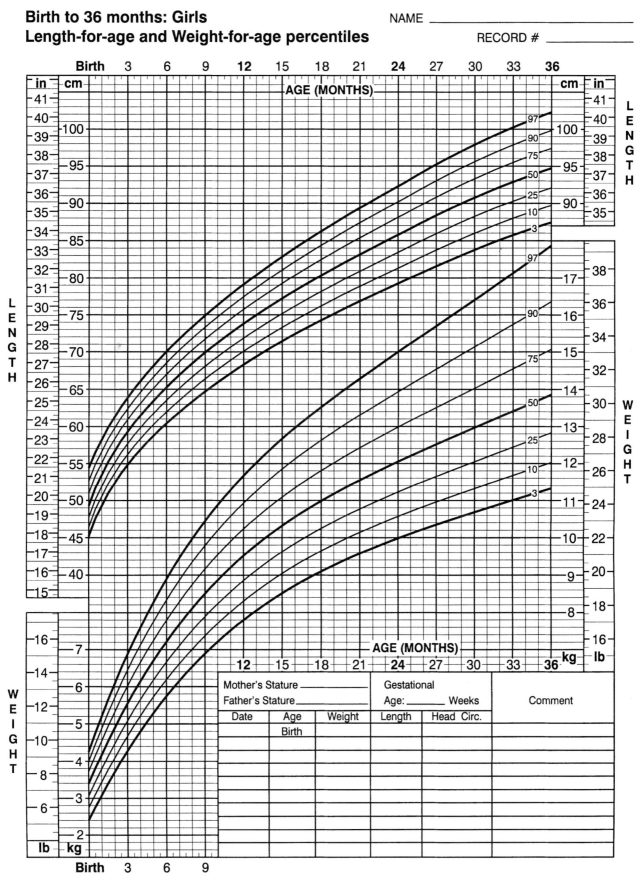

Figure 8-4   Growth Chart for Girls from Birth to 36 Months. Published May 30, 2000 (modified 4/20/01). Source: Developed by the National Center for Health Statistics in collaboration with the National Center for Chronic Disease Prevention and Health Promotion (2000). http://www.cdc.gov/growthcharts

2 to 20 years: Boys
Stature-for-age and Weight-for-age percentiles

NAME _____

RECORD # _____

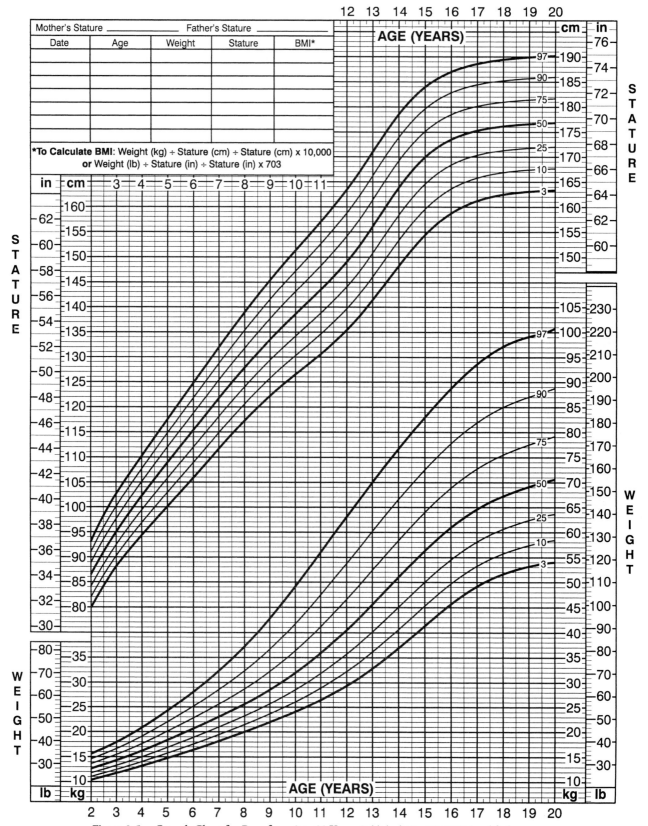

Figure 8-5   Growth Chart for Boys from 2 to 20 Years. Published May 30, 2000 (modified 11/21/00). Source: Developed by the National Center for Health Statistics in collaboration with the National Center for Chronic Disease Prevention and Health Promotion (2000). http://www.cdc.gov/growthcharts

2 to 20 years: Girls
Stature-for-age and Weight-for-age percentiles

NAME _____

RECORD # _____

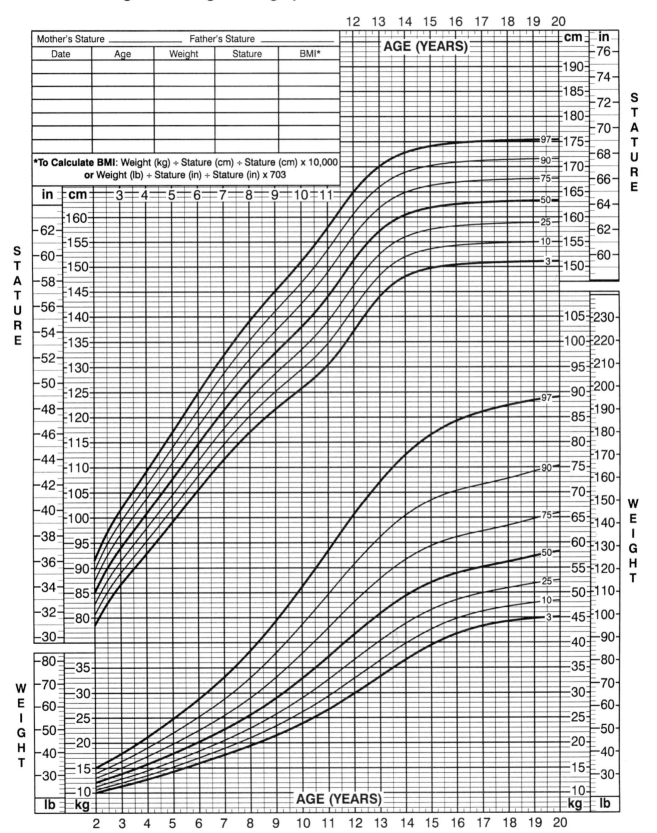

Figure 8-6   Growth Chart for Girls from 2 to 20 Years. Published May 30, 2000 (modified 11/21/00). Source: Developed by the National Center for Health Statistics in collaboration with the National Center for Chronic Disease Prevention and Health Promotion (2000). http://www.cdc.gov/growthcharts

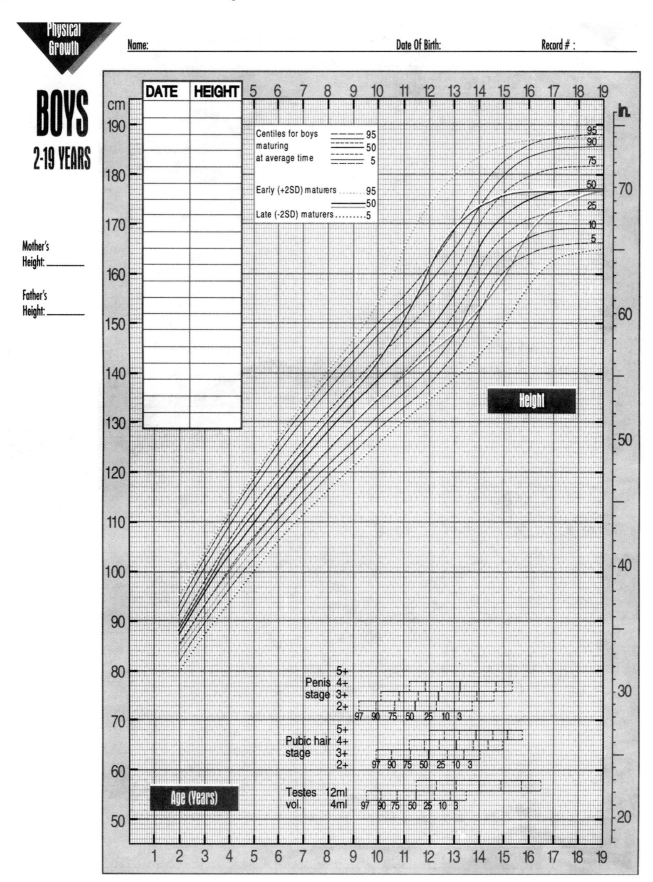

Figure 8-7 **Boys' Tanner Chart.** (From Tanner JM, Davis PSW: Clinical longitudinal standards for height and height velocity for North American children. J Pediatr 1985;144:267, The CV Mosby Company, Copyright 1985. Reproduced with permission Castlemead Publications.)

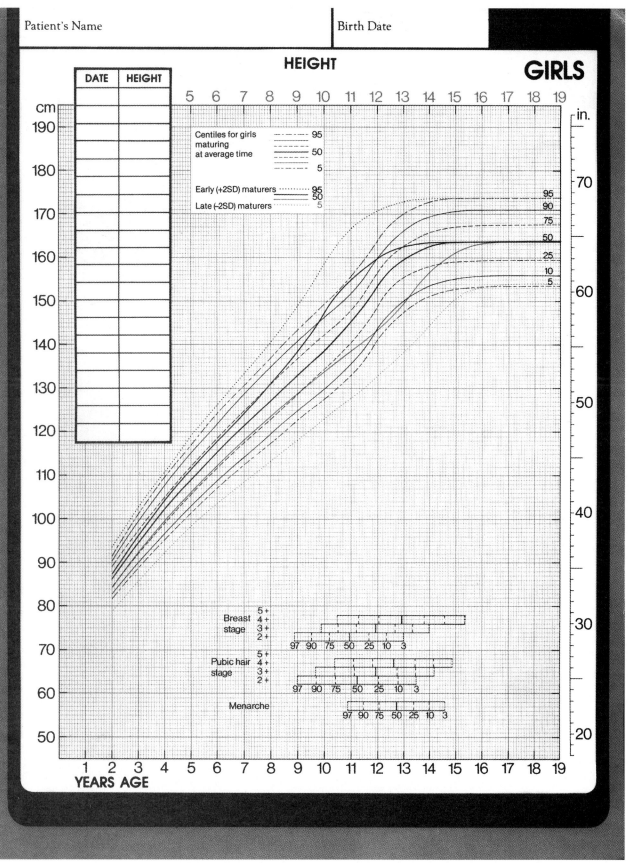

Figure 8-8   Girls' Tanner Chart. (From Tanner JM, Davis PSW: Clinical longitudinal standards for height and height velocity for North American children. J Pediatr 1985;144:267, The CV Mosby Company, Copyright 1985. Reproduced with permission Castlemead Publications.)

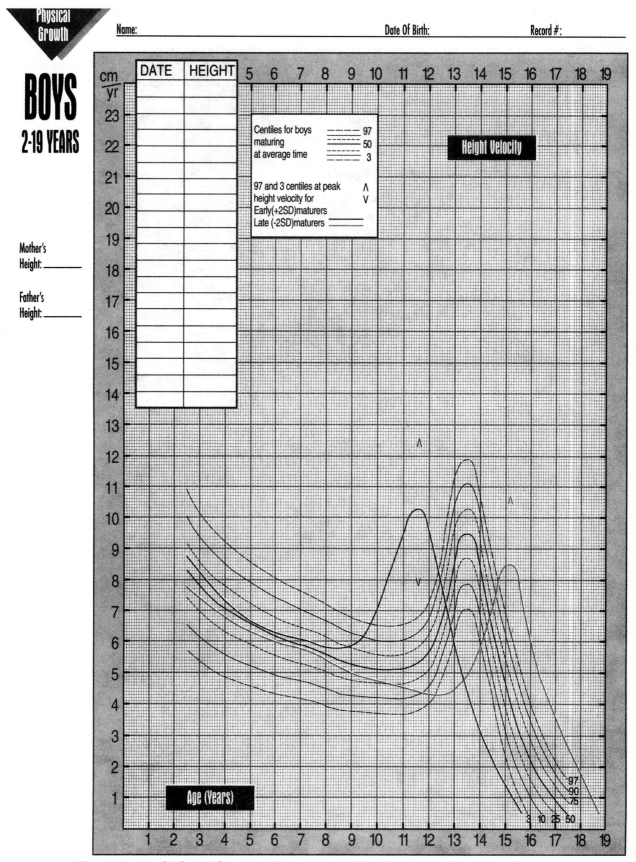

Figure 8-9   Boys' Velocity Chart. (From Tanner JM, Davis PSW: Clinical longitudinal standards for height and height velocity for North American children. J Pediatr 1985;144:267, The CV Mosby Company, Copyright 1985. Reproduced with permission Castlemead Publications.)

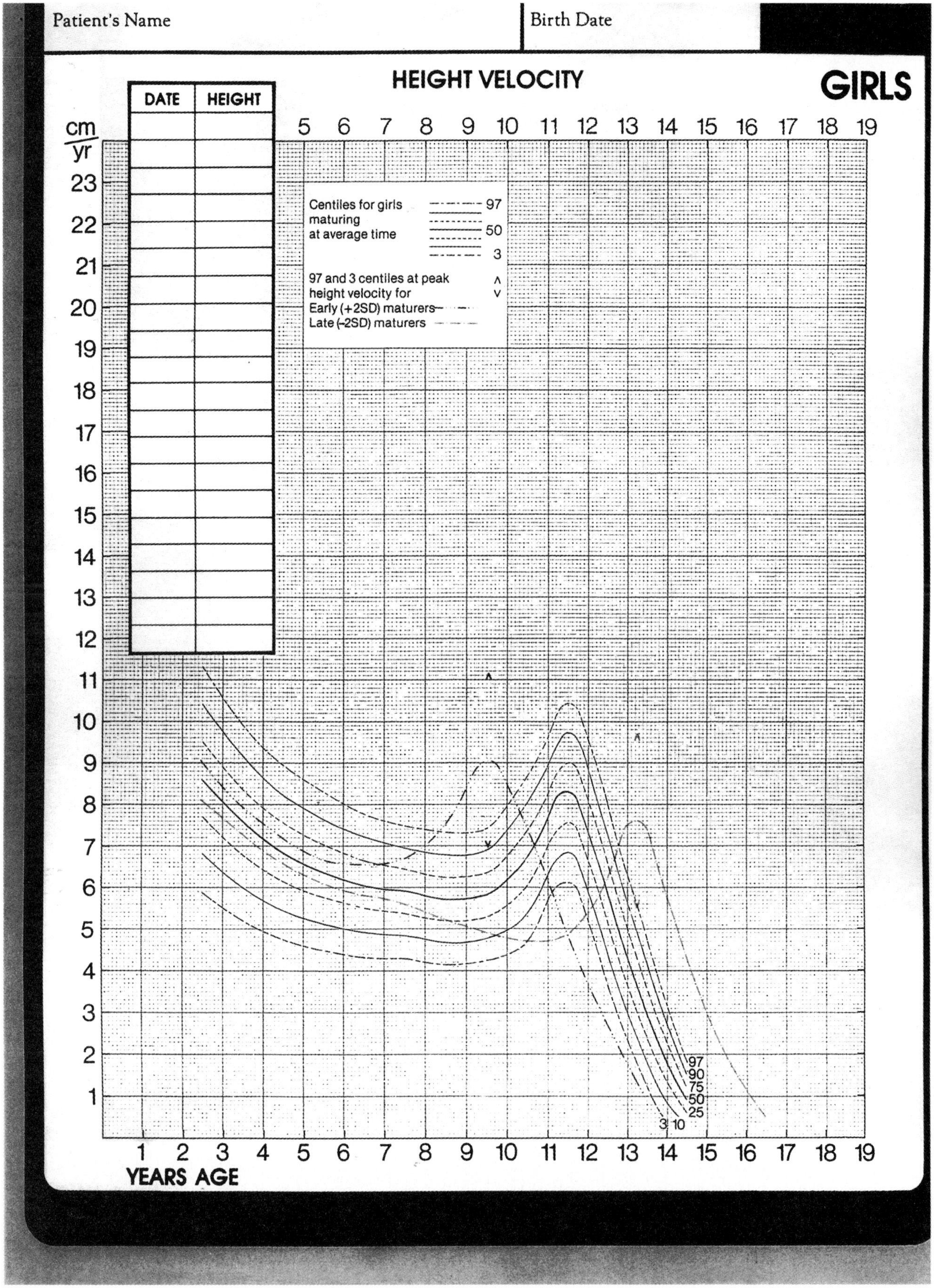

Figure 8-10 Girls' Velocity Chart. (From Tanner JM, Davis PSW: Clinical longitudinal standards for height and height velocity for North American children. J Pediatr 1985;144:267, The CV Mosby Company, Copyright 1985. Reproduced with permission Castlemead Publications.)

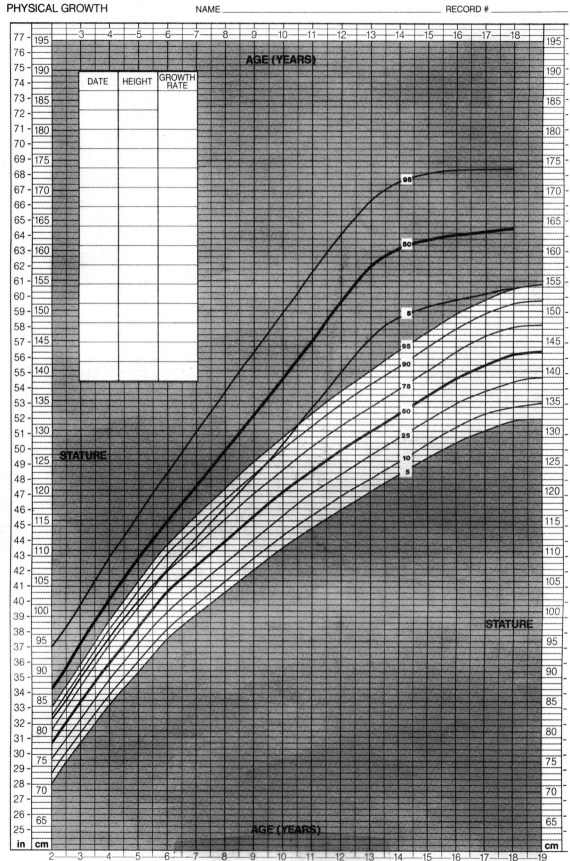

■ NORMAL GIRLS*
■ UNTREATED TURNER PATIENTS**

*Percentiles derived from National Center for Health Statistics
**Turner Percentiles from Lyon, A.J., Preece, M.A., and Grant, D.B.
Growth curve for girls with Turner Syndrome. Archives of Disease in Childhood 60: 932-935 (1985).

Figure 8-11 Growth Chart for Girls with Turner Syndrome. The top three lines represent normal girls; the remaining lines represent untreated Turner patients. (From Lyon AJ, Preece MA, Grant DB: Growth curve for girls with Turner syndrome. Arch Dis Child 1985;60:932, BMJ Publishing Group, copyright 1985.)

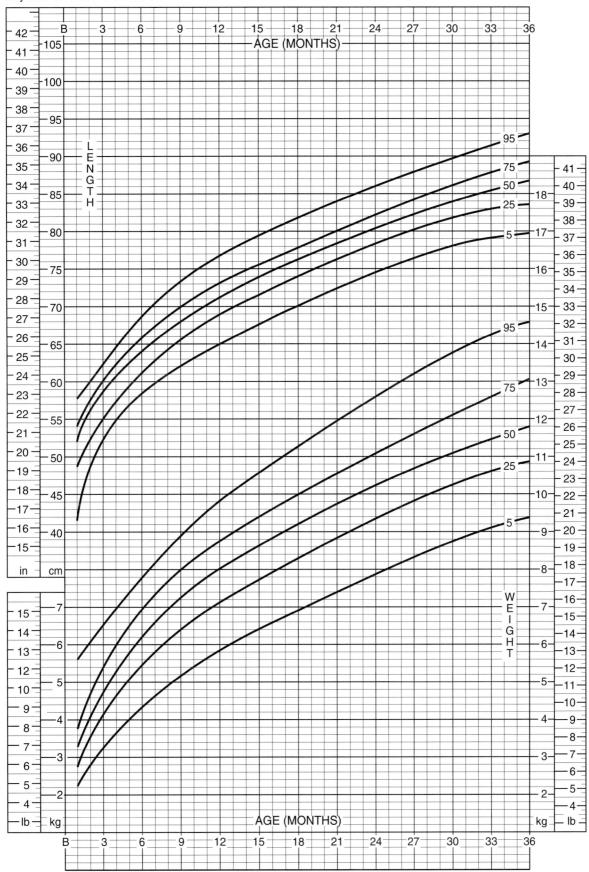

Figure 8-12   Growth Chart for Boys with Down Syndrome from 1 to 36 Months. (Reproduced with permission from Pediatrics 1988;81:102-110, Figures 5, 6, 7, and 8, copyright 1988.)

Girls with Down Syndrome:
Physical Growth: 1 to 36 Months

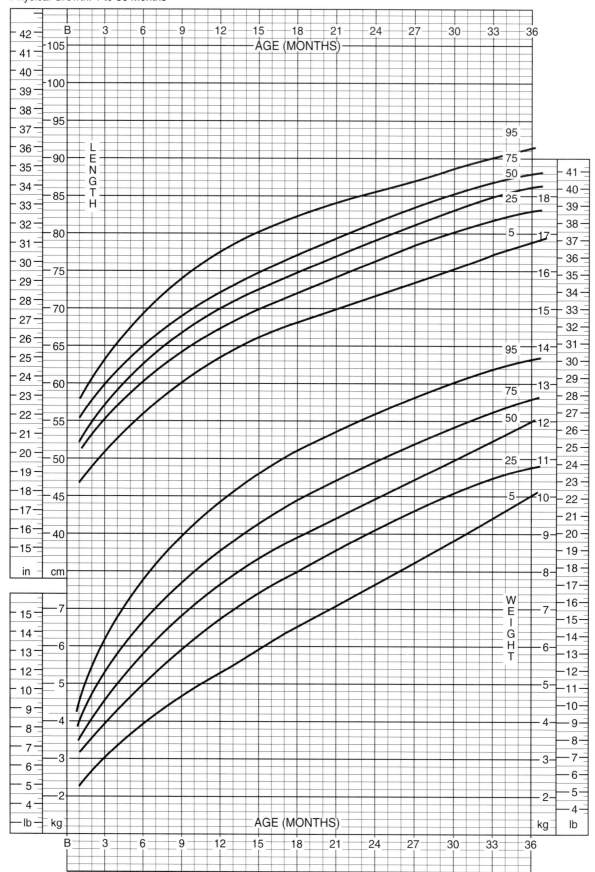

Figure 8-13   Growth Chart for Girls with Down Syndrome from 1 to 36 Months. (Reproduced with permission from Pediatrics 1988;81:102-110, Figures 5, 6, 7, and 8, copyright 1988.)

Boys with Down Syndrome:
Physical Growth: 2 to 18 Years

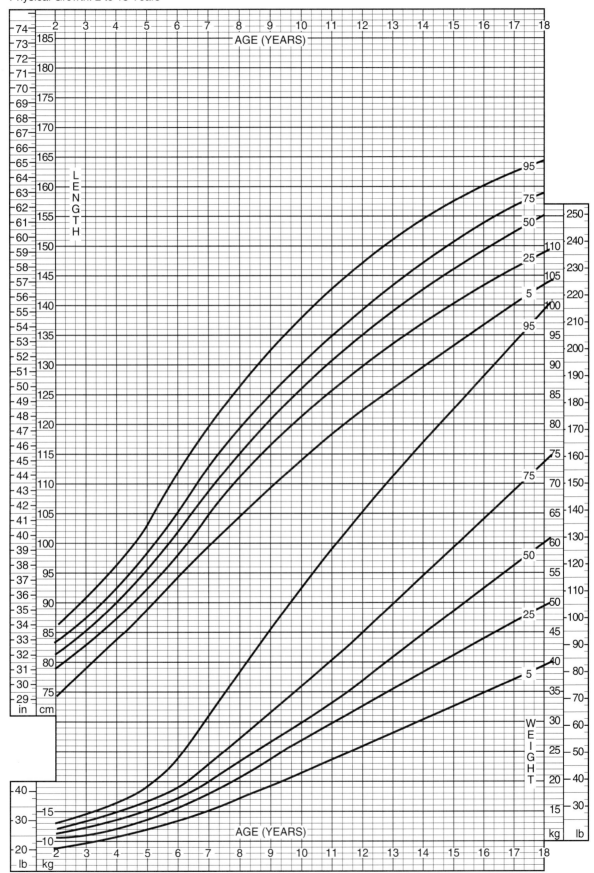

Figure 8-14   Growth Chart for Boys with Down Syndrome from 2 to 18 Years. (Reproduced with permission from Pediatrics 1988;81:102-110, Figures 5, 6, 7, and 8, copyright 1988.)

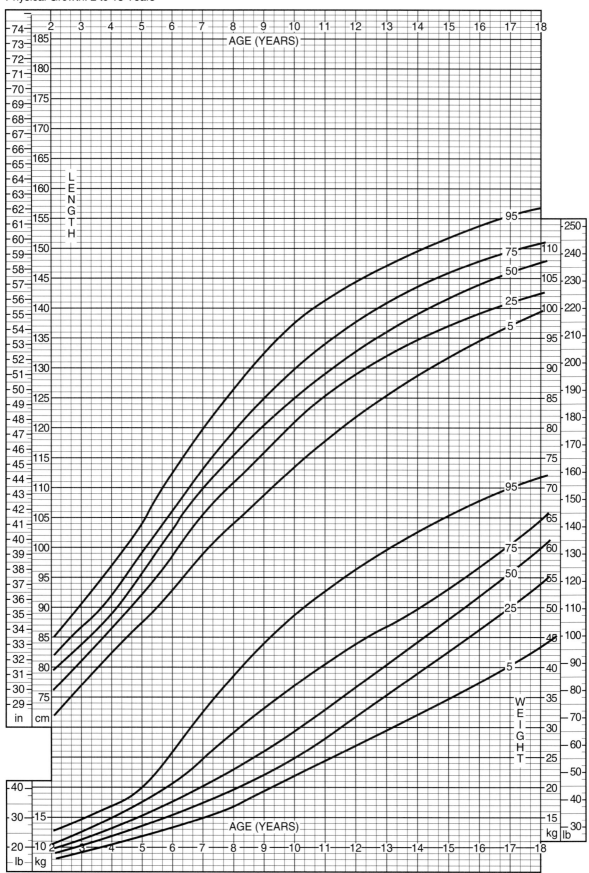

Figure 8-15   Growth Chart for Girls with Down Syndrome from 2 to 18 Years. (Reproduced with permission from Pediatrics 1988;81:102-110, Figures 5, 6, 7, and 8, copyright 1988.)

in determining appropriate heights for an individual child. The child's predicted adult height may be related to a parental target height or the mathematical average of the parents' heights with the addition or subtraction of 6.5 cm for boys and girls, respectively. Most children achieve within ±2 SDs of their midparental height, assuming the normal process of heredity and approximately similar environmental effects on growth in both generations. The 2-SD range for this calculated parental target height is about ±10 cm. For plotting purposes, on a boy's chart, the father's height is plotted straightforwardly, but the mother's height has to be approximately adjusted by adding 13 cm; this represents the average adult sex difference. In plotting the father's height on a girl's chart, 13 cm must be subtracted. The value midway between the father's and mother's plots represents the midparental height. Nevertheless, when a child's growth pattern deviates from that of parents or siblings, the possibility of an underlying pathological condition should be considered. When using parental height to evaluate a child's pattern of growth, there are some caveats. First, most of the time the parents' heights are obtained by their report and not by actual measurement, which often induces inaccuracies. Second, we assume that both of the parents grew up in environments that did not restrict their growth. Actual pathology in one or other of the parents disqualifies the use of their measurements.

Parental pubertal patterns provide the physician with insights into the likelihood that a child will enter puberty early or late in life. It is therefore important to obtain this information in addition to the parents' heights. Box 8-2 contains the formulas to calculate midparental heights in boys and girls.

Skeletal Maturation and Prediction of Adult Height

An estimate of tempo of growth and maturation is often important in the diagnosis and treatment of growth disorders, and the only available measurement at all ages from birth to adulthood is skeletal maturity, or *bone age*. The bone age represents an index of maturation that relates more closely than chronological age to growth. This is particularly obvious for patients who deviate significantly from the normal tempo of growth and puberty. The growth potential in the tubular bones can be assessed by evaluation of the progression of ossification within the epiphyses. The ossification centers of the skeleton appear and progress in a predictable sequence in normal children, and skeletal maturation can be compared with normal age-related standards. It is not completely clear what factors determine this normal maturation pattern, but genetic factors and multiple hormones, including thyroxine, GH, and gonadal

steroids, are involved (see Figure 8-2). During puberty, estrogen is the main determinant of skeletal maturation.

After the neonatal period, a radiograph of the left hand and wrist is commonly used for comparison with the published standards of Greulich and Pyle. Greulich and Pyle's *Radiographic Atlas of Skeletal Development* consists of two parts. The first contains two series of hand/wrist radiographs, one for boys and another for girls. Each radiograph is labeled with a skeletal age. The second part consists of drawings and descriptions of the successive stages of development of each of the individual bones, with bone ages assigned to each stage. The recommended method to evaluate the bone age using the Greulich and Pyle atlas is a bone-by-bone assessment, followed by final use of the mean age of all ratable bones. Bone age is an index of somatic maturation, and the skilled interpretation of bone age radiography can indicate with some accuracy the amount of bone growth remaining. Because the evaluation of bone age films is not a straightforward process, it may be convenient for the primary care physician to identify a radiologist with experience in reading and interpreting bone age films.

Obviously, final height cannot be determined until epiphyseal cartilages have closed. Because it takes such a long time to attain final height, in the clinical setting we attempt to predict the ultimate stature of patients to evaluate the likely effects of therapeutic modalities. The extent of skeletal maturation observed in an individual can be used to predict the ultimate height potential. Height gain during a given period of life is directly related to the increment in height and inversely related to the advancement in the bone age. Predictive evaluation of any endocrine condition or therapy on ultimate height must rely on studies of the rate of linear growth versus the rate of bone maturation. The prediction is based on the observation that the more delayed the bone age (relative to the chronological age), the longer is the time before epiphyseal fusion precludes further growth. The estimate of predicted adult height is useful both at the time of diagnosis of growth pathology for comparison with parent target range and during treatment. There are several methods to predict adult height, but the most commonly used one, based on Greulich and Pyle's, atlas, was developed by Bayley and Pinneau and relies on bone age, height, and a semiquantitative allowance for chronological age. The more advanced the bone age, the greater is the accuracy of the adult height prediction because a more advanced bone age places a patient closer to final height. Final height predictions are less accurate in patients showing marked deviations from the range of physiological variations in height or marked differences between bone age and chronological age. All methods of predicting adult height are based on data from normal children and do not accurately predict adult height in children with growth abnormalities. The predicted adult height of the child being evaluated is compared with the target range. If it falls anywhere within the range, the child is likely to be normal.

SHORT STATURE/GROWTH FAILURE

The Clinical Problem

The prospect of short stature worries parents, children, and pediatricians. "Heightism" refers to the psychosocial prejudice and discrimination against shorter individuals. The severity of heightism depends on both the degree of statural deficit and the general level of social tolerance in the local culture. The average heights of men and women in the United States, according to the 2000 National Center for Health Statistics, are 5 feet 9.5 inches and 5 feet 4 inches, respectively. Tall stature has been associated with success in multiple social arenas, as exemplified by salary and recruitment profiles, outcomes of presidential elections, life insurance policy values, and the social mores of men always being taller than their romantic partners. In one of the largest studies on heightism, all Swedish men born in 1976 and conscripted in 1994 were evaluated, excluding only those with growth-affecting disorders or missing data (final subject population, 32,887). Conscripts whose heights fell below −2 SDs were found to (1) have more psychiatric and musculoskeletal diagnoses, (2) more often be considered psychologically unsuitable for military service and less suitable for leadership positions, and (3) score lower on intellectual tests and assessments of psychological functioning during mental stress.

Two psychological phenomena may contribute to this outcome. First, by the halo effect, a person with one desired trait is assumed to possess other desired traits. Thus, short individuals enter each and every social interaction with one strike against them based on first impression. Because the desired physical trait is height in males but beauty in females, heightism affects males more than it does females. Also, in children, physical size is often interpreted as the main clue to their chronological age. Thus, an 8-year-old who is the size of an average 6-year-old is often treated by adults as a 6-year-old; the 8-year-old thereby loses out on the social, emotional, and cognitive developmental challenges and responsibilities appropriate to his or her age.

However, growth failure has significant medical implications far beyond the psychosocial aspects of heightism. Growth is the single most sensitive sign that something is amiss with a child. It is also very nonspecific. Consequently, as expanded in the following sections, the differential diagnosis of growth failure is as broad as the field of general pediatrics. Looking at it from another perspective, growth

failure is often the first and *only* sign of an underlying medical process. Prompt recognition, diagnosis, and treatment of the underlying pathophysiological process are equally imperative in children of both genders.

"Short stature" is defined as height below −2 SDs for age and gender (i.e., less than the third percentile for the population). "Dwarfism" refers to severe short stature, less than −3 SDs. "Midgets" have normally proportioned short stature. Inherent to these definitions is the comparison with an appropriate reference population. Along the same lines, growth failure can be defined as height less than 2 SDs below the parental target height. Thus, a child whose height is on the 25th percentile for age and gender of the general population may still have clinically significant growth failure if his or her genetic potential is at the 90th percentile. An abnormally slow growth velocity is another indication of growth failure. Between age 3 years and puberty, a growth rate below 5 cm/yr (2 in/yr) should prompt attention. Consequent to an abnormally slow growth velocity, downward crossing of percentile channels on the growth chart constitutes yet another definition of growth failure. This especially holds true after the age of 18 months. Before that age, many infants change channels from their birth size, which is primarily determined by extrinsic factors (pregnancy health, placental sufficiency, maternal health), to their own intrinsically determined curve, which they will track into adulthood. Whenever a child fulfills one of these definitions, summarized in Box 8-3, the differential diagnosis of growth failure should be investigated.

Differential Diagnosis of Short Stature/Growth Failure

Healthy but Short Children

Two main subgroups comprise the vast majority of short children, and neither indicates a pathological process (Box 8-4). *Familial short stature* (FSS) refers to normal growth

---

> **Box 8-3 Definitions of Growth Failure**
>
> - Height below third percentile (−2 SDs for age and gender)
> - Height significantly below genetic potential (−2 SDs below mid-parental target)
> - Abnormally slow growth velocity (<2 inches or 5 cm/yr from age 3 years to puberty)
> - Downwardly crossing percentile channels on growth chart (after the age of 18 months)

<table>
<tr><td colspan="1">

Box 8-4   Differential Diagnosis of Short Stature/Growth Failure

</td></tr>
</table>

l. Healthy but short children
   - Familial short stature
   - Constitutional growth delay
2. Nonorganic etiologies
   - Psychosocial deprivation
   - Nutritional dwarfing
     - Gross deficiencies: kwashiorkor, anorexia nervosa
     - Subtle macronutrient deficiencies: nonorganic failure to thrive (NOFTT), picky eater, fear of obesity, fear of hypercholesterolemia
     - Micronutrient deficiencies: iron, zinc
3. Intrinsic short stature
   - Small-for-gestational age
   - Genetic syndromes
     - Down syndrome
     - Turner syndrome
     - Prader-Willi syndrome
   - Achondroplasia/hypochondroplasia
4. Systemic diseases
   - Infectious: human immunodeficiency virus, tuberculosis
   - Cardiac
   - Renal: renal tubular acidosis, chronic renal insufficiency
   - Gastrointestinal: cystic fibrosis, inflammatory bowel disease, celiac disease
5. Endocrinopathies
   - Early puberty
   - Cortisol excess: endogenous and iatrogenic
   - Hypothyroidism
   - Poorly controlled diabetes mellitus
   - Inadequate growth hormone action
     - Growth hormone deficiency: isolated versus panhypopituitarism, congenital versus acquired
     - Growth hormone insensitivity: Laron types 1 and 2

leading to an inherited short adult height. These children track short growth channels with normal growth velocity and normal bone age; their growth curves parallel normal curves and their final heights are consistent with their midparental targets. Laboratory investigations, if done, are completely normal.

Constitutional growth delay (CGD) is the medical term for "late bloomers." Skeletal maturity in these children lags behind their chronological age, but they are otherwise completely normal. Thus, apart from a delayed bone age, laboratory investigations will be normal. Compared with their classmates matched for chronological age rather than bone age, these children appear relatively growth stunted. This deficit becomes most pronounced in the peripubescent years, when classmates enter puberty and undergo their pubertal growth spurts, whereas children with CGD persist at the slow prepubertal growth velocity. To worsen matters,

there is a slight growth deceleration before the onset of puberty. However, when the classmates have completed puberty and their growth plates have fused, the children with CGD will still be growing and will ultimately reach adult heights consistent with their midparental targets. Sometimes, CGD occurs superimposed on FSS, and these children can be significantly short.

Nonorganic Etiologies

"Nonorganic" etiologies refer to causes extrinsic to the infant or child and primarily involve socio-environmental and nutritional factors. Psychosocial dwarfing results from child abuse, neglect, and emotional deprivation. The growth failure is associated with an attachment and/or depressive disorder, and some of the children also develop a transient deficiency of GH or other anterior pituitary hormones. The primary treatment is removal from the harmful environment and placement into a nurturing home or hospital; dramatic catch-up growth ensues without the aid of exogenous hormonal therapies.

Inadequate nutritional intake is a major cause of growth failure worldwide. Gross nutritional deficiencies may be readily apparent, as in kwashiorkor or anorexia nervosa. However, they can also be more subtle. Suboptimal nutrition may result from ignorance of proper pediatric nutritional requirements (e.g., excessive fruit juice intake, overdilution of infant formula, or very imbalanced diets due to personal dietary beliefs), from improper feeding techniques, or from disturbances in the feeding dynamic (stressors or behaviors that have been likened to a separation disorder). In the 1980s, Fima Lifshitz and colleagues described the fear of obesity and the fear of hypercholesterolemia as two specific subtypes of nutritional dwarfing. In the face of the American obesity epidemic and the pervasive media emphasis on the beauty of thinness, some parents restrict their children's intake; in efforts to spare their children the ills of excessive dietary intake, they unwittingly do not provide adequate nutritional support to maintain normal growth. If the child is old enough, he or she may be the one restricting the intake, sometimes without the parents' knowledge. The hallmark of nonorganic failure to thrive and nutritional dwarfing, across the spectrum from severe to subtle, is a fall-off in the weight curve that precedes the fall-off in the height growth curve. Restoration of adequate nutrition promotes catch-up growth for both weight and height.

Growth failure can be caused by specific micronutrient, and not just macronutrient, deficiencies. The two most common culprits are iron deficiency and zinc deficiency. Microcytic anemia and acrodermatitis enterohepatica may be respective clues but do not always accompany the growth failure. Diet modification and micronutrient supplementation can correct these problems.

Intrinsic Short Stature

Some children are born with conditions that destine them to become short adults. Most children born SGA enjoy postnatal catch-up growth that normalizes their stature. However, about 10% never catch up. This subgroup remains significantly short (height <−2.5 SDs) and tends to demonstrate a low appetite, very lean body habitus, acceleration in bone maturation from mid-childhood, relatively early puberty, and increased incidence of impaired carbohydrate tolerance. It is not understood what distinguishes this subgroup from other SGA infants, but it is becoming increasingly clear that SGA describes a very heterogeneous group of disorders. A series of randomized multicenter studies of GH treatment have shown improvements in height SD scores in SGA children, even in those without documented GH deficiency. Thus, the FDA has recently approved GH treatment for SGA children who fail to manifest catch-up growth by age 2 years.

Short stature may also occur as part of a well-defined genetic syndrome. It is imperative that the growth of such children be plotted on growth curves specific for their syndromes; tracking a syndrome-specific channel provides a more realistic indication of the expected final adult height, whereas falling off a syndrome-specific channel maximizes the sensitivity of the growth curve as a tool for identifying underlying health problems. For example, children with trisomy 21 have short stature due to Down syndrome. They also have a higher incidence of thyroiditis. If a child with trisomy 21 is followed on a growth curve referenced to the general population, then all the pediatrician may see is that he or she is growing "below the curve." If the same child is plotted on a Down syndrome growth curve (see Figures 8-12 through 8-15), then it may become evident that the child has fallen across percentile channels. This can be the main clue that the child has developed thyroiditis, especially because the phenotypes of hypothyroidism and Down syndrome overlap significantly.

Turner syndrome is another genetic syndrome with a characteristic growth pattern, created by in utero growth retardation, altered postnatal skeletal development and the absence of the pubertal growth spurt. Girls with Turner syndrome are born generally at about −1 SD for the height and weight of their normal populations. Growth velocity is normal in the first 3 years of life but then decelerates significantly. Girls with gonadal failure not receiving estrogen replacement do not achieve the pubertal growth spurt heralded by estrogen effects on pituitary GH secretion. Although girls with Turner syndrome follow their syndrome-specific growth pattern overall (see Figure 8-11), underlying genetic influences still carry over. Thus, the girl's height percentile on the Turner syndrome growth curve correlates with her parental target on the normal population

growth curve, and the final heights of women with Turner syndrome vary by country in parallel to the heights of their general populations. Turner syndrome is classically attributed to a missing X chromosome (45,X karyotype), but various X chromosome abnormalities, including mosaicism, may also result in the Turner phenotype. The growth failure has recently been attributed specifically to haploinsufficiency of the *SHOX* gene (for Short stature HomeobOX; also called *PHOG* for pseudoautosomal homeobox-containing osteogenic gene), a gene at Xpter-p22.32 in the pseudoautosomal region of the X chromosome. Although girls with Turner syndrome do not have GH deficiency, their intrinsic skeletal dysplasia responds to GH therapy with significant improvement in final height. As such, Turner syndrome is an FDA-approved indication for GH treatment, and GH treatment has become part of the standard of care for Turner syndrome.

A second genetic syndrome that has achieved FDA approval as an indication for GH therapy is Prader-Willi syndrome (PWS). Because genetic testing has not achieved 100% sensitivity, PWS remains a clinical diagnosis based on major and minor criteria, with the hallmark of neonatal and infantile hypotonia, poor feeding and failure-to-thrive switching in early childhood to ravenous eating, central obesity, and global developmental delays. The lower caloric requirement and hyperphagia combined with other features like hypogonadotropic hypogonadism, short stature, and infantile temperature instability have suggested an underlying hypothalamic defect as the primary lesion. However, the growth deceleration occurs even in those children with normal results on GH testing. Other skeletal features of PWS are disproportionately small hands and feet, osteoporosis, and scoliosis. PWS results from deletion of the paternally imprinted chromosome 15q11-13; deletion of the maternally imprinted chromosome 15q11-13 leads to Angelman syndrome, which has a completely different phenotype.

Short stature may also result from a genetic condition that primarily affects skeletal development. Achondroplasia and hypochondroplasia result from mutations in the fibroblast growth factor receptor (FGFR)3. Achondroplasia can be inherited in an autosomal dominant fashion or arise by de novo mutation and occurs with an overall frequency of 1:15,000. Because FGFR3 is expressed in articular chondrocytes, its mutation results in disproportionately shortened limbs but near normal craniofacies. There is also caudal narrowing of the spine. Hypochondroplasia is less severe than achondroplasia, and thanatophoric dysplasia more severe, with many infants dying shortly after birth due to respiratory insufficiency. Genetically, the three conditions arise from mutations in different regions of the *FGFR3* gene; achondroplasia mutations map to the transmembrane domain, hypochondroplasia to the proximal tyrosine kinase domain and thanatophoric dysplasia-II to the distal tyrosine kinase domain. Trials of GH therapy in these conditions have worsened the disproportions. There are other types of chondrodysplasias, mapping to other loci, that disrupt endochondral ossification and skeletal growth.

Systemic Diseases

Growth failure frequently is the first and, for a time, the only manifestation of a myriad of systemic diseases. Virtually any chronic illness can delay growth; if the underlying condition can be adequately treated, catch-up growth occurs. As the differential is too broad for an exhaustive review, the more common conditions are discussed here.

Globally, infectious diseases constitute the largest subgroup of this category. Infection with the human immunodeficiency virus (HIV) has surpassed tuberculosis (TB) as the most common culprit. Infants born to HIV-infected women have a higher frequency of intrauterine growth retardation, even if the virus was not transmitted transplacentally. Growth failure is the most common clinical complication in perinatally infected children, as well as in pediatric infections. Preferential loss of lean body mass occurs despite normal resting and total energy expenditures. HIV-infected children with poor growth harbor higher viral loads than those with normal growth, and studies of HIV infection in children with hemophilia have shown growth failure to predate the lowering of CD4 counts and the onset of symptoms. No consistent endocrine abnormality has been documented in HIV-associated growth failure. Several studies have shown low IGF-I levels despite normal GH testing and another suggested resistance to IGF-I. Changes in thyroid and adrenal axis testing have been reported, especially due to glandular involvement by opportunistic infections.

Growth failure frequently accompanies congenital heart disease. Sometimes both occur as part of a genetic syndrome, such as Down, Turner, and Noonan syndromes, chromosome 22q deletion, and CHARGE association. At other times, growth failure may be a consequence of the congenital heart disease. The degree of growth failure depends on the type of cardiac lesion and is most severe in infants and children with congestive heart failure. Supranormal energy expenditures in infants and children with congenital heart disease make them particularly vulnerable to nutritional dwarfing, even when their caloric intakes may be nearly adequate for age. Chronic hypoxemia has also been suggested as a cause of the growth failure, as children with cyanotic congenital heart disease, especially those with pulmonary hypertension, are more growth stunted than those with acyanotic heart disease.

Renal disease is another major category of growth-stunting conditions. Growth failure may be the only clinical symp-

tom of renal dysfunction. For example, infants and children with renal tubular acidosis (RTA) commonly present with growth failure. RTA refers to impaired renal acidification that causes hyperchloremic metabolic acidosis and bicarbonaturia despite normal rates of acid production from the diet and metabolism. Different types of RTA have been classified according to the specific underlying defect. Treatment with alkali, correcting the metabolic acidosis, can improve the growth velocity and produce normal adult height in RTA type I (distal) and isolated type II (proximal). Significant growth failure is a major complication of chronic renal insufficiency (CRI). Growth failure is associated with adverse clinical outcomes in children with end-stage renal disease, such as more frequent hospitalizations and increased mortality, and likely serves as a marker for high-risk patients. The growth failure of CRI has been attributed to GH resistance, and recently, impaired JAK/STAT signaling has been demonstrated in a rat model of nonacidotic uremia. IGF bioactivity is further decreased by the impaired renal clearance of the IGFBPs. Despite the GH resistance, children with CRI respond to exogenous GH treatment with improved growth velocities and better adult heights. Thus, CRI (pretransplantation) was the first FDA-approved indication for GH therapy after replacement for pediatric GH deficiency.

Because nonorganic nutritional dwarfing is a major cause of growth failure, it should follow that gastrointestinal disease can also stunt growth. Any gastrointestinal disease that impairs nutritional intake and/or absorption causes "organic" nutritional dwarfing. Three gastrointestinal diseases bear mentioning in particular: cystic fibrosis (CF), inflammatory bowel disease (IBD), and celiac disease. That is because growth failure plays such an important part in the clinical presentations of these patients.

CF is an autosomal recessive disease, consisting of chronic obstructive lung disease and pancreatic exocrine deficiency, caused by mutations in the cystic fibrosis transmembrane regulator (CFTR), a cAMP-activated chloride channel. Poor growth may be the first presenting symptom, predating any pulmonary or gastrointestinal complications. Even if it is not the first presenting sign, growth failure frequently accompanies the other characteristic findings. The growth failure of CF has been attributed to the following: decreased energy intake and increased energy expenditure, malabsorption due to pancreatic insufficiency, chronic airway inflammation due to frequent infections, frequent and chronic glucocorticoid treatments, and even the primary CFTR defect itself (CFTR is expressed in the thalamus, hypothalamus, and amygdaloid nucleus—brain centers that regulate appetite, energy expenditure, and sexual maturation). In a longitudinal study of the National Cystic Fibrosis Patient Registry (n = 19,000), height-for-age below the fifth percentile at ages 5 and 7 years was a significant poor prognostic indicator of survival in both genders. However, earlier diagnosis, as with the Wisconsin Cystic Fibrosis Neonatal Screening Project, led to significantly greater growth, even after 4 years of age, despite similar nutritional therapy and a higher proportion of patients with pancreatic insufficiencies than in the group with the later diagnoses.

IBD represents a particular diagnostic challenge. Growth failure may predate by years the classic abdominal pain, bloody diarrhea, or other systemic manifestations of IBD. In fact, growth failure is present in up to 50% of children at the time of diagnosis. The growth failure of IBD may result from protein and calorie malnutrition, active inflammation, possible GH resistance and, later, medication effects. Serum IGF-I levels are low in IBD, as they are in many catabolic conditions, and sometimes lead to misdiagnoses; children presenting solely with growth failure may be misdiagnosed with GH deficiency and receive GH treatments before the classic GI symptoms declare the underlying disease. Optimal medical, surgical, and nutritional treatments can improve growth and raise IGF-I levels in children with Crohn disease, although a significant number continues to grow poorly. Reports of the adequacy of GH secretion in children with Crohn disease are conflicting, and the few studies evaluating the effectiveness of GH therapy in enhancing growth had mixed results.

Celiac disease is an autoimmune disease resulting in a permanent intolerance to wheat gliadins and related prolamines. Gluten peptides efficiently presented by celiac disease–specific HLA-DQ2– and HLA-DQ8–positive antigen-presenting cells trigger an immune response in the intestinal lamina propria; during inflammation, cells release tissue transglutaminase, a highly specific endomysial autoantigen. Classic descriptions of the disease consist of steatorrhea and malnutrition, but it is increasingly apparent that celiac disease occurs as a spectrum of clinical severity including asymptomatic individuals and isolated growth failure. Even if clinically silent, long-standing untreated celiac disease can predispose to other autoimmune diseases. Effective treatment consists of a gluten-free diet, which reduces the intestinal inflammation and leads to catch-up growth.

Endocrinopathies

Dysfunction of any hormonal system affects growth. Perhaps the most misleading growth paradox is that of early puberty. Early puberty, even when it is not early enough to fulfill the definition of precocious puberty, is associated with bone age acceleration. Thus, during childhood, these children appear tall for their chronological ages with height percentiles above expected from their parental targets. No one would surmise these individuals may ultimately experience short stature. However, the accelerated skeletal maturation heralds a premature termination of growth. If puberty commences early or proceeds with a very rapid tempo, the growth plates fuse early and the child loses out on years of the steady childhood growth of 5 cm/yr. The end result is that these children go from being taller than expected to final adult heights that fall short of their genetic targets (Figure 8-16). Gonadotropin-releasing hormone agonist therapy has been used to halt skeletal maturation and "buy time" for continued growth while the chronological age catches up to the bone age. Upon review, final height compromise and height gains from gonadotropin-releasing hormone agonist therapy in girls with borderline early pubertal onset (age, 6 to 8 years) are far less than originally believed. This topic is covered in more detail in the later section on overgrowth.

Growth failure due to cortisol excess is increasing in frequency. Although endogenous cortisol excess (Cushing syndrome) is still rare in the pediatric age range, iatrogenic cortisol excess from chronic glucocorticoid therapy is becoming fairly common. Cushing syndrome is divided into Cushing disease (corticotropin [ACTH]-dependent hypercortisolism) and ACTH-independent hypercortisolism, as described in detail in Chapter 10. Iatrogenic cortisol excess falls into the latter category; in fact, ACTH is often suppressed by the chronic high doses of glucocorticoids used as anti-inflammatory and immunosuppressive agents. The clinical features of Cushing syndrome and iatrogenic glucocorticoid excess are the same ("cushingoid phenotype"). The cushingoid phenotype is characterized by linear growth deceleration with accelerated weight gain leading to moon facies, truncal obesity, and buffalo hump formation. Violacious striae, plethora, increased bruisability, muscle wasting, osteoporosis, and hypertension are other common traits. Apart from inhibiting collagen synthesis and promoting protein catabolism, glucocorticoids suppress growth both centrally (inhibit GH secretion via augmented somatostatin tone and repressed GH synthesis) and peripherally (direct effects on the growth plates: inhibit chondrocyte proliferation and hypertrophic cell differentiation and influence local GH/IGF signaling). Although linear growth improves when the source of the excessive cortisol is removed, iatrogenic cortisol excess is clinically more challenging; discontinuation or significant reduction of the glucocorticoid therapy may result in flares of the underlying disease, which can be far more harmful than the growth failure. It was originally believed that growth would be protected by insufficient systemic absorption of the intranasal and inhaled glucocorticoids used to reduce airway inflammation in environmental allergies and asthma. Evidence has shown growth deceleration even at moderate doses, and although the effect on final height remains con-

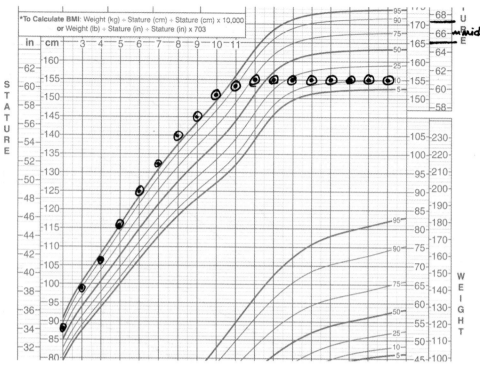

*To Calculate BMI: Weight (kg) ÷ Stature (cm) ÷ Stature (cm) x 10,000
or Weight (lb) ÷ Stature (in) ÷ Stature (in) x 703

Figure 8-16   The Growth Paradox of Early Puberty. An illustrative growth curve is shown for a girl with early puberty. During childhood her height exceeds her midparental target (75%) due to advanced skeletal maturation. However, early puberty with premature closure of the growth plates leads to early termination of growth and a final adult height that is below her genetic potential.

troversial, the FDA requires that labels on inhaled and intranasal steroids warn of a potential growth reduction.

Like cortisol excess, hypothyroidism can impede growth through both central and peripheral actions. Centrally, thyroid hormone stimulates pituitary GH gene expression. Peripherally, thyroid hormone stimulates chondrocyte IGF-I expression, directly promotes endochondral ossification, and is required for vascular invasion at the resorption front of the growth plate. Thyroid receptor knockout mice have decreased pituitary GH secretion, growth failure, retarded endochondral ossification, and disrupted growth plates. Also like cortisol excess, the linear growth failure of hypothyroidism is associated with increased weight gain (in hypothyroidism, this is due to reduced energy expenditure). Hypothyroidism is important in the evaluation and management of children with growth failure for two reasons. First, the incidence of primary hypothyroidism is far greater than GH deficiency, and the most common cause in the United States is chronic lymphocytic thyroiditis (Hashimoto thyroiditis). Thus, more children with growth failure can be successfully treated with L-thyroxine replacement therapy than with GH replacement therapy. Second, many children with GH deficiency also have dysfunction of other anterior pituitary hormones, including thyroid-stimulating hormone (TSH). If a child has unrecognized and untreated secondary or tertiary hypothyroidism, then his or

her growth response to GH treatment for his or her GH deficiency will be substandard. Hypothyroidism will be covered in detail in Chapter 9.

Growth failure can also be caused by poorly controlled diabetes mellitus. Insufficient insulin action leads to hyperglycemia, osmotic diuresis with glycosuria, lipolysis, and overall catabolism. Chronic glycosuria is tantamount to flushing the child's nutritional intake down the toilet. Unfortunately, some adolescent girls with type 1 diabetes mellitus learn that underdosing their insulin is an effective means of weight control. Long-term, linear growth also suffers. Severe diabetic dwarfing, usually associated with hepatomegaly, is called Mauriac syndrome. Improvement in the metabolic control can lead to catch-up growth. The maintenance of normal growth curves for both weight and height is one of the principal goals of pediatric diabetes management.

Inadequate GH action is the rarest entity of the differential of growth failure; 1:3500 children between the ages of 5 and 12 years have GH deficiency (GHD). Inadequate GH action can be divided into GHD (insufficient hormone) and GH resistance (decreased responsiveness to normal or high GH levels). GHD can be subdivided into congenital and acquired causes (Boxes 8-5 and 8-6). GHD can also occur as an isolated hormonal deficit or as part of multiple pituitary hormonal dysfunctions. These distinctions are more fluid, as loss of the pituitary hormones may

---

Box 8-5   Differential Diagnosis of Congenital Growth Hormone Deficiency

1. Idiopathic (the most common form)
2. Identified malformations
   - Congenital absence of the pituitary
   - Associations
     - Holoprosencephaly
     - Septo-optic-dysplasia
     - Midline defects (cleft lip, cleft palate)
3. Identified genetic mutations
   - Familial multiple anterior pituitary hormone deficiency (*Pit-1, PROP-1* mutations)
   - Familial isolated growth hormone deficiency (*GH* gene mutations)
4. Trauma: birth trauma/perinatal insult

---

accumulate with time, so a child with what appears to be isolated GH deficiency may later develop deficiencies of other pituitary hormones. Likewise, there may be a delay in clinical symptomatology such that not all congenital cases are diagnosed in infancy. Nonetheless, thinking of congenital versus acquired causes is helpful in developing the differential diagnosis.

The most common form of congenital GHD is idiopathic; i.e., a specific etiology is not identified, although the growing knowledge of genetics, molecular signaling pathways and organ development is making in-roads into clarifying this category. Of the identified causes, malformations and genetic mutations account for most of the inherent

---

Box 8-6   Differential Diagnosis of Acquired Growth Hormone Deficiency

1. Idiopathic (the most common)
2. Infection
   - Viral encephalitis
   - Bacterial or fungal infection
   - Tuberculosis
3. Vascular: pituitary infarction or aneurysm
4. Infiltration affecting pituitary gland or sella turcica
   - Histiocytosis
   - Sarcoidosis
5. Trauma
   - Child abuse or other closed head injury
   - Surgical resection/damage of the pituitary gland/stalk
6. Tumors
   - Craniopharyngioma
   - Medulloblastoma
   - Glioma
   - Pinealoma
7. Pituitary or hypothalamic irradiation
8. Chemotherapy

---

congenital GHD while other infants acquire GHD at the time of delivery due to birth trauma or asphyxia. The anterior pituitary gland develops from oral ectoderm, whereas the posterior pituitary, of neuroectodermal origin, contains the axonal projections from hypothalamic cells. Pituitary primordium appears at about 4 weeks of gestation, and at 8 weeks, the primary pituitary gland separates into the sellar and pharyngeal portions. Carefully regulated patterns of transcription factor expression, organized temporally and spatially, orchestrate the differentiation of the ectodermal field into distinct cell lineages that ultimately produce particular subsets of the different anterior pituitary hormones. The sella turcica, the bony pocket that supports the pituitary gland, constitutes a developmental boundary area of the cranial base, between notochord-dependent development posteriorly and neural crest cell migration–driven development anteriorly.

Malformations of the pituitary gland can be isolated or associated with other congenital malformations. The most severe isolated malformation is pituitary aplasia, in which the pituitary gland is completely absent. If undiagnosed and untreated, pituitary aplasia is usually fatal in the neonatal period due to adrenal insufficiency. Empty sella syndrome refers to a sella turcica that is filled with cerebrospinal fluid (CSF) on magnetic resonance imaging (MRI); the pituitary gland may be undetectable or present and abnormally small. It is not clear what comes first in those cases: pituitary gland hypoplasia with secondary filling of the sella by CSF or primary herniation of CSF through an incompetent sella diaphragm that compresses what otherwise would have been a healthy pituitary gland. GH deficiency is the most common endocrinopathy in empty sella syndrome. Other rare pituitary malformations include double pituitary glands or ectopic glands.

Pituitary malformations may occur with other midline defects. Holoprosencephaly, an embryological disruption in the midline cleavage of the forebrain, usually results in severe mental and motor delays with malformed or completely absent pituitary glands. Septo-optic-dysplasia (de Morsier syndrome) consists of optic nerve hypoplasia and variable hypoplasia of the septum pellucidum and corpus callosum. Thirty-seven percent of children with septo-optic dysplasia also have pituitary insufficiency, with GHD the most frequent of the hormonal deficiencies. Other midline defects associated with hypopituitarism include cleft lip or palate and solitary central maxillary incisor.

Although most congenital pituitary malformations occur sporadically, some familial cases have been reported. As the multiple factors involved in pituitary formation and development are better studied, many cases of glandular dysgenesis may ultimately turn out to be the results of specific genetic mutations. The molecular regulation of pituitary embryology is thoroughly reviewed by Dasen and Rosenfeld and is beyond the scope of this chapter. Mutation of transcription factors active early in the sequence of pituitary gland formation may result in gross glandular abnormalities; mutations in later transcription factors may result in poorly differentiated cells with impaired hormonal synthetic capabilities but grossly normal appearing pituitary glands. Two such mutations in particular bear discussion, as there have been reports clearly linking these mutations to clinical hormonal deficiencies: *POU1F1 (Pit-1)* and *PROP-1*. *POU1F1* (also called *Pit-1* and *GHF-1*) is a POU domain–containing transcription factor expressed in certain pituitary cells. It is required for the differentiation, survival, and proliferation of the somatotrophs, lactotrophs, and thyrotrophs, and it enhances transcription of the hormonal products of these cell lines (GH, prolactin, and TSHβ, respectively) by binding specific DNA sites in the promoters of these genes. *POU1F1* mutations leading to somatotroph, lactotroph, and thyrotroph insufficiencies have been demonstrated in the Snell and Jackson dwarf mice as well as in humans. Heterozygous *Pit-1* mutations in clinically symptomatic patients suggest dominant negative mutation activity. *PROP-1 (Prophet of Pit-1)* occurs one step ahead of *POU1F1* in pituitary development. *PROP-1*, a pituitary-specific paired-like homeodomain factor, is required for *POU1F1* gene expression as well as for generation of the gonadotrope cell lineage. Thus, patients with *PROP-1* mutations have the same deficiencies noted for patients with *POU1F1* mutations with additional deficiencies of the gonadotropins, luteinizing hormone, and FSH. Pedigrees with the *PROP-1* mutations demonstrate autosomal recessive inheritance of familial multiple anterior pituitary hormone deficiency (MAPD), characterized by significant growth failure, severe GH/IGF-1/IGFBP-3 deficiency, low free T_4 levels, low prolactin levels, and low FSH and luteinizing hormone with very low estradiol and testosterone levels but, in some individuals, normal cortisol levels. The Ames dwarf mouse is a model of *PROP-1* deficiency.

Mutations specific to GH production result in familial isolated GHD, which has been divided into three types based on the mode of inheritance. Type 1 is inherited as an autosomal recessive trait; it is further subdivided into 1A and 1B. GHD type 1A is caused by *GH1* gene deletions such that there is no endogenous GH production. Complete lack of GH, even prenatally, predisposes these individuals to immune intolerance of exogenous GH treatment, so they tend to develop anti-GH antibodies that can limit the growth response to GH treatment. In contrast, patients with GHD type 1B have low but detectable GH levels on provocative testing and maintain good growth responses to exogenous GH therapy. Mutations in the gene for the GHRH receptor have been identified in some patients with GHD type 1B. GHD type 2 is inherited in an autosomal dominant fashion and responds well to GH treatment. Mutations affecting the donor splice site of intron 3 of the *GH1* gene have been identified in some of these patients. Missplicing of GH produces a GH molecule that folds improperly and suppresses secretion of the wild-type GH encoded by the normal allele in a dominant negative manner. GHD type 3 follows an X-linked recessive inheritance pattern and sometimes is associated with agammaglobulinemia, another X-linked trait. These children respond well to GH treatment, so investigations for GHD should be pursued in children with agammaglobulinemia, rather than solely attributing their growth failure to frequent infections. Recently, polymorphisms in the *GH1* gene have been found to be associated with GH secretion and height.

Like congenital GHD, the most frequent etiology of acquired GHD is "idiopathic," and in acquired pituitary dysfunction, GH is the most commonly deficient hormone. The differential of pituitary gland injury/destruction is similar to the general pediatrics differential of most organ failures. Direct injury to the organ by infectious agents, in the case of the pituitary gland, may result from viral encephalitis, bacterial, fungal or tuberculous meningitis, and parasitic infections with *Cysticercus* and *Echinococcus* (also in acquired immune deficiency syndrome, *Toxoplasma*, and *Pneumocystis carinii*). The pituitary may become involved via hematogenous dissemination of the infectious agent or via contiguous spread of an infection, such as sphenoid sinusitis or cavernous sinus thrombophlebitis. It is important to monitor the growth of these children in the long term, because abnormal GH testing may not develop until years after the infectious insult.

The pituitary gland may also be consumed by sterile inflammatory processes. Lymphocytic hypophysitis, an autoimmune destruction of the anterior pituitary gland, occurs most commonly during pregnancy or the first postpartum year; it has been reported rarely in men and children. Other autoimmune endocrine dysfunctions are often associated, making this part of the polyglandular autoimmune syndromes. The inflammatory infiltration enlarges the pituitary gland, and then leads to fibrotic changes. Granulomatous involvement can be seen in sarcoidosis, which especially affects the hypothalamus and infundibulum. Langerhans cell histiocytosis (histiocytosis X), infiltration with large mononuclear Langerhans cells, also involves the hypothalamus, infundibulum, and posterior pituitary.

Vascular insults can also cause acquired hypopituitarism, including GHD. From 1% to 6% of unselected adult autopsies revealed small adenohypophyseal infarcts that were clinically silent; the majority of the gland must be lost to produce symptoms. Pituitary infarction has most commonly been attributed to obstetrical delivery; hypovolemic shock due to severe blood loss can be contributory, and Sheehan syndrome consists of postpartum hemorrhage and necrosis of the physiologically enlarged pituitary gland of pregnancy leading to postpartum hypopituitarism. Other causes include antepartum infarction in insulin-dependent diabetic women, hemodynamic changes during cardiac bypass surgery, infarction of a pituitary adenoma, and injury during mechanical ventilation. Pituitary apoplexy is the acute hemorrhagic infarction of a pituitary adenoma frequently followed by glandular involution. Because the posterior pituitary gland has its own blood supply, diabetes insipidus generally does not accompany anterior pituitary deficiencies caused by vascular events.

Trauma has the opposite predilection; severe head trauma, especially involving basal skull fracture, may shear the pituitary stalk. As the stalk contains the axonal connections between the hypothalamus and posterior pituitary, diabetes insipidus is the most common endocrinopathy incurred. However, with sufficient shearing forces, anterior pituitary dysfunction may also occur.

The single largest identifiable cause of acquired hypopituitarism (and again, GH is the most frequently affected of the hormones) is oncological. There are four potentially contributing mechanisms. First, tumors located in the sella, suprasellar region, or pineal gland may physically compress and destroy the glandular tissue or may secrete hormones that interfere with normal pituitary function. Second, during neurosurgical excision of the tumor, the pituitary and hypothalamus may become permanently injured. Third and fourth, irradiation and chemotherapeutic treatments for the tumor may also permanently impair hypothalamic and pituitary functioning. Hypopituitarism may result from irradiation and chemotherapy for physically distant malignancies as well. For example, total body irradiation in preparation for bone marrow transplantation includes the hypothalamus/pituitary within the direct radiation field, although the primary tumor may have been an abdominal mass that could not affect these glands by direct mass effect.

Perhaps the most common tumor causing pediatric acquired hypopituitarism is craniopharyngioma. Craniopharyngioma, a benign tumor derived from remnants of Rathke's pouch, has a bimodal distribution of age-related incidence, with a peak between ages 5 and 10 years and a second smaller peak between 50 and 60 years. Most craniopharyngiomas are suprasellar, and their presenting symptoms directly result from mass effects unique to their location: compression of the optic chiasm causes temporal hemianopsia, growth into the third ventricle causes hydrocephalus with severe headaches and vomiting, and distortion of the hypothalamus and pituitary can cause hormonal dysfunction, including growth failure evident at the time of presentation. The majority of craniopharyngiomas are cystic, and many contain calcifications that are apparent on computed tomography scanning. Because craniopharyngiomas are not encapsulated, curative resections may be challenging. The other more common pediatric tumors resulting in hypopituitarism are medulloblastomas and gliomas. Gliomas may involve both the optic tracts and hypothalamus directly, and 20% to 40% can be associated with neurofibromatosis. Pituitary adenomas are far less common in children than adults.

Because the number of pediatric cancer survivors is rising, there is an increasing appreciation of the late effects of cancer therapy. Nutritional insufficiencies, psychosocial stressors, and the malignant disease process itself may all contribute to the growth failure that frequently occurs. Irradiation may cause growth failure by inducing GH deficiency. GH deficiency is more likely with higher total radiation doses, larger fraction sizes administered over shorter periods, younger age at the time of irradiation, and longer intervals between the times of GH testing and irradiation. Irradiation may also cause growth failure by damaging the spine itself. Unfortunately, craniospinal irradiation leads to disproportionate growth, with decreased upper-to-lower body segment ratios, that is resistant to GH therapy. Chemotherapy also retards growth and bone age maturation. Chemotherapy-induced growth failure is evident in the absence of irradiation, such as acute lymphoblastic leukemia treated with intrathecal chemotherapy in lieu of cranial radiation. When chemotherapy is added as adjuvant treatment to craniospinal irradiation, the growth failure is even worse than with irradiation alone. In addition to effects on the GH axis, radiation and chemotherapy can cause hypothyroidism, precocious puberty, hypogonadotropic hypogonadism, or primary gonadal failure, all of which can adversely impact growth. Because hormonal deficits may not manifest until years after cancer treatment, long-term careful monitoring of the child's growth is an important component of cancer survivor care.

GH insensitivity is characterized by low IGF-I levels despite normal or high GH levels; although GH itself is normal and not deficient, its bioactivity is significantly reduced. Like GHD, GH insensitivity can be congenital or acquired. Congenital GH insensitivity results from genetic mutations downstream of GH in the GH axis, whereas acquired GH insensitivity can be caused by malnutrition or malabsorption, hepatic dysfunction, inflammatory disease, sepsis, or the development of anti-GH antibodies; these topics were discussed previously. Congenital GH insensitivity, or Laron syndrome, has been found to cluster in parts of the Middle East (Sephardic Jews, Arabs, and Druze patients) and Ecuador. Laron syndrome is classically caused by mutations in the GHR (called type 1 Laron syndrome). One family had a defect in the post-GHR signal transduction (called type 2), and there is one reported case of IGF-I gene deletion causing intrauterine growth retardation and postnatal growth failure. Patients with Laron syndrome have a characteristic phenotype with many features common to severe GHD: severe short stature (final height, 109 to 138 cm in men and 100 to 136 cm in women), underdeveloped sphenoid leading to prominent forehead but hypoplastic nasal bridge, sparse hair, high-pitched voice, small hands and feet, progressive adiposity with hypercholesterolemia, delayed bone age and osteoporosis, and reduced muscle strength. Hypogonadism is common with delayed puberty, although fertility is maintained. IGF-I is important for prenatal growth of the central nervous system, so the majority of patients with Laron syndrome have intellectual deficits of varying severities. Due to the phenotypic overlap with severe GHD, diagnosis of congenital GH insensitivity rests on abnormally low IGF-I (and IGFBP-3 levels) but normal or high GH levels (24-hour GH profiles in patients with Laron syndrome reveal GH pulsatility with normal numbers of GH peaks but greatly elevated peak amplitudes). An IGF generation test was devised to demonstrate insensitivity to exogenous GH. Because GHBP is derived from proteolytic cleavage of the extracellular GHR, and most of the type 1 Laron syndrome mutations occur in the GHR extracellular domain, serum GHBP concentrations in these patients are not measurable or decreased.

Initial Evaluation

Because the differential diagnosis of growth failure is so broad, the initial evaluation requires a thorough history and physical examination. Critical to these are accurate measurements of height and weight and correctly plotted growth curves. For any child who fits one or more of the criteria for growth failure listed in Box 8-3, the next step is a detailed history of both the child and his or her family. Key components of the history are listed in Box 8-7. It is important to establish the growth pattern inherent to the family for proper interpretation of the child's growth. Likewise, the family history may provide clues to an inherited condition for which growth failure is the first or only presentation in the child. A thorough review of systems, including neurological, is important to screen for the various conditions discussed in the differential diagnosis. Dentition history, as hallmarked by age of first tooth eruption and age at which the first primary tooth is lost, can be an additional clue. Dentition history can serve as a "poor man's bone age," indicating delays in skeletal maturation. Psychosocial health

---

> **Box 8-7   Key Elements in History Gathering for the Evaluation of Growth Failure**
>
> 1. Family history
>   - Parents' heights
>   - Parents' ages of puberty
>   - Family history of short stature (women <4 feet 11 inches or men <5 feet 4 inches)
>   - Family history of delayed growth or puberty (growth after high school, menarche at 14 years or older)
>   - Family history of endocrinopathies or systemic illnesses that may affect growth
> 2. Child's history
>   - When did growth failure begin?
>   - How psychosocially distressed is the child about his or her growth?
>   - Perinatal history
>   - Complications of pregnancy and delivery
>   - Birth weight
>   - Potential clues to etiology
>   - Hypopituitarism: hypoglycemia, prolonged jaundice, in boys micropenis
>   - Turner syndrome: lymphedema
>   - Prader-Willi syndrome or Down syndrome: hypotonia
>   - History or signs/symptoms of systemic illnesses
>   - In older children, any signs of puberty and age at which they commenced
> 3. Medication history, including nonprescription drugs and health-food store supplements
> 4. Dentition history
> 5. Psychosocial history

---

can be readily screened by inquiring about household composition and school performance. Like growth failure, a deterioration in school performance should be an instant "red flag" that something is amiss. For children in whom weight gain is more severely impaired or fall-off in weight gain precedes the decline in linear growth, a more detailed nutritional history should be sought. Rather than asking vague questions about overall diet, it is often more fruitful and efficient to list a typical day's intake, including both foods and drinks, specifying times, contents, and quantities.

A thorough physical examination is also required. Particular attention should be placed on the neurological examination, including confrontational testing of visual fields and visualization of the funduscopic discs, for the evaluation of potential brain tumors. Current dental age, scoliosis, and proportionality of limbs relative to height (or measurement of sitting height) are good skeletal indicators for every child; cubitus valgus and shortened fourth metacarpals are particularly notable in girls with Turner syndrome. A single central maxillary incisor or other midline defect should raise suspicion for hypopituitarism. The thyroid gland should be palpated in every child. Auscultation for respiratory or cardiovascular problems and a careful abdominal examination will also help screen for systemic diseases. Tanner staging is critical.

Again, due to the broad differential and the great sensitivity but poor specificity of growth failure as a sign, screening laboratory tests should be used to evaluate the multifaceted differentials discussed earlier and in Box 8-4. Such screening laboratory tests are listed in Box 8-8. Should the history and/or physical examination provide any clues to a potential etiology, then testing can be fine-tuned. For example, lymphadenopathy should raise the suspicion for infectious processes, and HIV infection testing and PPD placement should be pursued. Historic elements may suggest cystic fibrosis which would require sweat testing, and poor weight gain should prompt the additional measurement of tissue transglutaminase antibodies to rule out celiac disease. Hyperpigmentation and poor weight gain may suggest Addison disease, which can be evaluated by early morning (8 to 9 AM) cortisol and ACTH levels, whereas plethora, hypertension, striae, and excessive weight gain may suggest Cushing syndrome, which is best screened with a 24-hour urine collection for free cortisol to creatinine ratio. Although T_4 and TSH levels are reliable screens for hypothyroidism, if secondary or tertiary hypothyroidism is suspected, then a measurement of the free T_4 is a more sensitive test. Brain MRI with contrast should be obtained in any child with neurological signs or symptoms. Because the pituitary is so small, proper pituitary visualization will require extra fine slices of the region; lesions may be missed on standard brain MRI studies. Therefore, visualization of the pituitary gland must be specified to the radiologist when ordering the test to ensure an adequate study.

Box 8-8   Initial Screening Evaluation of Growth failure

1. General tests
   - Chemistries, including kidney and liver function tests
   - Complete blood cell count with differential
   - Sedimentation rate
   - Urinalysis
2. Genetic tests: chromosomes in *every* female
3. Endocrine tests
   - Thyroid function tests
   - Growth factors: IGF-I and IGFBP-3
4. Imaging studies: bone age (anteroposterior radiograph of left hand and wrist)

Evaluation by a Pediatric Endocrinologist

Due to inherent difficulties in diagnosing GHD, this evaluation should be deferred to a pediatric endocrinologist. However, it certainly behooves the primary physician to first effectively rule out any nonendocrine, systemic disease causes of growth failure. When making the referral, providing a copy of the child's growth curves is the single most helpful piece of data; this picture is worth a thousand words. Likewise, providing results of any laboratory evaluations will prevent unnecessary duplications and expedite care.

Because of its circadian rhythmicity, random GH measurements are useless (except in neonates before the sleep entrainment is established). Because blood work is usually obtained during the day, the period of lowest GH release, a random GH measurement cannot evaluate the adequacy of overall GH secretion. A helpful surrogate screening test is a random measurement of circulating IGF-I and IGFBP-3 levels. These levels do not alter significantly with time of day, and because their production is dependent on hepatic stimulation by GH, normal circulating IGF-I and IGFBP-3 levels suggest adequate GH action. However, circulating IGF-I and IGFBP-3 levels change with age and gender (they rise through childhood to peak during puberty and decline thereafter), so it is important to interpret the growth factor levels according to age- and gender-specific norms. Such normative data are provided in Table 8-1. Because growth factor production is also influenced by other factors, including hepatic function and nutritional status, low levels cannot be taken as bona fide evidence of GHD; further testing must be pursued.

Provocative testing has been developed as a means of bypassing the circadian rhythm of endogenous GH secretion. After an overnight fast (water is allowed ad libitum), the child is brought to the hospital for a few hours in the morning for administration of known GH secretagogues and serial measurements of the circulating GH levels before and after the stimulus. An in-dwelling blood-drawing intravenous catheter is used throughout the procedure to minimize the number of venipuncture procedures. In essence, the provocative tests force a GH peak to occur at a convenient time during the day when circulating levels can be readily measured, and the magnitude of that peak is judged as adequate or inadequate. Adequacy of peak amplitude depends on the method and patient age. The "normal" cutoff may be 10 or 7 ng/mL depending on whether the laboratory uses a polyclonal or monoclonal antibody GH assay. Because endogenous GH secretion is significantly less in adults than in children, diagnosing GHD in adults uses a lower cutoff value. Because 20% of healthy, GH-replete children can fail any given provocative test, to minimize the false failure rate, two tests are performed in tandem and

Table 8-1 Age- and Gender-Specific Norms for Circulating Insulin-Like Growth Factor-I (IGF-I) and IGF Binding Protein 3 Levels

Insulin-Like Growth Factor Binding Protein 3 Expected Values

Age	Term		Preterm*	
	Range (ng/mL)	Mean (ng/mL)	Range (ng/mL)	Mean (ng/mL)
NEWBORNS AND INFANTS				
Birth	0.4-1.7	0.9	0.3-1.4	0.9
2 mo	0.5-2.1	1.3	0.9-2.3	1.6
4 mo	0.6-2.4	1.4	0.4-2.2	1.5
6 mo	0.5-2.4	1.4	1.0-2.3	1.5
12 mo	0.8-3.0	2.1	1.0-2.8	1.8

Age (yr)	Range (mg/L)	Mean (mg/L)
CHILDREN		
1-4	1.4-3.0	2.1
5-6	1.5-3.4	2.4
7-8	2.1-4.2	3.0
9-11	2.0-4.8	3.3
12-13	2.1-6.2	3.8
14-15	2.2-5.9	4.2
16-18	2.5-4.8	3.8
ADULTS		
19-30	2.0-4.2	3.0
30-70	1.9-3.6	2.7

*Values from preterm infants were determined at these ages from expected gestation.

Insulin-Like Growth Factor-I (IGF-I)-Blocking Assay Expected Values

Age	Term		Preterm*	
	Range (ng/mL)	Mean (ng/mL)	Range (ng/mL)	Mean (ng/mL)
NEWBORNS AND INFANTS				
Birth	15-109	59	21-93	51
2 mo	15-109	55	23-163	81
4 mo	7-124	50	23-171	74
6 mo	7-93	41	15-132	61
12 mo	15-101	56	15-179	77

Age (yr)	IGF-I (ng/mL) in Males			IGF-I (ng/mL) in Females		
	Range	Mean	SD	Range	Mean	SD
CHILDREN						
1-2	30-122	76	23	56-144	100	22
3-4	54-178	116	31	74-202	138	32
5-6	60-228	144	42	82-262	172	45
7-8	113-261	187	37	112-276	194	41
9-10	123-275	199	38	140-308	224	42
11-12	139-395	267	64	132-376	254	61
13-14	152-540	346	97	192-640	416	112
15-16	257-601	429	86	217-589	403	93
17-18	236-524	380	72	176-452	314	69

*Values from preterm infants were determined at these ages from expected term gestation.

Continued

Table 8-1	Age- and Gender-Specific Norms for Circulating Insulin-Like Growth Factor-I (IGF-I) and IGF Binding Protein 3 Levels—cont'd					
	IGF-I (ng/mL) in Males			IGF-I (ng/mL) in Females		
Age (yr)	Range	Mean	SD	Range	Mean	SD
ADULTS THROUGH 80 YR						
19-20	281-510	371	76	217-475	323	75
21-30	155-432	289	73	87-368	237	74
31-40	132-333	226	62	106-368	225	71
41-50	121-237	160	42	118-298	205	60
51-60	68-245	153	48	53-287	172	55
61-70	60-220	132	34	75-263	180	51
71-80	36-215	131	46	54-205	156	46

Data reproduced with permission from Esoterix Endocrinology, Calabasas Hills, CA.

both must prompt inadequate peaks for the diagnosis of GHD to be made. GH secretagogues commonly used for these tests include arginine, clonidine, insulin-induced hypoglycemia, propranolol, glucagon, L-DOPA, and GHRH.

Inadequate GH peaks after stimulation imply that the pituitary gland cannot synthesize and/or release sufficient GH. However, if the lesion occurs at the level of the hypothalamus rather than the pituitary, the provocative testing may be misleading. The normal pituitary gland will release sufficient GH when provoked by the exogenous pharmacological stimuli, but actual GH secretion in the patient remains inadequate due to defective endogenous signaling. This secondary GH deficiency is called neurosecretory GHD and can be tested by serial measurements of circulating GH concentrations, every 20 minutes from 8 PM to 8 AM. Controversy persists about whether it is the number and amplitude of the GH peaks or the integrated overnight GH level that serves as the best marker for GHD. Clearly, the overnight GH testing is the most invasive and involved procedure, requiring overnight hospitalization and the largest blood collection of all the GH studies. Historically this was the first and, for a time, the only test for GHD. Currently, it is reserved as a last-line test for those children who "pass" the provocative tests but raise a high clinical suspicion of GHD. Recognizing neurosecretory GHD is important because these patients will respond to GH therapy with significant improvements in final height, similar to children with classic GHD. In contrast, short children with normal GH functioning do not significantly improve their final heights with GH treatment.

All children diagnosed with GHD should undergo pituitary MRI. To enhance the sensitivity for detecting pituitary lesions, the MRI must be used with gadolinium-enhanced and extra fine slices through the pituitary gland. Imaging is important to diagnose a pituitary malformation or acquired mass lesion. Whenever there is gross glandular abnormality, formal testing of the function of all the pituitary hormone axes must

be pursued, and any and all deficiencies must be replaced therapeutically to achieve an optimal growth response.

Overall Approach to the Patient

The overall approach to the evaluation of short stature/growth failure involves a series of decision points. First, the physician must determine if the child does or does not have short stature/growth failure. Tantamount to answering this question are accurately measured heights and weights correctly plotted on the appropriate growth curves. Any child who fulfills at least one criterion listed in Box 8-3 warrants further investigation.

The second decision point is ruling out those children who are short but healthy. Three major clues are helpful here, beyond a benign history and normal thorough physical examination. The first critical piece of data is the genetic target height based on the parents' heights. If the child is short but channeling the midparental target with a normal growth velocity, then he or she has familial short stature and further intervention is not warranted. The second major clue is the bone age, because the bone age improves the ability to predict final height. Most endocrinopathies and many growth-impairing systemic diseases are associated with delayed bone ages. If the bone age is delayed beyond 2 SDs below the mean for age and gender, the child must be further evaluated. If the bone age is delayed within 2 SDs and the predicted final height concurs with the parental genetic target, then the child most likely has constitutional delay of growth. A normal growth velocity is reassuring that there is no ongoing process that is holding back the child's linear growth.

The third decision point is distinguishing primary linear growth impairment from a problem in adequate weight gain. The child often appears to be underage for both height and weight. A review of the child's previous growth curves is critical to see if a fall-off in weight gain preceded the linear growth decline. If so, the subsequent decision tree should focus on nutritional issues. In that case, the next decision is whether the child has "organic" or "nonorganic" nutritional dwarfing. *Organic* causes include diseases of the gastrointestinal system, which should be actively sought through a thorough review of symptoms, physical examination, and laboratory studies. *Nonorganic* causes can be surmised from a careful dietary history. Also, if an acute fall-off is noted, the clinician should inquire about major psychosocial stressors that may have occurred at that time (e.g., parental divorce, death in the family, change in residences, new school, issues with peers). Frequently, change in appetite, diet, or activity, manifesting as poor weight gain, can be the sign of underlying depression or anxiety. For children whose growth failure is weight driven, rather than height only, formal evaluation by a gastroenterologist or pediatric dietitian may be more effective than an evaluation by a pediatric endocrinologist.

The fourth decision point involves ruling out systemic diseases, including genetic syndromes. Thorough history and physical and neurological examinations are required. Subsequent laboratory and/or radiological evaluations are determined on the basis of the signs detected on the history and physical examination. Screening chemistries, including renal and liver functions, complete blood cell counts with differentials, and sedimentation rates are helpful in everyone.

For those children whose projected final heights fall below their genetic targets and/or demonstrate abnormally slow growth velocities, endocrinopathies should be considered. Thyroid functions must be evaluated. Because of the complexities involved in the correct diagnosis of GHD, such patients should be referred to a pediatric endocrinologist.

Treatment

Treatment of short stature/growth failure should target the underlying cause. Sometimes, as in a patient with familial short stature or constitutional growth delay, the proper treatment consists solely of education and reassurance. An exhaustive review of the treatments for the nutritional and systemic problems discussed in the preceding sections and listed in Box 8-4 is beyond the scope of this chapter. Therapies for each of the endocrinopathies are covered in the relevant chapters of this book; therefore, this section focuses on GH therapy.

GH therapy for the replacement of GHD in short children has been practiced since the 1960s. From 1963 to 1985, the National Hormone and Pituitary Program (NHPP) of the National Institutes of Health (NIH) provided cadaveric human GH to about 8000 American children and other children worldwide. This program was terminated in 1985, when three young men died of Creutzfeldt-Jakob disease (CJD), a latent prion-mediated neurodegenerative disease. In a 1999 follow-up, the tally was up to 22 CJD deaths in the United States (diagnosis confirmed in 19) and an additional 6 in overseas recipients (5 in New Zealand and 1 in Brazil). Also, there have been 62 CJD cases in France, 32 in England, 1 in Holland, and 1 in Australia in recipients of cadaveric GH from the national pituitary programs of their respective countries.

Fortunately, at the same time the NHPP was closed, advances in molecular biology techniques allowed the production of recombinant human GH (rhGH). The human GH gene was subcloned into nonpathogenic bacteria that mass-produce the human GH, which is then highly purified. All of the current commercially available rhGH results from this synthetic process, which eliminates all infectious risks, and produces a peptide identical in structure to the 22-kDa major circulating isoform of endogenous human GH (all brands except Protropin, which has an additional amino-terminal methionine residue). After the CJD scare, rhGH has been closely monitored through extensive postmarketing surveillance databases, and more than 110,000 patient-years of experience worldwide reveal a very safe adverse effect profile. Benign increased intracranial pressure (pseudotumor cerebri) has been reported in 0.07 to 1.6:1000 patient-years of rhGH treatment for idiopathic GHD; it is readily reversible with immediate cessation of the rhGH treatment. rhGH can then be safely restarted at a lower dose. Another observed fluid-shift phenomenon is peripheral edema, which most notably caused carpal tunnel syndrome in adults treated with pediatric rhGH doses. As a result, current recommended rhGH replacement doses for adult GHD are far lower than pediatric doses, and this adverse effect now occurs far less frequently. Because rhGH accelerates growth, scoliosis and slipped capital femoral epiphysis (SCFE) can occur similarly to that seen in the normal pubertal growth spurt. Gynecomastia has been reported in some prepubertal boys receiving rhGH, and children with nevi tend to experience increases in the number and size of nevi but no malignant transformation. Because GH is an insulin counterregulatory hormone, rhGH therapy increases insulin resistance. Most children maintain euglycemia via a compensatory increase in insulin production. Finally, the greatest concern is that long-term treatment with a growth-promoting hormone may increase the occurrence of cancer. Careful inspection of the databases shows a cancer incidence equivalent to that of the normal population. It is important to note that many of the children receiving rhGH develop GHD due to an underlying condition that already predisposes them to cancer, such as a prior malignancy. Several case-control studies have found a higher risk of cancer (e.g., prostate, lung, colorectal) in individuals with higher serum IGF-I levels; higher IGFBP-3 levels were associated with lower cancer risk. These associations do not prove causation, and the relative importance of circulating versus local IGF-I levels in carcinogenesis remains unclear. rhGH therapy raises circulating levels of both IGF-I and IGFBP-3. To safeguard rhGH use, especially as it is becoming more pharmacological and less physiological, IGF-I and IGFBP-3 levels should be routinely monitored in rhGH recipients and rhGH dose should be titrated to prevent supraphysiological IGF-I levels.

In addition to the enhanced safety, the switch from cadaveric GH to rhGH has revolutionized its accessibility. The less-pure cadaveric GH was administered by intramuscular injections. rhGH can be administered subcutaneously, which is less painful. Compliance is further facilitated by the development of various administration devices that are more child-friendly than the needle-and-syringe route. Because the supply of cadaveric GH was very limited, GH treatment was initially restricted to modest doses in children with severe GHD. In contrast, rhGH production is theoretically limitless, subject only to financial considerations, so its introduction has allowed investigations into optimal dosing regimens and alternative indications beyond replacement for GHD. For example, studies have shown better height gains when the same weekly total dose is divided into nightly rather than thrice-weekly doses. Thus, to best mimic endogenous GH production, rhGH is administered in nightly subcutaneous injections. A sustained-release rhGH polymer has been developed to enhance compliance by reducing administration frequency, and its optimal dosing paradigms are being worked out. High-dose rhGH in pubertal children, inspired by the physiological increase in normal endogenous GH production that is induced by puberty, has been shown to safely increase height gains without the need for pubertal delay with GnRH-analog therapy. Further dosing and effectiveness trials are ongoing. The current FDA-approved indications for rhGH therapy are listed in Box 8-9.

OVERGROWTH

The child whose height is greater than +2 SDs is less likely to be the subject of evaluation than the one whose height is less than −2 SDs, but it is equally important to identify those situations where tall stature is the result of an underlying pathology. To study the overgrowth syndromes in this chapter, we classify them in two groups: those that affect fetal growth and those that present with postnatal overgrowth (Box 8-10).

Prenatal Onset of Overgrowth

The most common cause of large size at birth is maternal diabetes mellitus. The birth of an excessively large infant should lead to evaluation for maternal (or gestational) diabetes even in the absence of clinical symptoms or family history. The infant of the diabetic mother is large, more so in weight than in length, and frequently presents with hypoglycemia. The infant's size is directly related to the extent of hyperglycemia in the mother. Body fat is increased, and hepatomegaly may be present. Similarly, but far less common, genetic mutations causing congenital hyperinsulinism can also produce large-for-gestational age newborns. The mechanism responsible for overgrowth in both cases is the elevated fetal insulin levels; during intrauterine growth, insulin acts as a growth factor, causing overgrowth.

Other, more rare, causes of large-for-gestational age infants are the Sotos, Weaver, Marshall-Smith, and Beckwith-Wiedemann syndromes. All of these syndromes may present with dysmorphology in addition to macroso-

---

Box 8-9 Current Food and Drug Administration–Approved Indications for Recombinant Human Growth Hormone Therapy

1. Linear growth
   - Pediatric growth hormone deficiency
   - Chronic renal insufficiency
   - Turner syndrome
   - Small-for-gestational age
   - Idiopathic short stature
2. Metabolic effects
   - Adult growth hormone deficiency
   - AIDS cachexia
   - Prader-Willi syndrome (also improves linear growth)

Box 8-10 Differential Diagnosis of Overgrowth

1. Prenatal onset of overgrowth
   - Maternal diabetes
   - Sotos syndrome
   - Weaver syndrome
   - Marshall-Smith syndrome
   - Beckwith-Wiedemann syndrome
2. Postnatal onset of overgrowth
   - Familial (constitutional) tall stature
   - Obesity
   - Precocious puberty
   - Hyperthyroidism
   - Klinefelter syndrome
   - XYY syndrome
   - Marfan syndrome
   - Homocysteinuria
   - Excessive growth hormone secretion

mia, and they tend to share several other characteristics. First, overgrowth is commonly present at birth and persists into postnatal life. Second, both weight and length are involved. Third, most of the overgrowth syndromes are associated with various anomalies. Fourth, mental deficiency is often a feature. Finally, some of these syndromes are associated with neoplasia.

Sotos syndrome (also known as cerebral gigantism) is characterized by increased birth length and weight, excessive growth during the first 4 years of life, advanced bone age, and distinctive facial features including macrodolichocephaly, ocular hypertelorism, and prominent mandible. Most patients have nonprogressive neurological dysfunction manifested by unusual clumsiness and mental retardation. GH secretion and serum IGF-I levels are normal in children with Sotos syndrome. Most cases are sporadic, but familial occurrence has been documented. The diagnosis can be suspected at birth, but follow-up over months or years usually confirms it. Weaver syndrome can be difficult to differentiate from Sotos syndrome because they share many characteristics. Weaver syndrome presents with persistent overgrowth of prenatal onset, accelerated skeletal maturation, distinctive craniofacial appearance, developmental delay, widened distal long bones, broad thumbs, and camptodactyly. There is mild hypertonia, developmental lag, progressive spasticity, and often a low-pitched or hoarse cry. Little is published regarding serum GH and IGF-I concentrations in Weaver syndrome. The distinction between these two syndromes may be very difficult to make and is beyond the scope of this chapter. Patients with Marshall-Smith syndrome also have accelerated growth and maturation in utero, advanced bone age, and prominent foreheads, which can be confused with Weaver syndrome. However, children with Marshall-Smith syndrome are more severely retarded and usually have significant and persistent respiratory difficulties. Nothing is published regarding circulating GH or IGF-I concentration in this syndrome.

The prototypic congenital macrosomia syndrome is Beckwith-Wiedemann syndrome. The most consistent features are overgrowth, hemihypertrophy, macroglossia, umbilical defects ranging from hernia to omphalocele, and earlobe pits. Hyperplasia of various visceral (especially the kidney) and endocrine (especially pancreatic β cells) organs is the rule. Hypoglycemia can be present in 30% to 50% of these infants and tends to spontaneously resolve after several months. Excessive fetal, neonatal, and childhood growth ultimately leads to early epiphyseal fusion, without an increase in adult height. These children are predisposed to embryonal intra-abdominal tumors in early childhood, most commonly, Wilms tumor and adrenocortical carcinoma. The syndrome is caused by alterations in chromosome region 11p15.5, which is subject to imprinting. Duplications, translocation/inversion, or uniparental disomy causes an imbalance between the function of growth-promoting genes such as IGF-II and tumor suppressor genes on this imprinted region. An association between Beckwith-Wiedemann syndrome and disordered regulation of IGF-II gene transcription has been reported, but no consistent abnormality of the GH-IGF axis has been identified. The paternally derived gene for IGF-II is overexpressed and the maternally transmitted gene is not active.

Postnatal Onset of Overgrowth

As in the case of the child with growth failure, crossing up height percentiles between infancy and the onset of puberty is an indication for further evaluation. Such growth pattern can indicate a serious underlying pathological condition, but it is important to evaluate the child with tall stature in the context of familial growth and pubertal patterns. The differential diagnosis of tall stature in childhood includes familial tall stature, obesity, thyrotoxicosis, excessive GH secretion, sexual precocity, and genetic or chromosomal disorders such as the Marfan, XYY, and Klinefelter syndromes. In the following sections we discuss each of these conditions.

Familial (Constitutional) Tall Stature

This category includes tall children who mature at a usual rate and reach puberty and tall adult stature at a usual age. The family history generally reveals this to be a familial tendency, hence the designation "familial tall stature." Children are typically normal size at birth and a high-normal growth rate is established by 3 years of age. Thus the child typically crosses the height percentiles during the first 3 years of life and thereafter maintains a height-attained channel above and closely parallel to the 95th percentile. There usually are no associated problems other than the psychological impact of being unduly taller than the peers.

Genetic tall stature in otherwise normal children can be diagnosed by the family history of tall stature, after the exclusion of Marfan syndrome and homocysteinuria. When a family history of tall stature is available, support and reassurance are frequently all that are required. The evaluation consists of assessing stature, bone age, pubertal stage, and psychological impact of the tall stature. A predicted adult height should be determined. The prediction of adult height evaluating pubertal status and bone age in the older child usually obviates the need for hormonal therapy. Societal attitudes toward tall individuals appear to discourage treatment except in extreme circumstances. In some cases, this normal variant can be quite serious and even devastating in the tall girl and, less commonly, in the tall boy.

Therefore, management, if used, is indicated by the psychological needs of the patient.

Therapy indications and modalities vary widely between different centers and practitioners and different countries. When necessary, therapy is aimed at the acceleration of puberty to cause premature epiphyseal fusion. The earlier the intervention, the more likely it is that the adult height can be decreased. In girls, high-dose estrogen is used to advance skeletal maturation and fusion while interfering with longitudinal growth. Potential risks of estrogen therapy include thrombosis, hyperlipidemia, glucose intolerance, nausea, mild hypertension, and weight gain. Although evidence indicates that estrogen therapy can reduce adult height as much as 3.5 to 7.3 cm below the predicted, the results cannot be ensured. In boys, therapy is more controversial. Androgens have been used to accelerate skeletal maturation, presumably via aromatization to estrogen, but at the price of rapid virilization. The use of estrogen or androgens in otherwise normal children must be weighed against the known (and unknown) potential toxicity of such therapy.

Obesity

Overnutrition during childhood typically accelerates growth slightly and advances skeletal maturation in a manner comparable with height age. This association is so characteristic that the linear growth pattern is the single most important "test" in the evaluation of children with obesity. Those with exogenous (nutritional) obesity maintain robust linear growth, whereas those with short stature or linear growth fall-off should be evaluated for an underlying pathological condition. IGF-I levels are normal in the presence of low GH levels. The mechanisms involved in the overgrowth of children with obesity include the effects of elevated insulin levels (due to obesity-induced insulin resistance) cross-reacting with IGF-1R. Early activation of adrenarche and pubarche is common. Increased aromatization of adrenal androgens by fat tissue causes advancement of bone maturation and, as a result, adult height is normal.

Precocious Puberty

Sexual precocity as a cause of overgrowth is obvious when gonadarche or adrenarche, reflecting excessive sex steroids, is present. However, the adolescent growth spurt precedes the clinical findings of gonadarche and adrenarche in some instances, particularly in females. Therefore, when a child's growth velocity is accelerating rapidly, bone age determinations are mandatory. Advanced skeletal maturation prompts consideration of a diagnosis of sexual precocity. Precocious puberty, centrally or peripherally mediated, results in accelerated linear growth in childhood, mimicking the pubertal growth spurt. Skeletal maturation is accelerated so these children become tall but stop growing prematurely and the final height is frequently compromised (Figure 8-16). However, slowly progressive forms of precocious puberty do not necessarily deleteriously affect adult height. Diagnostic evaluation and therapy for precocious puberty are discussed elsewhere in this book.

Hyperthyroidism

Another example in which linear growth is only mildly accelerated is hyperthyroidism. Hyperthyroidism results in a moderate acceleration of linear growth with a rather striking acceleration of skeletal maturation during infancy, an age when it is extremely rare. In later childhood or in adolescence, when it is relatively more common, there is moderate acceleration of both growth and skeletal maturation. Such patients are seldom evaluated because of the change in growth rate; other symptoms predominate. For further discussion and treatment of this condition please refer to Chapter 9.

Genetic and Chromosomal Disorders

Genetic and chromosomal disorders are known causes of tall stature. Hyperploidy of sex chromosomes predisposes to tall stature. The most common of these disorders is Klinefelter syndrome (47,XXY), which is the most common sex chromosome disorder, affecting 1:500 males. Affected males carry an additional X chromosome, which results in male hypogonadism, androgen deficiency, and impaired spermatogenesis. Some other characteristics include gynecomastia, small testes, sparse body hair, tallness (long-legged proportions), and infertility. In children with Klinefelter syndrome, the tendency toward tall stature becomes evident starting at 5 to 6 years of age; of note, however, men with Klinefelter syndrome usually have normal adult stature. The definite diagnosis of Klinefelter syndrome is made with a karyotype, but a careful history and physical examination, with the hallmark being small, firm testes, would provide sufficient diagnostic clues to make the practitioner suspect the diagnosis. Therapy for patients with Klinefelter syndrome consists of testosterone replacement to correct the androgen deficiency and give the patients appropriate virilization. This therapy cannot reverse infertility.

Children with 47,XYY syndrome are normal sizes at birth, with no congenital defects. The mean adult height in one series was 189 cm, and in other series, final heights of the patients have been greater than the heights of their siblings. Genitalia are normal and plasma testosterone concentrations are in the high-normal ranges. The average IQ is reduced. The diagnosis can be made only by karyotype.

The prototypic genetic syndrome associated with tall stature is Marfan syndrome, an autosomal dominant connective tissue disorder. Marfan syndrome has diverse and even seemingly unrelated manifestations in different organs arising from a single mutation in the fibrillin gene *(FBN1)* at chromosome 15q21. Organs involved include the skeleton, eyes, cardiovascular system, skin, integument, lungs, and muscle tissue. Diagnosis of Marfan syndrome is largely clinical and pragmatic. Classically, Marfan syndrome is characterized by hyperextensible joints, dislocation of the lens, kyphoscoliosis, mitral valve prolapse, and aortic dilatation and dissection. Patients with Marfan syndrome have long, thin bones that result in arachnodactyly and moderately tall stature with long-legged proportions. Because of the possible lethal complications of the cardiovascular manifestations of Marfan syndrome, awareness of the classic features for early diagnosis by the primary physician is important. Among causes of sudden death among competitive athletes, Marfan syndrome trails behind only hypertrophic cardiomyopathy, congenital anomalies of the coronary arteries, and occlusive coronary disease. Any situation that results in greater catecholamine release increases inotropy and, as a result, the impulse of blood ejected into the aorta, with the risk of dissection of the aorta. Therefore, it is recommended that patients avoid situations of considerable emotional or physical stress. It is currently recommended that all patients with Marfan syndrome be considered for β-adrenergic blockade, because this is believed to have a protective effect from both aortic dilatation and dissection, but this has yet to be conclusively proved. Techniques for repairing all aspects of cardiovascular disease in Marfan syndrome have undergone rapid evolution and today, corrective surgery for the mitral valve and the aortic root (dissected and not dissected) carries a lower risk for the majority of the patients. In regard to the tall stature, treatment with estrogen or testosterone has not been systematically tested for efficacy or toxicity, so its use to reduce ultimate height should be done with caution.

Homocysteinuria, an autosomal recessive disorder of methionine-homocysteine metabolism, is associated with marfanoid features but may also involve mental retardation, seizures, joint contractures, and a tendency for thromboembolism. Early diagnosis by amino acid studies and dietary treatment can prevent mental retardation.

Excessive Growth Hormone Secretion

Acromegaly or pituitary gigantism is considered last because it is quite rare in the pediatric population. It is usually due to a pituitary somatotroph adenoma or to somatotroph hyperplasia. GH-secreting tumors have been reported in multiple endocrine neoplasia and McCune-Albright syndrome and in association with neurofibromatosis and tuberous sclerosis. If the oversecretion of GH occurs before epiphyseal fusion, it results in rapid growth

and attainment of adult heights to greater than the expected genetic potential. Clinical manifestations of acromegaly also include soft tissue swelling and enlargement of the nose, ears, and jaw, with coarsening of facial features, pronounced increases in hand and foot size, diaphoresis, and menstrual irregularities. Neurological complications may ensue from the anterior pituitary mass or the thickened skull, or both, giving rise to visual impairment, headaches, or paresthesias. Long-term excessive GH production may result in diabetes mellitus, hypertension, or cardiac decompensation.

In patients with acromegaly, IGF-I levels are elevated. Basal GH levels may be normal or increased but fail to suppress normally by administration of glucose. Often in acromegaly there are high prolactin and phosphate levels. The diagnosis should be completed with radiological evaluation of the pituitary by MRI. The goals of treatment in acromegaly are to return GH secretion to normal, correct the clinical symptoms and signs, reverse mass effects of the tumor such as headache and visual abnormalities, and preserve other anterior pituitary functions. The definition of cure is a reduction in the serum IGF-I level to normal for age and sex and the return of a normal GH response to oral glucose.

Treatment for GH-secreting pituitary adenomas includes surgical resection, pituitary radiation, and medical therapies with dopamine agonist or somatostatin analogues. The use of somatostatin analogues (to suppress GH secretion) is a somewhat effective treatment for acromegaly, but surgical excision is the definitive therapy.

Diagnostic Evaluation of Tall Stature

A tall child whose height parallels the 95th percentile and has tall parents, no dysmorphic features, a normal tempo of puberty, and normal bone age often does not need further investigations. However, chromosomal disorders, Marfan syndrome, homocysteinuria, and occasionally, excessive GH can simulate the clinical picture of familial tall stature. The finding of dysmorphic features, micro-orchidism, or intellectual impairment in a tall child suggests the need for chromosome analysis and more comprehensive metabolic and genetic evaluations.

A tall child with advanced skeletal maturation and progressive deviation above the 95th percentile should be evaluated for precocious pubertal development, including clinical assessment of primary and secondary sexual characteristics, as well as evaluation for the possibility of central nervous system disorders. Because hyperthyroidism may mimic these findings, the clinical examination includes evaluation for goiter, ophthalmological abnormalities, and hypermetabolism. Exogenous obesity, in the absence of dysmorphic features or intellectual impairment, may also cause this pattern of tall stature. In the absence of puberty or symptoms or signs suggestive of a hypothalamic disturbance, the tall stature virtually excludes an endocrine basis. If the bone age is significantly advanced, screening should start with determination of estradiol, testosterone, dehydroepiandrosterone sulfate, gonadotropins, and possibly serum human chorionic gonodotropin. Screening for excessive GH secretion should be initiated with random IGF-I level. The definitive test for the diagnosis of GH excess is failure of serum GH to become suppressed after an oral glucose load.

CONCLUSION

More is being learned about the hormonal regulation of growth at the systemic and cellular levels. However, endocrinopathies comprise only a fraction of the causes of growth failure and overgrowth conditions. Recognition of a growth disturbance, either reduction or acceleration, is an important clinical clue for the primary physician. This can be achieved only by the systematic and precise plotting of regular, accurate measurements onto appropriate growth charts. In the growing child, the growth curve constitutes a vital sign every bit as much as pulse and blood pressure.

MAJOR POINTS

Normal Physiology
Growth hormone stimulates hepatic production of IGF-I, and both have direct actions on the growth plate.

Growth Evaluation
Accurate measurements using adequate techniques and instruments are important.
Use of appropriate growth chart (gender specific, condition specific) and plotting techniques (use of correct age) are needed.
Consider genetic potential when evaluating a child's height.

Short Stature/Growth Failure
Growth failure is a very sensitive, yet nonspecific, sign of a child's overall health.
The differential diagnosis of short stature/growth failure is very broad, including healthy children. Endocrinopathies constitute only a minority.
The initial evaluation of short stature/growth failure starts with accurate measurement and plotting on the appropriate growth chart. A thorough history and physical examination are needed before proceeding to screening laboratory or radiological studies.
Diagnosing growth hormone deficiency should be deferred to a pediatric endocrinologist.

MAJOR POINTS—Cont'd

Overgrowth

Prenatal Onset of Overgrowth
Gestational diabetes is a common cause; a large-for-gestational age infant may require glucose monitoring. Congenital hyperinsulinism should be considered.
Genetic disorders are most likely to be associated with other anomalies and mental deficiency, and overgrowth usually persists postnatally.

Postnatal Onset of Overgrowth
Exogenous obesity is becoming a common cause of postnatal overgrowth.

SUGGESTED READINGS

Arpadi SM: Growth failure in children with HIV infection, J Acquir Immun Defic Synd 25 Suppl 2000;1:S37.

Beker LT, Russek-Cohen E, Fink RJ: Stature as a prognostic factor in cystic fibrosis survival, J Am Diet Assoc 2001;101:438.

Blum WF, Cotterill AM, Postel-Vinay MC, et al: Improvement of diagnostic criteria in growth hormone insensitivity syndrome: solutions and pitfalls. Acta Paediatr Suppl 1994;399:117.

Bourguignon JP: Linear growth as a function of age at onset of puberty and sex steroids dosage: therapeutic implications, Endocr Rev 1988;9:467.

Cohen MM Jr: Overgrowth syndromes: an update, Adv Pediatr 1999;46:441.

Cox LA: Auxology, J Pediatr Endocrinol 1994;7:135.

Dasen JS, Rosenfeld MG: Signaling and transcriptional mechanisms in pituitary development, Annu Rev Neurosci 2001;24:327.

Frost HM, Schonau E: On longitudinal bone growth, short stature, and related matters: insights about cartilage physiology from the Utah paradigm, J Pediatr Endocrinol Metab 2001;14:481.

Greulich WW, Pyle SI: Radiographic Atlas of Skeletal Development of the Hand and Wrist. 2nd ed. Stanford, CA, Stanford University Press, 1959.

Growth Hormone Research Society: Consensus guidelines for the diagnosis and treatment of growth hormone (GH) deficiency in childhood and adolescence: summary statement of the GH Research Society, J Clin Endocrinol Metab 2000;85:3990.

Haffner D, Schaefer F, Nissel R, et al: Effect of growth hormone treatment on the adult height of children with chronic renal failure, N Engl J Med 2000;343:923.

Kaplowitz PB, Oberfield SE, Drug and Therapeutics and Executive Committees of the Lawson Wilkins Pediatric Endocrine Society: Reexamination of the age limit for defining when puberty is precocious in girls in the United States: implications for evaluation and treatment. Pediatrics 1999;104:936.

Lipman TH, Hench K, Logan JD, et al: Assessment of growth by primary health care providers, J Pediatr Health Care 2000;14:166.

Maggioni A, Lifshitz F: Nutritional management of failure to thrive, Pediatr Clin North Am 1995;42:791.

Moshang T Jr, Grimberg A: The effects of irradiation and chemotherapy on growth, Endocrinol Metab Clin North Am 1996;25:731.

Pyeritz RE: The Marfan syndrome, Annu Rev Med 2000;51:481.

Sharek PJ, Bergman DA: The effect of inhaled steroids on the linear growth of children with asthma: a meta-analysis, Pediatrics 2000;106:E8.

Smyth CM, Bremmer WJ: Klinefelter syndrome, Arch Intern Med 1998;158:1309.

Tanner JM, Davies SWD: Clinical longitudinal standards for height and height velocity for North American children, J Pediatr 1985;107:317.

Tuvemo T, Jonsson B, Persson I: Intellectual and physical performance and morbidity in relation to height in a cohort of 18-year-old Swedish conscripts, Horm Res 1999;52:186.

Zeitler PS, Travers S, Kappy MS: Advances in the recognition and treatment of endocrine complications in children with chronic illness, Adv Pediatr 1999;46:101.

THYROID

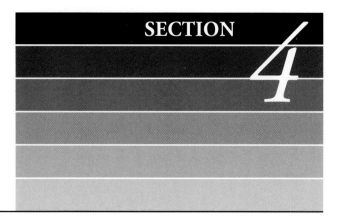

SECTION

4

CHAPTER 9

Thyroid Disorders in Children

WILMA C. ROSSI

NEIL CAPLIN

CRAIG A. ALTER

FETAL THYROID DEVELOPMENT AND FUNCTION

The human adult thyroid gland has two lobes connected by a narrow central isthmus. Embryological development of the thyroid begins on day 24 of gestation as a *diverticulum,* which is an endodermal downgrowth of the primitive pharyngeal floor. The developing thyroid descends in the ante-

rior neck and reaches its adult position opposite C5-7 by the seventh week of gestation. This migration from the posterior pharynx to the base of the anterior neck can be interrupted at any point causing an ectopic thyroid gland. Ectopic thyroid gland is the most common cause of congenital hypothyroidism.

Thyroid hormone production is limited until the 18th to 20th week of gestation. The production of thyroxine (T_4) gradually increases throughout gestation. The production of triiodothyronine (T_3) is dependent on the maturation of a hepatic deiodinase that converts T_4 to T_3 starting at about 30 weeks' gestation. Thus infants born before a gestational age of 30 weeks are unable to make T_3, which is the more active of the two hormones in the periphery. Although once thought to be impermeable to thyroid hormone, the placenta is freely permeable to T_4. Thus maternal T_4 is available throughout gestation. This provides protection for the fetus with hypothyroidism and explains why newborns with congenital hypothyroidism generally have minimal symptoms of hypothyroidism.

Within 30 minutes of delivery, an abrupt rise in the infant's serum thyroid-stimulating hormone (TSH) occurs as of results of the change in environmental temperature. TSH levels can reach as high as 70 µU/ml in the first 12 hours of life. This TSH surge causes a marked increase in the concentrations of both serum T_4 and T_3 by 24 to 48 hours of life. This explains why newborn thyroid screening tests performed before 48 hours of life are frequently falsely positive with an elevation of TSH and depression of T_4 that can be misinterpreted as congenital hypothyroidism. Screening for congenital hypothyroidism is most accurate if performed after 48 hours of life.

Premature infants also have a TSH surge at birth, but it is of lesser magnitude than that of the term infant. As a result, the serum T_4 and T_3 levels are also lower. Preterm infants may have low T_4 levels without elevation of the TSH up to a gestational age of 36 weeks. This is thought to reflect immaturity of the hypothalamic-pituitary-thyroid axis. Sick preterm infants may have very low serum T_4 levels that may be due to a protective mechanism to decrease their overall metabolism. It has been suggested that giving these infants thyroid hormone might improve their condition and neurological outcomes; however, some studies have shown that thyroid hormone may increase oxygen requirements and actually worsen long-term outcome. Thyroid hormone is not recommended in these infants unless they have an elevated TSH level indicating a failing thyroid or proved deficiency of TSH due to hypothalamic or pituitary hypofunction.

THYROID HORMONES

Thyroid hormones have broad effects on development and metabolism; these effects include changes in oxygen consumption, protein, carbohydrate, lipid, and vitamin metabolism.

The thyroid gland secretes the active thyroid hormones, T_3 and T_4. T_4 is more abundant in the circulation but T_3 is more active in the periphery. T_3 is directly secreted by the thyroid and is also produced by peripheral deiodination of T_4. Peripheral production of T_3 can be inhibited by a variety of drugs, including propylthiouricil (PTU), dexamethasone, propranolol, iodinated contrast material, and amiodarone.

TSH is a glycoprotein hormone secreted by the anterior pituitary. TSH acts on the thyroid gland via cell surface receptors to stimulate cell growth, iodine uptake and organification, and thyroid hormone synthesis and release. Thyrotropin-releasing hormone (TRH) is a tripeptide synthesized in the hypothalamus by neurons in the supraoptic and supraventricular nuclei. TRH reaches the anterior pituitary via the pituitary portal venous system. It acts via cell surface receptors on pituitary TSH-secreting cells and prolactin-secreting cells to cause synthesis and secretion of TSH and prolactin. TRH secretion is pulsatile in its secretion and shows a circadian rhythm causing a TSH peak in the early hours of the morning.

The synthesis and secretion of thyroid hormones by the thyroid gland are regulated by the hypothalamus and pituitary via a feedback loop. TRH stimulates secretion of TSH by the anterior pituitary. TSH acts on the thyroid to stimulate many steps in thyroid hormone synthesis. In turn, thyroid hormones exert negative feedback control over TSH and TRH secretion. High levels of thyroid hormones inhibit TRH and TSH secretion, and low levels stimulate TSH secretion. High levels of thyroid hormones also inhibit the actions of TRH on TSH-secreting cells of the anterior pituitary gland. Acute and chronic disease,

dopamine and dopamine agonists, somatostatin, and glucocorticoids also inhibit TSH secretion.

Thyroid hormone synthesis occurs in the colloid of the thyroid follicle and requires multiple steps in its production: the uptake of iodide by active transport, thyroglobulin (TG) biosynthesis, oxidation and binding of iodide to TG, and coupling of two iodotyrosines into iodothyronines. If any of these steps are blocked, thyroid hormone synthesis does not occur. This occurs in genetic disorders called *dyshormonogenesis* and is one of the less common causes of congenital hypothyroidism.

Thyroid hormones are stored in TG in the colloid of thyroid follicles. The hormones remain bound to TG until secreted. TG is a glycoprotein secreted by the follicular cells. TG serum levels and their increase after TSH stimulation constitute a useful index of the functional state of the gland. TG is absent in athyreosis. It should be absent after treatment for thyroid cancer that requires that all thyroid tissue be ablated. A rise in the TG after thyroid ablation indicates that there is residual thyroid tissue, which is a risk for cancer recurrence.

Thyroid hormones are bound to plasma proteins. The major serum thyroid hormone-binding proteins are thyroid-binding globulin (TBG), thyroxine-binding prealbumin (TBPA), and albumin. TBG binds 75% of serum T_4, whereas TBPA and albumin bind only 20% and 5%, respectively. Deficiencies and excesses of thyroid binding proteins produce changes in the values of serum total thyroid hormones, because the assays for total hormones measure both free and bound T_4 and T_3. Measurement of free hormone or an estimate of the binding capacity such as T_3 uptake (T_3U) helps to differentiate between pathologically abnormal thyroid hormone levels and abnormalities in the binding proteins that are variants of normal.

Iodine is essential in the production of thyroid hormone. Dietary sources of iodine include milk, meat, vitamin preparations, some medications such as cough syrups, and iodized salt. The recommended daily intake of iodine is 100 μg for adults and adolescents, 60 μg to 100 μg for children, and 30 to 40 μg for infants less than one year. Although it is rare in North America, iodine deficiency is the leading cause of hypothyroidism worldwide. Its effects are most pronounced if iodine deficiency is present early in life, when it results in intellectual impairment.

THYROID FUNCTION TESTS

Thyroid function studies are commonly performed in the primary care setting for a variety of indications. The practitioner is frequently faced with some component of the results listed as "out of range." Thyroid tests should be evaluated within the clinical setting for which the tests were obtained.

In most circumstances, assessment of the hypothalamic-pituitary-thyroid axis can be performed by measurement of the plasma TSH. If the TSH is normal, it is unlikely that the patient has thyroid dysfunction. Mild abnormalities of thyroid function tests are common and can be difficult to interpret. These tests and some of the factors accounting for abnormal results are discussed later. Occasionally, specific additional tests of the thyroid axis such as antithyroid antibodies, anti-TSH receptor antibodies (TRAb), plasma TBG, plasma TG concentrations, and reverse T_3 (rT_3) are indicated. These tests are usually done is specific circumstances, such as in as differentiating nonthyroidal illness (NTI) or for surveillance in following thyroid carcinoma.

T_4 and T_3

The measurement of circulating levels of thyroid hormones is complicated by the high degree of protein binding of T_4 and T_3 in the circulation. These binding proteins are subject to variations in quantity and binding potential that may be hereditary or acquired resulting in variations in the total thyroid hormone concentration. When measuring total T_4 and T_3, it is helpful to measure an estimate of the serum binding capacity simultaneously. (See discussion of T_3U and free thyroxine index [FTI] later in this section.) Levels of serum total T_4 and T_3 vary with age. Normal values according to age for T_4 are shown in Table 9-1.

Because the free hormone is the biologically active component, its measurement theoretically provides the most useful assessment of thyroid function. Most of the free hormone assays correct for moderate variations in thyroid-binding proteins but may give inaccurate results in the presence of extreme variations in the concentrations of these proteins. Conditions that may interfere with the free T_4 assay include severe congenital TBG abnormalities and the presence of T_4 or T_3 autoantibodies. As reference ranges

vary among methods, results must be compared with the reference range of the laboratory performing the test.

The free T_4 value should always be interpreted together with the TSH concentration and in relation to the clinical findings. Patients taking exogenous L-thyroxine have higher free and total T_4 for equivalent TSH and T_3 compared with controls. Premature infants and patients with critical and NTI require special care in the interpretation of free T_4 values, as discussed subsequently.

The determination of T_3 is most useful in evaluating and monitoring hyperthyroidism. It is not useful in the evaluation of suspected hypothyroidism. However, T_3 is extraordinarily low in NTI and, in conjunction with reverse T_3, helps in differentiating NTI from central hypothyroidism.

T_3 Uptake and Free Thyroxine Index

The T_3U (also known as T_3RU) and FTI tests are methods of estimating thyroid binding. Most assays of T_3U are inversely proportional to the degree of concentration of thyroid-binding protein. Therefore, an increased T_3U represents a decreased concentration of binding proteins. Clinical examples include congenital deficiency of TBG, the use of androgens, corticosteroids, phenytoin, salicylates, and any protein-losing state such as the nephrotic syndrome. Persons with such conditions have decreased total T_4, increased T_3U, and normal TSH.

Decreased T_3U represents an increase in thyroid-binding proteins as seen in pregnancy, estrogen therapy, hepatitis, congenital TBG excess, acute intermittent porphyria, and dysalbuminemia. Persons with these conditions have increased total T_4, decreased T_3U, and normal TSH.

The product of the T_3U and serum total T_4 is the FTI. This is a calculation that attempts to correct the total T_4 for the plasma thyroxine–binding capacity. It reflects the free T_4 but is not a direct measure of it. Current T_3U and FTI tests are prone to error in the presence of significant abnormalities of TBG and thyroid hormone autoantibodies, with some medications, and in the setting of NTI. When performing diagnostic studies, it is usual to perform either a free T_4 or a combination of total T_4 and T_3U. Although free T_4 may be more specific, total T_4 is often more readily available and less costly.

Table 9-1	Normal T_4 Values for Children by Age (Esoterix Endocrinology Laboratory)	
Age	**Range (μg/dL)**	**Mean (μg/dL)**
1-3 days	8.2-19.9	14.6
1 wk	6.0-15.9	12.0
1-12 mo	6.1-14.9	9.8
1-3 yr	6.8-13.5	9.3
3-10 yr	5.5-12.8	8.6
11-18 yr	4.9-13	8.0
Adults	4.2-13.0	8.0

Thyroid-Stimulating Hormone

When the hypothalamic-pituitary-thyroid axis is intact, circulating TSH provides a sensitive measure of thyroid function. TSH is sensitive to changes in free T_4. Until the late 1980s, TSH assays were not able to differentiate between the low and normal ranges for TSH. Therefore, these assays could used only when the TSH was expected to be elevated, such as in primary hypothyroidism. Currently, third-generation assays are available with lower detection limits of 0.01 to 0.02 μU/ml. These highly sensitive assays allow for a reliable distinction to be made between low and normal TSH values and can be used alone as screening tests for both hypothyroidism and hyperthyroidism.

Causes of elevated TSH include primary hypothyroidism, drugs (lithium, iodine, dopamine antagonists, spironolactone), TSH-producing adenoma, and resistance to thyroid hormone (RTH) (discussed later in this chapter). Causes of a low TSH include hyperthyroidism, L-thyroxine administration, hypopituitarism, starvation, critical illness, severe depression, and drugs (dopamine, bromocriptine, serotonin antagonists, glucocorticoids, somatostatin, opiates, α-adrenergic antagonists).

Thyroid Autoantibodies

Commercial assays are available for anti-TG antibodies, thyroid peroxidase antibodies (TPO, formerly measured as antimicrosomal antibodies), and TRAb. TPO can be useful in the evaluation of patients suspected of having autoimmune thyroid diseases such as Hashimoto thyroiditis. TPO occur more frequently and correlate more closely with the likelihood of developing thyroid function abnormalities but do not necessarily indicate the presence of thyroid dysfunction. They occur more frequently in females and increase in frequency with increasing age. They are found in up to 10% of the population. Anti-TG antibodies are less useful than TPO but may be included in commercial panels of thyroid antibodies.

TRAb may stimulate or block the TSH receptor. TRAb are found in 95% of patients with Graves disease. Stimulating TRAb can cross the placenta in late gestation and produce transient neonatal hyperthyroidism, whereas blocking TRAb can cause transient neonatal hypothyroidism.

Thyroid Function Tests in Nonthyroidal Illness

Alterations in thyroid function tests are common in patients with severe illness unrelated to the thyroid. They may be due to the NTI per se, drugs administered for treatment of the NTI, or associated pituitary or hypothalamic disease. This condition is also referred to as the *euthyroid sick syndrome*. Measurement of serum TSH, free T_4, free T_3, and rT_3 yields the most accurate information in the setting of NTI. The most common pattern observed is a low T_3, T_4, and free T_3 but a normal or low free T_4, normal or elevated rT_3, and normal TSH. Patients with low free T_4 and normal or low TSH are more likely to have central hypothyroidism, which is usually due to transient hypofunction of

the hypothalamic-pituitary axis in serious illness. A serum TSH level above 20 to 25 μU/ml is likely to reflect primary hypothyroidism. Accompanying findings of goiter, low free T_4, and positive TPO help establish the diagnosis of primary hypothyroidism. However, TSH can also be elevated in the recovery phase of NTI. The abnormalities of thyroid function testing indicative of NTI (i.e., very low T_3, elevated reverse T_3, normal TSH, and low or low-normal T_4) do not require treatment with thyroid hormones.

THYROID DISEASES OF THE NEWBORN

Thyroid diseases of the newborn must be analyzed, with the unique physiology of the gland both prenatally and in the newborn period, as reviewed earlier, kept in mind. It is important to remember that the TSH surge, which occurs in the first 24 hours of life, increases a very low concentration of T_4 into the normal range by the second postnatal day. Newborn thyroid tests must be considered in light of this normal physiology or they will be subject to interpretation errors.

Congenital Hypothyroidism

Congenital hypothyroidism (CH) affects in approximately 1:4000 live births. It occurs more frequently in girls, with a female-to-male ratio of 2:1. The prevalence in black infants is lower and in Latino infants higher than in white infants. Newborn screening programs were established in the 1970s to diagnose CH as early as possible in the newborn period. Newborn screening is universal in North America as well as in many other parts of the world.

The purpose of newborn screening is to identify infants with serious medical disorders who, if treated in the newborn period, can avoid devastating outcomes. Because CH can cause severe mental retardation unless treated early, newborn screening is clearly warranted in this disorder. The vast majority of infants with CH are diagnosed through newborn screening programs. An efficient screening program can identify the hypothyroid newborn by 3 weeks of age. This allows them to be treated early and to achieve improved, if not completely normal, neurological development.

Screening programs use dried blood spots on filter paper to perform thyroid tests. Programs are organized in one of two ways depending on the local preference. Some programs in North America perform an initial T_4. If the T_4 is in the lowest 10% to 20% of results obtained on a given day, a TSH is performed. An alternative method of screening is to measure TSH on all infants and recommend further evaluation on those infants with elevated levels. TSH screening gives a lower false-positive rate because only newborns with abnormal TSH are considered suspect. In interpreting primary T_4 screening, low normal T_4 values are considered potential cases of CH. Because many of these children are normal, the false-positive rate is higher. The disadvantage of primary TSH screening is that it does not identify children with hypothalamic or pituitary hypothyroidism (i.e., deficiencies in TRH or TSH).

The normal TSH is less than 20 to 25 µU/ml after the first 24 hours of life. This is higher than the normally accepted TSH levels for older infants and reflects the postnatal TSH surge. TSH levels greater than 50 µU/ml are consistent with CH and must be treated as a pediatric emergency. Infants should be evaluated immediately, preferably by a pediatric endocrinologist, so that the need for immediate treatment can be determined. TSH levels in the mid-range of 25 to 50 µU/ml often reflect transient

hypothyroidism but require prompt further evaluation. Initial confirmatory testing should include, at minimum, a serum T_4 and TSH. An algorithm for evaluation of the newborn with possible CH based on newborn screening test results is shown in Figure 9-1. Evaluation and treatment of CH are discussed later.

There are several problems with newborn screening that can cause confusion in the interpretation of screening results; these are listed in Table 9-2. TBG deficiency is a normal variant of thyroid physiology. Because T_4 measures both free T_4 and that bound to TBG and other binding proteins, TBG deficiency presents with a low T_4 in the newborn screen if T_4 is measured primarily. Because TSH is always normal in this condition, a primary TSH screening program does not demonstrate TBG deficiency. Free T_4, TBG, and T_3U are useful in clarifying this diagnosis. In TBG deficiency, the TBG is low and the T_3U is elevated,

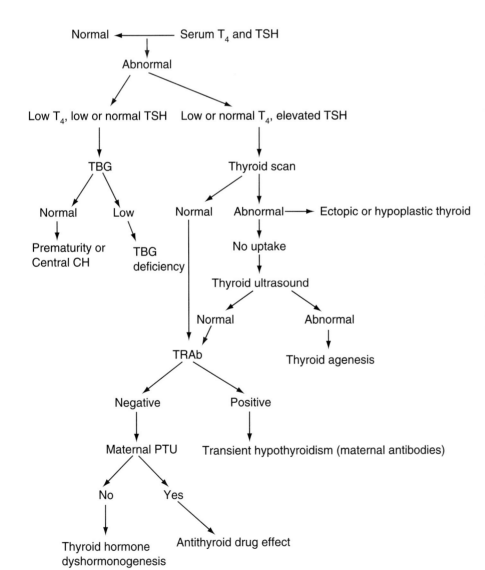

Figure 9-1 Evaluation of the newborn who fails congenital hypothyroidism screening. TBG, thyroxine-binding globulin; TSH, thyroid stimulating hormone; TRAb, anti-TSH receptor antibodies; CH, congenital hypothyroidism.

Table 9-2 Potential Problems in the Interpretation of Newborn Screening Tests for Congenital Hypothyroidism

CONDITION	TEST RESULT	DEFINITIVE TEST
TBG deficiency	Low T_4, normal TSH	Normal free T_4, low TBG
Early screening (<24 hours of age)	Low or normal T_4, elevated TSH	Normal repeat T_4 and TSH >24 hours of age
Prematurity	Low T_4, normal TSH	T_4 normalizes as infant matures

reflecting the decrease in binding proteins. Screening newborns less than 24 hours of life generate what appear to be abnormal thyroid tests because the T_4 will be low with an elevation of the TSH as it surges to bring the T_4 into the normal postnatal range. Premature infants' thyroid tests must be considered as a separate category. Premature infants normally have low T_4 and normal TSH levels; this reflects the immaturity of the hypothalamic-pituitary axis. The thyroid function tests slowly approach normal as the premature infant matures and should be in the normal range for a term infant by gestational age of 36 weeks.

Newborn screening is essential in the early diagnosis of CH because the signs and symptoms of the condition in the newborn period are mild and occur infrequently. Box 9-1 lists the clinical findings in CH. If untreated in the newborn period, most of these findings do not become apparent until 2 to 3 months of age. Initiation of therapy at that time does not prevent the neurological devastation that this disorder will have already caused.

The various etiologies of CH are listed in Box 9-2. They are either permanent forms or transient forms of the disorder. One of the permanent disorders and the most common form of CH is thyroid dysgenesis, representing 80% of

Box 9-1 Clinical Findings in Congenital Hypothyroidism in the Neonate

Postmature	Rough, dry skin
Large-for-gestational age	Mottled skin
Hypotonia	Jaundice
Constipation	Other congenital anomalies
Pallor	Congenital heart disease
Hypothermia	Chromosomal
Hoarse cry	abnormalities
Feeding or sucking	Microcephaly
difficulty	Unilateral clubfoot
Large tongue	Bilateral subluxation of the
Umbilical hernia	hip
Widened posterior	
fontanels	

cases. Most cases are sporadic, although familial cases have been reported and may be autosomal dominant or recessive. Thyroid-specific transcription factors play a role in thyroid development, and mutations of theses factors have been found in cases of thyroid dysgenesis. The thyroid gland can be aplastic, hypoplastic, or ectopic, with the latter being the most common form of thyroid dysgenesis. Ectopic glands result from a disruption in the migration of the fetal thyroid tissue from the pharynx to the neck. These glands are functional but do not produce adequate amounts of thyroid hormone lifelong. They can be missed during newborn screening if the gland functions adequately in the newborn period. Ectopic glands may not fail until later in childhood when the child presents with an ectopically placed goiter. When it is in the neck, it is often confused with a thyroglossal duct cyst. If the ectopic gland is lingual, a large mass may appear at the base of the tongue, which is the goitrous gland. Ectopic glands should not be removed. Treatment with L-thyroxine therapy quite effectively reduces the size of these misplaced goiters.

Another permanent form of CH is thyroid dyshormonogenesis, comprising about 10% of the cases. It is usually associated with a goiter or an easily palpable thyroid gland at birth. Thyroid hormone cannot be produced due to a disruption in the pathway of thyroid hormone synthesis. (See Box 9-2 for specific types of dyshormonogenesis.)

Central hypothyroidism, which comprises about 5% of cases of CH is another permanent form of CH. It is due to defects in the production of TRH and/or TSH. This can be an isolated defect or exist in conjunction with other hypothalamic-pituitary abnormalities. It should be considered in infants who have low serum T_4 levels and low or normal TSH levels on screening tests. As mentioned, a primary TSH screening program does not diagnose central hypothyroidism because the TSH is not elevated.

Transient CH comprises 10% of cases and can be caused by several different etiologies, although in most cases, an etiology is not found. Maternal antithyroid drugs such as propylthiouracil (PTU) and methimazole cause temporary hypothyroidism in the newborn because these drugs cross

Box 9-2   Causes of Congenital Hypothyroidism

PERMANENT FORMS OF CONGENITAL HYPOTHYROIDISM

DYSGENESIS

Aplasia
Hypoplasia
Ectopia

DYSHORMONOGENESIS

TSH unresponsiveness
Iodide trapping defect
Organification defect
Defect in TG
Iodotyrosine deiodinase deficiency

CENTRAL HYPOTHYROIDISM

Hypothalamic-pituitary anomaly
Panhypopituitarism
Isolated TSH deficiency

TRANSIENT FORMS OF CONGENITAL HYPOTHYROIDISM

DRUG INDUCED

PTU
Methimazole
Iodine

IODINE DEFICIENCY

MATERNAL ANTIBODY INDUCED

IDIOPATHIC

the placenta. Infants born to mothers who are deficient in iodine can have transient hypothyroidism. The hypothyroidism can be severe if the mother is also hypothyroid because the maternal-fetal transfer of thyroxine is minimal in this situation, putting the infant brain at risk for hypothyroidism. Maternal iodine ingestion is another drug-induced form of transient CH. Mothers who have autoimmune thyroid disease may transfer blocking TRAb across the placenta to the fetus. If the thyrotropin receptor is blocked, thyroid hormone synthesis cannot proceed. Radionuclide imaging in affected infants will not demonstrate the existence of the thyroid gland because the radionuclide cannot be taken up by the blocked TSH receptor. In this case, ultrasonography is useful in demonstrating that a thyroid gland exists. Transient CH can be idiopathic and is sometimes termed *transient hyperthyrotropinemia* (elevation of the TSH). Because hypothyroidism is potentially harmful to infants even if it is a temporary condition, infants with low serum T_4 and increased TSH levels should be treated with L-thyroxine until it is certain that the condition has resolved and they are able to make thyroid hormone normally.

Although RTH is not generally considered a form of CH, it may be discovered through newborn thyroid screening because the TSH can be elevated in this condition. The T_4 is in the upper range of normal to higher than normal. This condition is discussed separately in detail.

Figure 9-1 is a flow diagram for the evaluation of the newborn with possible CH based on newborn screening test results. The initial step in the evaluation of these new-borns is to repeat thyroid function tests. These tests must be interpreted specifically for the newborn period (see Box 9-2 for normal values of T_4 in full-term infants for the first months of life). They should include either free T_4 or total T_4 and T_3U. The T_3U is indicated as an indirect measure of thyroid binding proteins so that the total T_4 can be interpreted in light of any possible deficiency of thyroid binding proteins. Free T_4 measures free hormone only and does not depend on binding proteins. If T_3U is elevated with low total T_4, TBG should be measured to diagnose possible TBG deficiency. TSH should be repeated to determine if the elevation might have been transient. Thyroid imaging is useful in determining the etiology of CH. It cannot be performed if the infant has been taking L-thyroxine for more than 1 week because this drug will inhibit TSH and interfere with the uptake of the radionuclide scanning agent. Obtaining a thyroid scan should never delay the initiation of therapy. Further delineation of the etiology of the hypothyroidism can be determined after the child is 2 to 3 years old and no longer at risk for damage to the developing central nervous system. ^{99m}Tc scanning delineates anatomy and is simpler to perform in the newborn because it requires only a small intravenous injection of the technetium for adequate imaging. ^{123}I scanning is more difficult technically in the newborn but has the advantage of also delineating thyroid gland function, because ^{123}I scans measure thyroid uptake as well as demonstrate anatomy. This is useful in determining if the infant has a form of thyroid dyshormonogenesis. Thyroid ultrasonography is helpful in determining if a thyroid gland exists when radionuclide imaging fails to demonstrate a thyroid gland that may be suppressed due to maternal thyroid antibodies or antithyroid drugs or is unable to take up the tracer as in certain forms of dyshormonogensis.

The treatment for CH is L-thyroxine 10 to 15 μg/kg/day. L-Thyroxine is available only in tablet form. It is unstable in solution and should not be formulated into a suspension by the pharmacist. The tablets can be crushed and mixed with a small amount of breast milk, formula, or water and fed to the infant from a spoon or dropper. Parents should be instructed in giving the medication properly so that all of the particles of the tablet are administered at each dose. The goal of treatment with L-thyroxine is the normalization of the free T_4 or T_4 and/or the decrease of the TSH to less than 20 μU/ml by 3 weeks of age. Continued follow-up of treated children should monitor growth and development and should maintain the free T_4 or T_4 in the upper half of the normal range for age with a normal TSH. (Consult Box 9-2 for age-related T_4 values.) Note, however, that in some children, especially those with athyreosis, TSH may remain elevated for months despite adequate treatment that achieves a normal T_4 due to a resetting in utero of the pituitary-thyroid feedback threshold.

Unless the infant's hypothyroidism is clearly permanent, such as when there is a known ectopic gland, a trial off medication should be considered at the age of 2 to 3 years to determine if the hypothyroidism is permanent. This is done only if the infant has not required increasing doses of L-thyroxine and the TSH has not risen above 10 μU/ml after the age of 12 months. Because the thyroid gland has been suppressed with therapy, children may become temporarily hypothyroid when treatment is discontinued. A valid trial off therapy requires a 6-week interval off medication before thyroid tests are repeated to allow the thyroid gland to escape from suppression. If the thyroid tests are normal off therapy, transient hypothyroidism is confirmed. The patient may remain off therapy. If the TSH is elevated, permanent hypothyroidism is definitively diagnosed and therapy should be resumed on a lifelong basis.

The outcome in children diagnosed with CH by newborn screening programs and treated early is much better than that in children diagnosed and treated later in infancy. Infants who have had rapid normalization of T_4 and have had the T_4 maintained in the upper half of the normal range for age in the first year of life have the best prognosis regarding their neurological development. The New England Congenital Hypothyroidism Collaborative found that children diagnosed by newborn screening were no different with respect to their performance in elementary school than matched controls. Other authors, however, have found that infants who had severe hypothyroidism as manifested by extremely elevated TSH levels and delayed maturation of the epiphyseal growth plates on bone age radiography are at greater risk for decreased cognitive function even if treated early. These infants were likely to have been hypothyroid in utero. Overall intelligence can by diminished by 6 to 19 intellectual quotient (IQ) points. Milder cognitive defects and behavior problems can be seen in less severe CH. There is speculation that very early diagnosis and treatment with higher initial doses of L-thyroxine, as is currently recommended, may lead to better outcomes in the next generation of children with CH.

Another factor that influences outcome in children with hypothyroidism is the degree of compliance with treatment. Children who have had long and/or frequent intervals of hypothyroidism can have significant developmental delay. Noncompliance in adolescents with CH is common and has been shown to decrease both IQ and performance on psychometric testing results. Parents of children with CH must understand the importance of making sure that L-thyroxine is given daily as prescribed. It is essential that these children have careful medical follow-up to ensure that they are receiving their medication in the appropriate amounts to maintain a euthyroid state and achieve normal growth and development.

Hypothyroidism in Infancy due to Giant Hemangioma

A relatively uncommon form of hypothyroidism that can threaten infant brain development is associated with large hemangioma. The infants have normal newborn screening tests because their hypothalamic-pituitary thyroid axis is normal. However, as the hemangioma grows, there is increased "consumption" of free T_4 because of increased type D3 deiodinase within the hemangioma. The D3 deiodinase converts the T_4 to reverse T_3 and T_3 to T_2. Reverse T_3 and T_2 are biologically inactive. These children then develop biochemical changes of primary hypothyroidism, including an elevated TSH and low free T_4. The differentiating biochemical tests from primary hypothyroidism are the low T_3 levels and high rT_3 levels. NTI is excluded by the lack of serious illness and the elevated TSH. The consumption of T_4 reverses as the hemangioma shrinks in size (often by age 1 to 2 years). However, to protect brain development, thyroid hormone replacement is necessary during the period of decreased T_4 and elevated TSH. Newborn infants with large hemangioma should be followed prospectively with thyroid function testing.

Disorders of Thyroid-Binding Proteins

Abnormalities of thyroid-binding proteins may become apparent in the newborn period when a primary T_4 newborn thyroid screening program is used. These conditions are normal variants. Infants are euthyroid and do not require treatment. TBG deficiency and excess are X-linked conditions. T_4 and T_3 is decreased with TBG deficiency and elevated in TBG excess. Free T_4, free T_3, and TSH are normal in both conditions and the infant is euthyroid. TBG can be measured to diagnose these conditions definitively. Familial dysalbuminemic hyperthyroxinemia is an autosomal dominant condition caused by an abnormal albumin that binds to T_4 with increased affinity. The total T_4 is increased but the total and free T_3, free T_4, and TSH are all normal. The infant is euthyroid and does not require treatment.

Congenital Hyperthyroidism

Although hyperthyroidism in the newborn is rare, it is important to recognize infants with this condition immediately because it can cause serious and life-threatening complications. Cases of congenital hyperthyroidism should be immediately referred to a pediatric endocrinologist for management.

Neonatal Graves Disease

Neonatal Graves disease, which is due to transplacental passage of stimulatory TRAb, occurs in infants born to mothers who have Graves disease. Because stimulatory TRAb may be present in maternal circulation even if the mother is not hyperthyroid during the pregnancy, a history of Graves disease in the mother should alert the physician to an at-risk newborn. From 2% to 3% of infants born to mother who have Graves disease are affected. Infants at the greatest risk are those born to mothers with significantly elevated TRAb. Mothers with Graves disease can transmit either stimulatory or blocking TRAb, both antibodies, or neither antibody to their newborns. The type of antibody transmitted influences thyroid function in the newborn. There are reported cases of individual mothers with Graves disease who have had infants from different pregnancies who were euthyroid, hypothyroid, or hyperthyroid depending on whether or not antibodies crossed the placenta and which type of antibody was present.

Not all infants with neonatal Graves disease present with hyperthyroidism immediately after birth. They may be euthyroid initially. If maternal blocking TRAb are present, the infant may be transiently hypothyroid because blocking antibodies can mask the effect of stimulatory antibodies. When blocking TRAb degrade, the infant manifests symptoms of hyperthyroidism as the effect of the stimulatory antibodies predominate. Mothers who are treated for hyperthyroidism during pregnancy with PTU can also have infants who are hypothyroid immediately after birth but become hyperthyroid during the first postnatal week as the PTU effect wanes.

The clinical signs and symptoms of neonatal Graves disease are presented in Box 9-3. The presence of a goiter should alert the physician to thyroid dysfunction. Symptoms such as irritability, poor feeding, tachycardia, and hypertension may not be present in the first few days of life. Because the consequences of untreated hyperthyroidism in the newborn are so serious, infants born to mothers with Graves disease or a history of Graves disease should be followed carefully for the first several weeks of life for signs and symptoms of hyperthyroidism. Serial thyroid function tests should be performed. Affected infants have elevated T_4 and T_3 and suppressed TSH. TRAb are typically positive in both the mother and the infant.

The treatment for neonatal Graves disease is PTU 5 to 10 mg/kg/day given orally and taken in divided doses every 8 hours. β-Blockade with propranolol 2 mg/kg/day orally taken in divided doses every 6 hours alleviates cardiac manifestations of the disease. For severely hyperthyroid infants, Lugol solution of potassium iodide, 1 drop orally every 8 hours, is given to block thyroid hormone synthesis. Rapid correct of hyperthyroidism is desired; however, care must be taken to avoid overtreatment, with resultant hypothyroidism. Despite titration of PTU, it may be difficult to achieve a euthyroid state in the infant without the addition of L-thyroxine at replacement doses. This allows the gland to be maximally suppressed without the risk of hypothyroidism.

The course of neonatal Graves disease is self-limited. The process resolves when maternally transmitted TRAb degrades; this generally takes 3 to 12 weeks. Treatment can be discontinued when thyroid function returns to normal.

Autosomal Dominant Hyperthyroidism

Autosomal dominant hyperthyroidism is a permanent condition that is not autoimmune in origin. TSH receptor genes in this condition have been shown to have autosomal dominant gain of function mutations. Infants present

Box 9-3	Clinical Findings in Congenital Hyperthyroidism
Irritability	Tachycardia
Poor feeding	Hepatosplenomegaly
Poor weight gain	Jaundice
Diarrhea	Craniosynostosis
Insomnia	Cardiac failure
Goiter	Death
Proptosis	

similarly to those with neonatal Graves disease. They should be treated with antithyroid medications before thyroidectomy.

ACQUIRED THYROID DISEASE IN CHILDREN

Presentation of Clinical Thyroid Disease

Disorders of the thyroid are frequently sought in children because of concerns of either the gland structure or abnormal thyroid hormone activity. Because many of the symptoms of thyroid disease are not specific, the clinician is often faced with the dilemma of interpreting thyroid function studies and deciding whether any abnormalities represent true disease. This section focuses on clinical abnormalities that result in hypothyroidism and hyperthyroidism and presents algorithms to assist in the workup of suspected thyroid disease.

Hypothyroidism

Acquired hypothyroidism in children is more common in adolescent girls but may be seen in either sex, and presents as early as infancy. Children present with either characteristic symptoms (Box 9-4) or as a result of a battery of screening studies for many nonthyroidal conditions. Thyroid studies are typically included in laboratory work-up panels of many specialists, including gastroenterologists, psychiatrists, immunologists, and hematologists.

The signs and symptoms of hypothyroidism are listed in Box 9-4; lethargy and decreased activity are the most frequent signs. Poor growth velocity with an increasing weight for height is frequently seen, although overt obesity is rare. In contrast, obese children without hypothyroidism commonly have an accelerated growth velocity. Other symptoms of hypothyroidism include dry skin and hair, cold

intolerance, constipation, decreased appetite despite good weight gain, and flat affect. In contrast to the poor concentration and school performance seen in hyperthyroidism, hypothyroidism typically spares academic performance and occasionally improves the teacher's perception of the child's work. Hypothyroidism may delay puberty, although in rare cases it induces sexual precocity.

There are several causes of hypothyroidism in children, but most cases are due to chronic lymphocytic thyroiditis (Hashimoto thyroiditis, CLT). Other etiologies include errors in thyroid hormone synthesis (dyshormonogenesis), drugs, infection, infiltration, iodine deficiency, and iatrogenic causes such as radiation exposure (Box 9-5).

Chronic Lymphocytic Thyroiditis

Hashimoto described CLT in 1912 as a diffuse lymphocytic infiltrative condition with fibrosis, parenchymal atrophy, and eosinophilic changes in some of the acinar cells. The damaged gland loses the ability to store iodine and becomes inefficient at making L-thyroxine. Other names given to this disease include Hashimoto thyroiditis, autoimmune thyroiditis, and thyroiditis. Although characteristically found in middle-aged women, it is seen frequently in the pediatric population. CLT is an autoimmune disorder with a destructive attack by the immune system on the thyroid gland, in contrast to the stimulatory effect seen in Graves disease.

CLT occurs in two varieties: goitrous and atrophic. The goitrous form is more common and is associated with a diffusely enlarged gland. The thyroid enlargement is caused by either stimulation by elevated TSH or autoimmune invasion by lymphocytes. In contrast, the atrophic form leads to a small gland and often severe clinical hypothyroidism.

Antibodies directed against the thyroid are commonly found in CLT, but their absence does not rule out the diagnosis. Most clinical laboratories measure both antibodies directed against thyroid peroxidase and antibodies against thyroglobulin, a protein involved in the synthesis of thyroxine in the thyroid gland. TPO antibodies are more

---

Box 9-4   Clinical Features of Hypothyroidism

HISTORY	SIGNS
Lethargy	Poor growth velocity
Decreased activity	Goiter
Weight gain (despite low appetite)	Nonpalpable or atrophic thyroid (severe)
Dry skin	Decreased pulse
Cold intolerance	Delayed bone and dental age
Constipation	
Delayed puberty	
Precocious puberty (rare)	

Box 9-5   Causes of Hypothyroidism

Chronic lymphocytic thyroiditis (Hashimoto)	Central/tertiary
	Iatrogenic
Thyroid dyshormonogenesis	Thyroid hormone resistance
Drugs	
Infection	
Infiltration	
Iodine deficiency	

commonly found than are antibodies to thyroglobulin. These antibodies are not responsible for causing the thyroid destruction and only serve as markers of the presence of CLT. The level of antibody elevation does not correlate with thyroid function, and therefore decisions to treat should not be based on the level of antibodies. However, in some children with atrophic hypothyroidism, TRAb are responsible for some of the autoimmune destruction of the thyroid gland. These antibodies prevent TSH from binding to the TSH receptor but lack the stimulatory effect seen in Graves disease.

Studies of the incidence of autoimmune thyroid disease vary depending on the population studied. In one study, 3% of Japanese children aged 6 to 18 years showed the presence of thyroid antibodies. There is a strong predilection for females. Peak incidence of pediatric cases is in adolescence, although autoimmune thyroiditis may occur as early as infancy. Thyroid antibodies (either to thyroid peroxidase or to thyroglobulin) are present in over 95% of children with CLT and serve as markers of autoimmune disease. TPO antibodies are more sensitive and specific. Autoimmune thyroid disease is seen in association with type 1 diabetes mellitus, Down syndrome, Turner syndrome, Klinefelter syndrome, polyglandular endocrine failure including adrenal insufficiency, and other autoimmune conditions, such as celiac disease, vitiligo, alopecia, and others (Box 9-6). In 30% to 40% of cases of CLT, there is a family history of autoimmune thyroid disease, either Graves disease or CLT. Approximately 20% of children with type 1 diabetes have thyroid antibodies, of which only a fourth have a rise in TSH. Ten percent of children with polyglandular failure (autoimmune polyendocrinopathy candidiasis ectodermal dystrophy [APS-1 or APECED]) have CLT. The coexistence of CLT and diabetes mellitus with and without adrenal insufficiency has been referred as both Schmidt syndrome and APS-2. Schmidt syndrome is more common in older children or in young adults, in contrast to APS-1, which is more common in younger children.

CLT presents most commonly with a diffusely enlarged thyroid in an asymptomatic child, but a variety of presentations are possible (Box 9-7). These include cases of mild to severe hypothyroidism, with the most severe cases typically presenting without a goiter. The pathogenesis of the latter form of CLT has been postulated to be the result of a burnt-out thyroid gland; however, more recent information suggests the pathogenesis to be distinct from goitrous CLT. Blocking antibodies to TSH are occasionally found in the nongoitrous form of CLT. Occasionally, CLT is detected only as the result of a search for a variety of autoimmune diseases. The presence of antibodies in these cases serves as a marker for the autoimmune process but does not signify a need for treatment.

Rarely, a child with CLT presents with thyrotoxicosis, or "hashitoxicosis." Mechanisms for this temporary hyperthyroidism include the release of thyroid hormone from a damaged gland and the coexistence of thyroid-stimulating antibodies.

Physical examination of a child with suspected CLT focuses initially on the general energy level of the child. The pulse rate is a useful screen for hypothyroidism and hyperthyroidism. A child with hypothyroidism typically has a pulse rate lower than that previously documented. The skin is assessed for dryness as well as low temperature. The thyroid can be examined by several methods. Some prefer palpation while standing behind the child. The neck can be extended to highlight the thyroid for visual inspection, but often a slight flexion of the neck makes palpation easier. The thyroid should be distinguished from surrounding structures such as adipose pads, lymph nodes, and surrounding musculature and cartilage. The thyroid is typically diffusely involved, although asymmetry of the lymphocytic invasion may lead to an asymmetric thyroid gland. Multinodular gland can be seen, but if a child has a uninodular enlargement, thyroid cancer must be ruled out. The thyroid gland in CLT is typically painless and of rough consistency ("pebbly") and may be firm but not typically "rock hard."

Any child with suspected hypothyroidism should have TSH and thyroid antibodies measured. With a higher initial

---

Box 9-6   Conditions Associated With Autoimmune Thyroid Disease

Down syndrome	Klinefelter syndrome
Type 1 diabetes	Celiac disease
Turner syndrome	Polyglandular failure
Addison disease	Vitiligo
Any autoimmune condition	Alopecia

Box 9-7   Presentation of Chronic Lymphocytic Thyroiditis

Goiter and euthyroid (normal TSH)
Goiter and compensated hypothyroidism (normal T_4, elevated TSH)
Goiter and hypothyroidism
Atrophic thyroid, severely hypothyroid
Hyperthyroid (hashitoxicosis)
Alternating hypothyroidism and hyperthyroidism
Incidentally detected as part of a medical work-up

index of suspicion, or if the screen shows any abnormalities, free T_4 or T_4 plus T_3U should be assessed. Negative thyroid antibodies do not rule out CLT, and markedly positive thyroid antibody levels do not need to be followed longitudinally as they do not correlate with a need to treat with L-thyroxine. Although in hypothyroidism the decision to treat with L-thyroxine is clear, more often the practitioner is faced with a child who is euthyroid and has a goiter or one with only a mild elevation of TSH. There is no strong evidence that treatment is necessary in a child who is euthyroid with goiter and a normal TSH. Treatment does not typically result in shrinkage of the gland. In those with a mild degree of elevation of TSH but a normal T_4 level (compensated hypothyroidism), the decision to treat is subject to controversy. TSH assays vary, but normal values range typically between approximately 0.3 and 6. Many children with a mild elevation of TSH (i.e., <10 μU/ml) revert to normal thyroid studies over time, in the absence of treatment. Most children with a TSH level between 5 and 10 have no symptoms, other than a mild goiter, and treatment is not indicated. Thyroid function tests should be repeated in 3 to 6 months. Even with TSH levels between 10 and 20 μU/ml, most children have no clinical symptoms other than thyromegaly. Children with TSH over 10 μU/ml should be treated with L-thyroxine. In severe hypothyroidism (i.e., TSH > 50 μU/ml), treatment with L-thyroxine should be initiated at a low dosage and a pediatric endocrinologist should be consulted. Referral of children presenting with a euthyroid goiter or compensated hypothyroidism (normal T_4, but mildly elevated TSH) should be based on the comfort level of the primary care physician. If no treatment is initiated, repeat thyroid function tests should be done in 3 to 6 months. If treatment is initiated, they should be done in 1 to 2 months. An algorithm detailing the evaluation of a child with a diffuse goiter is shown in Figure 9-2.

After initial treatment with L-thyroxine, some children with hypothyroidism experience of shedding of hair such as on pillows or after hair brushing. Weight often decreases for

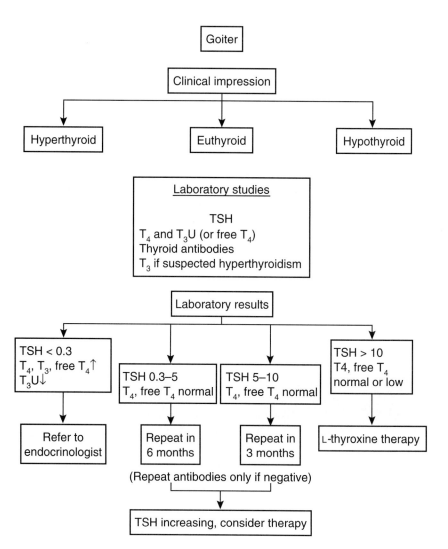

Figure 9-2   Algorithm of work-up of a child with a diffusely enlarged thyroid.

up to 6 months while growth accelerates. During this time, the appearance of the previously hypothyroid child often changes dramatically.

Other Causes of Hypothyroidism

Iodine Deficiency

Since the addition of iodine to salt in the 1920s, iodine deficiency has been become rare in industrialized societies. However, worldwide, iodine deficiency remains a problem. A particularly troublesome situation is when a pregnant mother is iodine deficient; not only are both the infant and mother hypothyroid, but also there is insufficient maternal-fetal transfer of thyroxine to protect the infant brain. Iodine, in excess, transiently halts thyroid hormone release but is overcome typically within several days. In an infant exposed to a procedure requiring large amounts of iodine to cleanse of the skin, there is occasion transient hypothyroidism.

Thyroid Dyshormonogenesis

As described in the section on congenital hypothyroidism, thyroid dyshormonogenesis refers to a deficiency of any of the enzymes responsible for thyroid hormone synthesis. Thyroid dyshormonogenesis is transmitted as an autosomal recessive disorder. Severe deficiency can result in CH, but milder deficiencies result in presentation at any age in childhood. A typical presentation is that of a child with a goiter due to increased TSH but in the absence of thyroid antibodies. The goiter is smoother that that found in CLT. Work-up may show normal or low free T_4 and increased TSH. Thyroid scan, if performed, shows diffuse uptake without the patchiness sometimes seen in CLT. If a child is diagnosed with thyroid dyshormonogenesis, siblings should be screened given the risk of 1:4.

Medications Causing Hypothyroidism

Some medications affect the thyroid-pituitary axis by altering TSH, T_4-to-T_3 conversion, T_4 release, or T_4 synthesis. Anticonvulsants such as diphenylhydantion and carbamazapine affect the thyroid hormone axis by stimulating thyroid hormone breakdown, although the TSH remains normal or slightly elevated. Lithium, used commonly to treat bipolar disorder, can cause thyromegaly and even induce myxedema. Lithium slows thyroid iodine transport and decreases thyroid hormone release. Although much less frequently, lithium can also cause thyrotoxicosis. Cobalt inhibits iodide binding by the thyroid via an unknown mechanism. One child had cobalt excess from ingestion of magnets that resulted in hypothyroidism. Gamma interferon can also induce hypothyroidism via an unknown mechanism. Amiodarone used for certain cardiac conditions can inhibit the conversion of T_4 to T_3 and cause hypothyroidism. Octreotide and growth hormone can decrease TSH release, although frank hypothyroidism is rare. Medications that affect the thyroid are shown in Table 9-3.

Hypothyroidism due to Radioablation or Surgery

When Graves disease is treated with radioablation or surgery, hypothyroidism typically follows. After radioablation, however, it may take several months or longer before the thyroid gland is injured sufficiently to cause hypothyroidism. Radiation therapy of the neck or neck and spine for cancer treatment, such as used in Hodgkin disease, frequently leads to primary hypothyroidism. The algorithm for treatment with L-thyroxine is similar to that in CLT, but recovery is not likely and hence a child with a mild increase in TSH should be treated. Furthermore, many clinicians prefer to treat the hypothyroid thyroid cancer survivor with doses of L-thyroxine high enough to decrease the TSH to the low-normal range to prevent the development of thyroid cancer. This must be balanced with the potential risk of osteoporosis similar to that seen in hyperthyroidism.

Central Hypothyroidism (Secondary and Tertiary Hypothyroidism)

The term *central hypothyroidism* refers to hypothyroidism caused by decreased TRH or decreased TSH. *Secondary hypothyroidism* implies the hypothyroidism is due to TSH deficiency, whereas *tertiary hypothyroidism* refers specifically to hypothyroidism due to decreased TRH. The diagnosis should be suspected when there are clinical symptoms suggestive of hypothyroidism, such as unexplained lethargy, increased weight gain, and constipation, in a child with known organic brain disease. Central hypothyroidism in a child with an intact central nervous system is very rare. Most cases are due to brain tumors and radiation therapy. Laboratory diagnosis rests on demonstration of decreased free T_4 or free T_4 index. A child with low T_4 but increased T_3U implies a binding protein deficiency, and not hypothyroidism. The TSH is not diagnostic, as levels can be low, normal, or mildly increased in the face of a low free T_4 level.

Table 9-3 Medications Affecting the Thyroid Gland

Medications	Thyroid Effects
Lithium	May cause hypothyroidism, rarely hyperthyroidism
	Blocks iodide transport, decreases thyroid hormone release
Iodide	Inhibits thyroid hormone release transiently
Estrogens	Increases thyroid-binding globulin (results in increased T_4, T_3, decreased T_3U, normal TSH and free T_4)
Anticonvulsants (carbamazapine, phenobarbital, diphenylhydantoin)	Stimulates thyroid hormone degradation Lowers T_4 and T_3 levels, TSH remains normal or slightly increased

Treatment goals are to restore T_4 to the mid- to high-normal range and to reverse the clinical symptoms. Any child diagnosed with central hypothyroidism requires a search for other pituitary hormone deficiencies, as well as magnetic resonance imaging of the pituitary and hypothalamus.

Thyroid Hormone Resistance

RTH refers to a syndrome of reduced responsiveness of target tissues to thyroid hormone. There is persistent elevation of T_4 and T_3, in association with nonsuppressed serum TSH without a known factor altering thyroid hormone physiology. The clinical presentation of RTH is variable, but the common features of the syndrome are elevated serum levels of T_4 and T_3, normal or slightly increased TSH levels, absence of the usual symptoms and metabolic consequences of thyroid hormone excess, and a goiter. RTH can occur globally, or selectively in various tissues, depending on the genetic defect. Inheritance is commonly autosomal dominant. Familial occurrence of RTH has been documented in approximately 75% of cases.

Children and adults with RTH show partial resistance; complete resistance would be fatal. Refetoff's original description of RTH included deaf mutism, severe developmental delay, poor linear growth, short stature, and delayed bone age. This form of RTH (Refetoff syndrome) is rare whereas less complete resistance is more common. Evaluation of subjects with RTH revealed that about one half have some degree of learning disability with or without attention deficit–hyperactivity disorder (ADHD). 25% have an IQ of less than 85, although mental retardation (IQ <60) has been found only in 3% of cases. Impaired mental function was found to be associated with impaired or delayed growth in 20% of subjects, but growth retardation alone is rare (4%). Despite the high prevalence of ADHD in patients with RTH, the occurrence of RTH in children with ADHD is very rare. In one study, none of the 330 children studied with ADHD had thyroid abnormalities. Thus, data do not support a genetic linkage of RTH with ADHD.

Clinically, children with RTH can present with signs of hypothyroidism (generalized resistance) or with signs of hyperthyroidism such as hyperactivity and poor concentration. A diffuse goiter is seen in both varieties due to TSH-induced thyroid growth.

Hyperthyroidism

Hyperthyroidism in children is nearly always due to Graves disease. Other causes include hot nodules, subacute thyroiditis, the hyperthyroid phase of Hashimoto thyroiditis (hashitoxicosis), and hyperthyroidism due to a constitutively activated TSH receptor (Box 9-8). Hyperthyroidism is occasionally seen in association with the McCune-Albright syndrome and with central RTH.

The symptoms of hyperthyroidism are listed in Box 9-9. Children with hyperthyroidism present with hyperactivity, emotional lability, poor school performance due to poor concentration, weight loss despite excellent appetite, failure to thrive, palpitations, and tremors. Difficulty sleeping, increased bowel movements (although not typically diarrhea), heat intolerance, diaphoresis, and periods of fatigue are common. Proptosis, or bulging out of the eyes, is sometimes seen, although it is typically mild. Interestingly, although school performance is typically maintained in severe hypothyroidism, it is adversely affected in hyperthyroidism. Many of these symptoms are not specific to the thyroid, but the recent onset of any of these symptoms should alert the primary care physician to screen for hyperthyroidism.

Other clues to the diagnosis include a family history of thyroid or other autoimmune diseases. Children with type 1 diabetes or certain genetic syndromes such as Down syndrome are at risk for both CLT and Graves disease.

Graves disease, like Hashimoto thyroiditis, is an HLA-associated autoimmune disease. It is unusual in children under age 5 years, but it may occur even in infancy. Incidence is higher in females. Infants with hyperthyroidism may develop craniosynostosis and possibly brain damage.

Physical examination reveals many clues to the diagnosis of hyperthyroidism and Graves disease. A general sense of the child's activity level is important because hyperthyroid children typically have difficulty sitting still. Vital signs reveal tachycardia, widened pulse pressure, and occasionally increased temperature and blood pressure. The heart rate should be compared with previous readings. The growth curve may show normal linear growth with concomitant weight loss. The skin is often warm. Examination of the eyes may reveal proptosis, a sign specific to Graves disease. Lid lag and eye prominence are seen in all forms of hyperthyroidism. The thyroid is smooth and diffusely enlarged in Graves disease due to diffuse antibody stimulation of the gland. Heart murmurs are sometimes appreciated, as well

Box 9-8 Causes of Hyperthyroidism

Graves disease
Hot nodule
Thyrotoxic phase of CLT
Subacute thyroiditis
Exogenous over-medicated
Toxic multinodular goiter
Iodide induced
Tumors with excessive human chorionic gonadotropin
TSH–secreting tumor
TSH receptor mutation
McCune-Albright syndrome
Central thyroid hormone resistance

as thyroid bruits. Tremors are often seen. Pretibial edema, found occasionally in adults with Graves disease, is rare in children.

Laboratory assessment of children with hyperthyroidism should include T_4 and T_3U (or free T_4), T_3, and TSH. TSH is suppressed in this condition. T_3 is vital, as about 5% of children will have a predominant elevation of T_3 with either an upper normal or only slightly elevated T_4. This is known as *T_3 toxicosis*. Thyroid antibodies (anti-TG and anti-TPO) are found in many children with Graves disease and do not help distinguish Graves disease from the thyrotoxic phase of CLT. Thyroid-stimulating immunoglobulin (TSI) may be assessed with a functional assay. If a child has overt features of hyperthyroidism with a significant goiter and especially with proptosis of the eyes, then measuring TSI is not necessary, given it is an expensive test.

An elevated T_4 or T_3 without a suppressed TSH is unlikely to be due to hyperthyroidism. Estrogen (i.e., birth control pills or pregnancy) increases TBG levels. The body then raises the T_4 to high levels to generate normal free T_4. Given that girls do not always reveal the use of oral contraceptive pills, caution must be made in overinterpreting an isolated elevated T_4 and T_3. Free T_4, free T_3, or T_3U is helpful in further evaluating these patients.

If the diagnosis is uncertain, a thyroid scan reveals diffuse and high uptake of radioactive iodine in Graves disease. In contrast, uptake with a hot nodule or subacute thyroiditis is low.

Treatment options in Graves disease in children consist of medical thyroid suppression, radioiodine ablation, or surgical thyroidectomy. Because a significant percentage of children go into remission, medical therapy is the first line of therapy. Since the 1940s, thiocarbamides have been used to block the formation of thyroid hormone. Methimazole and PTU are commonly used in the United States, and carbimazole is used in Europe. These drugs do not affect the underlying mechanism that is causing the hyperthyroidism. Rather, they inhibit thyroid peroxidase. PTU also inhibits T_4-to-T_3 conversion in peripheral tissues. Methimazole has a longer half-life and is typically given once or twice daily, whereas PTU is given 2 or 3 times daily. Some physicians advocate oversuppression and add L-thyroxine. The latter approach is used because of preliminary data showing a better rate of remission with this approach. However, other studies have not shown the same benefit. Sometimes antithyroid medications cause a marked suppression in T_4 levels, and replacement with L-thyroxine therapy is the easiest way to achieve normal test results. In more severe cases of hyperthyroidism, a β-blocker such as propranolol is useful in controlling the adrenergic symptoms such as tachycardia and palpitations. The β-blocker is used until a euthyroid state is achieved, which may take 1 month or longer.

Initially, the medications are given at a higher dose, often twice the maintenance dosage, until levels are controlled. Because it is difficult to assess the precise dosage needed to achieve a euthyroid state, thyroid levels are initially monitored frequently (monthly). It should be noted that the TSH concentration may not return to normal until several months later and thus is not useful initially in monitoring therapy. The size of the goiter often decreases with therapy. An enlarging gland may indicate overtreatment and a rise in TSH. Treatment with medications continues until they are declared ineffective, compliance becomes an issue, side effects emerge, or the physician decides to attempt a trial without medication.

Side effects of antithyroid medications include rashes, urticaria, arthralgias, and decreased white blood cell (WBC) count and are found in 5% to 14% of children. More severe reactions include hepatitis, a lupus-like syndrome, thrombocytopenia, and agranulocytosis. Many practitioners switch from one medication to another when side effects emerge. Children must be warned that if they develop fever and severe sore throat, a WBC count is in order. Some advocate baseline WBC counts and liver function tests because hyperthyroidism itself can lower the WBC count and alter liver function.

Medication has its limitations due to side effects and difficulties in dosing several times per day. In addition, titration of the dosage of antithyroid medications is difficult due to fluctuating body requirements. Radioactive iodine is gaining popularity not only as a method of treating those in whom medication is problematic but also as initial therapy. However, permanent hypothyroidism is a disadvantage of this therapy. After radioactive ablation is used to treat a child with Graves disease, the thyroid needs to be monitored frequently. Complete destruction of the gland may take months to more than 1 year. Occasionally, eye disease becomes worse after radioablation of the thyroid gland. The female child should be educated that she still may produce antibodies that can stimulate the thyroid. Thus, consultation with an endocrinologist should be considered during any future pregnancy.

Surgery is an effective modality of treating children with Graves disease, especially when the gland is too large for radioablation. In addition to the horizontal scar on the neck, other potential side effects are unintentional removal of or injury to the parathyroid glands and damage to the laryngeal nerves. Thyroid surgery should only be performed by a surgeon experienced in the pediatric thyroid. Even in experienced hands, the complication rate for thyroidectomy is 1% to 2%.

Referral to a pediatric endocrinologist is warranted in children with hyperthyroidism.

Acute thyroiditis, or infectious thyroiditis, is caused by invasion of the thyroid by bacteria, mycobacterium, fungi, or other organisms. It is rare in pediatrics. Children present with a painful thyroid and fever.

Subacute thyroiditis, or DeQuervain thyroiditis, is thought to be of viral origin and last weeks to months. In the first few months, hyperthyroidism may be seen due to leakage of thyroid hormone in a damaged gland. A thyroid scan shows decreased radioactive iodine uptake, in contrast to that seen in Graves disease. In time, hypothyroidism frequently develops.

Evaluation of a Diffusely Enlarged Thyroid

Enlargement of the thyroid is one of the most common referrals to a pediatric endocrinologist. According to two large studies of more than 7000 children without risk factors for the development of thyromegaly, the incidence of a goiter was 3% to 7%. None of the children had overt symptoms of hyperthyroidism or hypothyroidism.

A diffusely enlarged thyroid is most commonly due to TSH-induced thyroid growth or to lymphocytic or colloid infiltration. Cysts and neoplasia present as focal nodules and are discussed later in this chapter. Other rare causes include granulomatous and iron infiltration. Frequently, a presumed thyroid enlargement is actually local fat, muscle, or an anatomical malformation such as a thyroglossal cyst.

The initial step in the evaluation is to determine the nature of the goiter. A focal enlargement should be worked up for potential malignancy, as discussed later in this chapter. After determining that the thyroid is diffusely enlarged, the clinician should determine whether the child is euthyroid, hypothyroid, or hyperthyroid.

Most patients found to have a goiter are euthyroid. The two most common diagnoses to consider are simple colloid goiter and CLT. A granular or pebbly gland on examination is suggestive of CLT. In CLT, the thyroid is enlarged because of lymphocytic infiltration or due to TSH stimulation of the gland. Simple colloid goiter (adolescent goiter, nontoxic goiter) is due to infiltration of enlarged colloid follicles. Thyroid function is always normal. Other causes of a diffusely enlarged gland are shown in Box 9-10. Dietary goitrogens such as cabbage and soybeans may also cause thyromegaly without resulting in hypothyroidism.

Work-up consists of assessing thyroid function (TSH, T_4 and T_3U, or free T_4) and thyroid antibodies (TPO and anti-TG). As assays for free T_4 improve and become readily available, free T_4 measurements may replace total T_4. Positive antibodies establish autoimmunity and thus CLT as the diagnosis. If antibodies are negative, then many diagnoses are possible, including CLT. A smooth goiter, normal TSH, and negative thyroid antibodies in an adolescent patient point to colloid goiter as the diagnosis. An algorithm for the work-up of a diffuse goiter is shown in Figure 9-2.

If a child appears hypothyroid (see Box 9-4), then CLT is likely; however, dyshormonogenesis should be considered, as well as other diagnoses listed in Box 9-5. Thyroid function tests (TSH, T_4 and T_3U, or free T_4) confirm the hypothyroidism, and positive thyroid antibodies verify the diagnosis of CLT. It should be recalled that in children with severe hypothyroidism and CLT, there often is no goiter.

If a child with a goiter has a hyperthyroid appearance confirmed by thyroid function assessment, the diagnosis is usually Graves disease. Rarely, CLT presents with hyperthyroidism (hashitoxicosis). A nodule, which is overproducing thyroid hormone, is rare in the pediatric population and presents as a focal, not diffusely enlarged thyroid gland.

THYROID NEOPLASIA

Although multiple thyroid nodules are seen often as part of the underlying process of autoimmune thyroid disease in children, single thyroid nodules are uncommon. These nodules must be fully evaluated, because the risk for malignancy in solitary thyroid nodules in children is relatively high. Most thyroid nodules in children are hypofunctional. Those that are functional can produce a variety of hormones, including T_4, T_3, and calcitonin. Children with soli-

---

Box 9-10 Differential Diagnosis of a Diffusely Enlarged Thyroid

Autoimmune	Iodine deficiency
CLT	Drugs
Graves disease	Thyroid resistance
Simple colloid goiter	TSH-secreting adenoma
Compensatory goiter (increased TSH)	Inflammatory conditions
Dyshormonogenesis	Acute thyroiditis
Goitrogens	Subacute thyroiditis
	Granulomatous infiltration

tary nodules should be referred to a pediatric endocrinologist for evaluation.

Risk factors for malignancies of the thyroid are listed in Box 9-11. There is a female predominance. Patients younger than 20 years are more likely to have a malignant solitary thyroid nodule than is an adult. Radiation exposure is a significant risk. Children exposed to the Chernobyl radiation accident have 100 times greater risk than that of the general population for thyroid cancer after 10 years. Children who received radiation therapy to the neck to treat childhood malignancies are also at increased risk for thyroid cancer. A history of prolonged iodine deficiency, hypothyroidism with elevation of TSH, and Graves disease are also risk factors. A family history of medullary thyroid carcinoma (MCT) or multiple endocrine neoplasia (MEN) increases the risk for thyroid malignancy. Genetic testing is essential in MEN because in genetically predisposed individuals the risk of MCT is 100%. ^{131}I ablation therapy for hyperthyroidism is not a risk factor in the development of thyroid malignancies in adults and is unlikely to increase the risk of thyroid neoplasia in children. Clinical features of nodules that are more likely to be malignant are hardness, pain, pressure symptoms, increasing size, and associated lymphadenopathy.

In the evaluation of solitary thyroid nodules, thyroid function tests should be performed. They are usually normal, but in hyperfunctioning nodules, the patient may be thyrotoxic. If the patient is hypothyroid, it is likely that there is an autoimmune process occurring in the thyroid and thyroid autoantibodies are usually elevated. Calcitonin levels are high in MCT. Thyroid ultrasonography is useful to evaluate possible thyroid cysts. If the thyroid mass is completely cystic with no solid component, radionuclide imaging is not needed. However, any solitary nodule that is not a cyst should be evaluated by radionuclide imaging with ^{123}I to determine thyroid uptake. A hypofunctioning, or

"cold," nodule takes up less of the tracer than the normal thyroid tissue. A hyperfunctioning, or "hot," nodule has increased ^{123}I uptake. An isofunctional, or "warm," nodule has normal uptake. Other studies that may be needed in the evaluation of thyroid nodules are aspiration and cytology and excisional biopsy. An algorithm for the assessment of solitary thyroid nodules is presented in Figure 9-3.

Thyroid Nodules: Benign Versus Malignant

Thyroid nodules can be cystic, solid, or a combination. Thyroid cysts are easily diagnosed on ultrasonography. Pure cysts are usually benign. Any solid component in a cystic nodule is suspicious and should prompt further evaluation as for solid nodules. Pure cysts should be aspirated and cytology performed. If the cytology is suspicious for malignancy, the cyst should undergo biopsy during thyroid lobectomy. If the cytology result is negative, the cyst can be observed. Thyroid cysts frequently recur, necessitating surgery.

Solid thyroid nodules can be classified based on their uptake of radioactive tracer. Hyperfunctioning (hot) nodules have a low risk of malignancy. The risk is greatest if the nodule is larger than 3 cm or the patient is thyrotoxic. A T_3 suppression test can be performed to determine if the TSH is suppressible. In this test, T_3 is given to the patient for 10 days and the ^{123}I uptake is measured before and after T_3 administration. If the ^{123}I is decreased after the T_3 is given, the nodule is TSH dependent and less likely to be malignant. Nonsuppressible nodules in which the ^{123}I uptake does not decrease after T_3 are TSH independent and function autonomously. They are at greater risk of malignancy. Nodules larger than 3 cm, those in thyrotoxic patients, and those that are TSH independent should be excised.

Hypofunctioning (cold) solitary thyroid nodules have about a 30% to 50% risk of malignancy in children compared with a 7% risk in adults. Because of concern about the high risk of malignancy, excision has been the standard treatment for cold nodules in children. In recent years, more experience has been gained using fine needle aspiration (FNA) and cytology in the evaluation of solitary cold nodules in children. The quality of the specimen and the skill of the pathologist evaluating it are critical. FNA should be done only by experienced practitioners. It should not replace clinical suspicion of malignancy in determining treatment. If the clinical suspicion is low and the cytology result is negative for malignant cells, suppression of the nodule with L-thyroxine is indicated. Failure to decrease in size by at least 50% on suppressive therapy indicates that the nodule is autonomous and more likely to be malignant. Although it is possible that a malignant nodule could suppress with L-thyroxine, it is unlikely that the malignancy will progress during the period of suppression.

Box 9-11 Risk Factors for Malignancy in Thyroid Nodules

<20 years old	Hard nodule
Single nodule	Lymphadenopathy
Pain	History of prolonged TSH elevation
Hoarseness	
Pressure symptoms	History of prolonged iodine deficiency
Enlarging nodule	
Fixed nodule	History of radiation exposure
	History of Graves disease
	Family history of MTC
	Family history of MEN

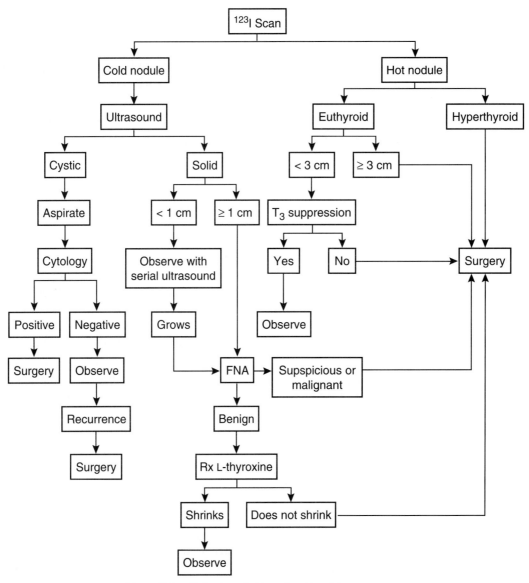

Figure 9-3   Evaluation of solitary thyroid nodules.

Excisional biopsy, which necessitates lobectomy, is indicated in all thyroid nodules that are suspicious for malignancy. In patients with a history of radiation exposure and a benign nodule, treatment with L-thyroxine after lobectomy should be considered to decrease the risk of the development of another nodule. Without radiation exposure, there is no evidence to indicate that L-thyroxine treatment is helpful in reducing recurrences, and no further treatment is needed.

Thyroid Cancer

Classification of thyroid cancers is shown in Box 9-12. The risk of thyroid cancers in North American children is 1:1 million per year. Although children have a higher incidence of metastatic disease, their risk of death from thyroid can-

cer is lower than that in adults. Risk factors for thyroid malignancy have been discussed and are listed in Box 9-11. The clinical presentation of thyroid cancer is not usually dramatic; an asymptomatic nodule is typically the only finding. The nodule may be soft or firm and usually is

Box 9-12   Types of Thyroid Malignancies

Papillary adenocarcinomas
Follicular adenocarcinoma
Mixed papillary and
   follicular carcinoma
Medullary carcinoma
Lymphoma

Sarcoma
Histiocytoma
Anaplastic tumor
Metastatic tumor

mobile. Hardness, pain, hoarseness, and fixation are ominous clinical signs of malignancy. Cervical lymphadenopathy may be present. Metastases to the lung and lymph nodes are frequent. All patients with thyroid nodules should be evaluated for the possibility of thyroid cancer. In patients with additional risk factors, biopsy should be considered as an early diagnostic procedure.

Papillary and Follicular Carcinoma

Papillary thyroid carcinoma is the most common form of thyroid cancer and comprises 80% of cases. It can be bilateral and present with multiple nodules. It is less aggressive than in adults and generally progresses slowly, and it frequently metastasizes to lymph nodes. The most common distant metastases are to lung and bone.

Follicular carcinoma is rare in children. The prognosis worsens with increased capsular invasion by the tumor. As with papillary carcinoma, nodules can be bilateral and multifocal. Distant metastases and vascular invasion are more common than lymph node metastases. Follicular adenoma and carcinoma can be difficult to differentiate histologically. Some thyroid cancers are mixed papillary and follicular, having the features of both, but these typically behave like papillary carcinoma even if the predominant cell type in the tumor is follicular.

The treatment for papillary and follicular thyroid carcinoma in children is total thyroidectomy including resection of the paratracheal lymph nodes. The surgery carries the risk of laryngeal nerve paralysis and hypoparathyroidism.

Despite "total" surgical thyroidectomy, some residual thyroid tissue remains. Many centers advocate radioablation with ^{131}I followed by complete suppression with L-thyroxine therapy. Suppression should achieve a TSH level at the lowest end of the normal range. If radioablation is used to eradicate remaining thyroid tissue, TG levels can be used for posttreatment surveillance. TG levels should remain low on suppressive thyroid hormone therapy. However, follow-up should include measurement of TG, as well as periodic ^{123}I whole body scanning after withdrawal of thyroid hormone or pretreatment with recombinant TSH.

Medullary Thyroid Carcinoma

MCT is rare, consisting of only 5% of cases of thyroid cancer. It occurs more frequently in adolescent girls. The incidence of this cancer was greater when the use of radiation of the head and neck in children was commonplace.

MCT in children at present is usually of the familial type. The origin of the tumor is neural crest tissue with parafollicular (C) cell hyperplasia. Inheritance is autosomal dominant. A germline mutation in the RET proto-oncogene has been identified in this disease. MCT can be part of MEN syndrome types 2A and 2B, or it can occur without other endocrinopathies (familial medullary thyroid carcinoma). When associated with MEN type 2A, the patient is at risk for pheochromocytoma and parathyroid hyperplasia. The characteristic phenotype in MEN type 2B includes large lips, long thin facies, and marfanoid habitus. Associated conditions in type 2B are pheochromocytoma, mucosal neuromas, and ganglioneuromas.

Clinical findings in MCT are often lacking; many cases are discovered when family members of index cases are screened. There is a 50% incidence in family members. Patients may have a thyroid nodule; however, even without a clinically apparent nodule, microscopic malignancy can be present. Increased calcitonin secretion by C cells measured randomly or in response to stimulation with pentagastrin is diagnostic and an indication for thyroidectomy. Genetic testing is replacing dynamic stimulation with pentagastrin. A mutation of the RET proto-oncogene is found in greater than 90% of cases of hereditary MCT and 25% of sporadic cases.

The treatment for MCT is total thyroidectomy followed by ^{131}I ablation. L-Thyroxine therapy is given in replacement (not suppressive) doses after thyroidectomy. Patients with a family history of MEN 2A or 2B should be initially evaluated for MCT at the age of 4 to 5 years and annually thereafter. If they are RET proto-oncogene positive or if they have random or stimulated elevation of calcitonin, prophylactic thyroidectomy is warranted. Evaluation for possible pheochromocytoma must be done preoperatively because failure to treat this condition can lead to intraoperative hypertension and sudden catecholamine release followed by postoperative hypovolemic shock. Patients should be monitored for pheochromocytoma annually.

Other Thyroid Malignancies

Other malignancies of the thyroid are very rare and include anaplastic cancer, lymphoma, sarcoma, histiocytoma, and metastatic tumors.

MAJOR POINTS

Thyroid function tests are age related. Adult normal ranges are not appropriate for interpreting thyroid tests in children.

TSH is the most useful screening test for thyroid dysfunction.

An abnormal newborn screening test for congenital hypothyroidism should be evaluated prompted. Patients with significantly elevated TSH levels (>50 µU/ml) should be referred to an endocrinologist immediately.

Continued

MAJOR POINTS—Cont'd

Conditions that cause false-positive newborn screening for congenital hypothyroidism include TBG deficiency, prematurity, and performing the screening at less than 24 hours of age.

The best prognosis for normal neurological development in congenital hypothyroidism is achieved if the T_4 is normalized rapidly and maintained in the upper half of the normal range for age in the first year of life.

A diffusely enlarged thyroid does not necessarily imply a need to treat with L-thyroxine.

School performance is typically maintained in hypothyroidism, but even mild hyperthyroidism can result in a marked decline.

Total T_3 is valuable in the evaluation of suspected hyperthyroidism but not in hypothyroidism.

Children with thyroid-stimulating hormone of 5 to 10 μU/ml are usually asymptomatic and in most cases can be followed without thyroid hormone replacement.

Although multiple thyroid nodules are common and are usually part of the underlying process of autoimmune thyroiditis, single thyroid nodules are uncommon in children and should be fully evaluated for possible malignancy.

SUGGESTED READINGS

American Academy of Pediatrics: Newborn screening for congenital hypothyroidism: recommended guidelines, Pediatrics 1993;91:1203.

Dayan CM: Interpretation of thyroid function tests, Lancet 2001;357:619.

Delange F: Neonatal screening for congenital hypothyroidism: results and perspectives, Horm Res 1997;48:51.

Koch CA, Sarlis NJ: The spectrum of thyroid diseases in childhood and its evolution during transition to adulthood: natural history, diagnosis, differential diagnosis and management, J Endocrinol Invest 2001;24:659.

Kraiem Z, Newfield RS: Graves' disease in childhood, J Pediatr Endocrinol Metab 2001;14:229.

Lafferty AR: Thyroid nodules childhood and adolescence: thirty years of experience, J Pediatr Endocrinol Metab 1997;10:479.

LaFranchi S: Congenital hypothyroidism: etiologies, diagnosis, and management, Thyroid 1999;9:735.

New England Congenital Hypothyroidism Collaborative: Correlation of cognitive test scores and adequacy of treatment in adolescents with congenital hypothyroidism, J Pediatr 1994;124:383.

New England Congenital Hypothyroidism Collaborative: Elementary school performance of children with congenital hypothyroidism, J Pediatr 19990;116:27.

VanVliet G: Neonatal hypothyroidism: treatment and outcome, Thyroid 1999;9:79.

VanVliet G: Treatment of congenital hypothyroidism, Lancet 2001;358:86.

ADRENAL GLAND

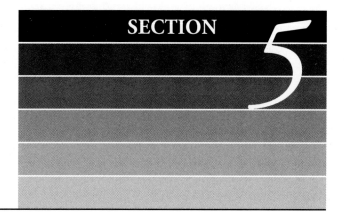

CHAPTER 10

Disorders of the Adrenal Gland

MARIA J. HENWOOD

LORRAINE E. LEVITT KATZ

ADRENAL GLAND STRUCTURE AND FUNCTION

Embryology

Fetal Adrenal Gland

The fetal adrenal cortex is derived from celomic mesothelium near the developing gonads. Steroid-producing cells appear in the cortex by the sixth week of gestation. By the 10th week, both the fetal zone and the adult zone synthesize steroid hormones under the influence of adrenocorticotropic hormone (ACTH). Degeneration of the fetal zone begins during the eighth month of gestation. Concurrently, the adult zone begins a long process of differentiation into the three zones that comprise the mature adult cortex. This differentiation is not complete until approximately age 3 years.

Anatomy

The adrenal gland consists of the cortex, which is responsible for steroid hormone synthesis, and the medulla, which produces catecholamines. Three zones comprise the mature adrenal cortex: the zona glomerulosa, the zona fasciculata, and the zona reticularis. The outermost region, the zona glomerulosa, constitutes 15% of the cortical volume and is responsible for synthesis of mineralocorticoids, of which aldosterone is the principal end product. The middle region, the zona fasciculata, comprises 75% of the cortex. The innermost region, or zona reticularis, contributes only

10% to cortical volume. The fasciculata and reticularis function together to synthesize glucocorticoids (principally cortisol) and androgens. Basal secretion of steroids is primarily the job of the zona reticularis, whereas stress steroidogenesis occurs in the zona fasciculata.

Physiology

Adrenal steroidogenesis requires an intact hypothalamic-pituitary-adrenal (HPA) axis. Corticotropin-releasing hormone (CRH) is secreted by the hypothalamus and stimulates the pituitary gland to secrete ACTH. ACTH in turn stimulates the adrenal cortex to produce three classes of hormones: mineralocorticoids, glucocorticoids, and androgens. Several enzymatic reactions occur during normal synthesis of these hormones, but the process begins when ACTH facilitates the conversion of cholesterol to pregnenolone, the essential first and rate-limiting step in steroid biosynthesis (Figure 10-1).

Mineralocorticoids

Regulation of mineralocorticoid secretion is complex in that it is intimately linked to extracellular fluid electrolyte concentration, extracellular fluid volume, blood volume, arterial pressure, and multiple aspects of renal function. Four factors are essential to the regulation of aldosterone secretion. Increased extracellular potassium concentration (1) and increased activity of the renin-angiotensin system (2) increase aldosterone secretion. Increased extracellular sodium concentration (3) causes a slight decrease in aldosterone secretion. ACTH (4) is essential for secretion of aldosterone but exerts little control over the rate of secretion.

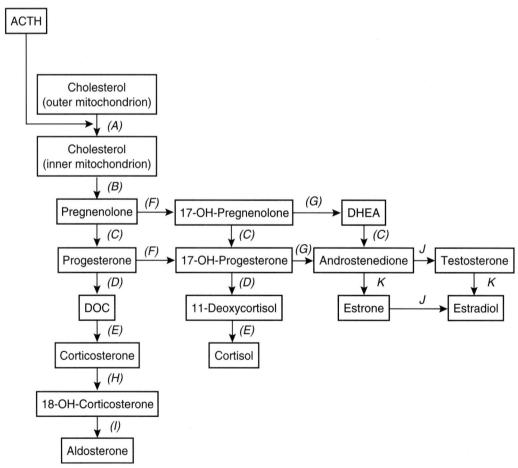

Figure 10-1   Steroid Synthesis in the Adrenal Gland. *A,* Steroidogenic acute regulatory;
B, 20,22-desmolase or side chain cleavage; *C,* 3β-hydroxysteroid dehydrogenase; *D,* 21-hydroxylase;
E, 11β-hydroxylase; *F,* 17-α-hydroxylase; *G,* 17,20-lyase; *H,* 18-hydroxylase; *I,* 18-oxidase;
J, 17β-hydroxysteroid dehydrogenase; and *K,* aromatase. The reactions catalyzed by enzymes
17β-hydroxysteroid dehydrogenase and aromatase occur primarily in the gonads. DOC,
deoxycorticosterone; DHEA, dehydroepiandrosterone.

The net effect of aldosterone is to promote sodium retention and potassium excretion in the distal convoluted tubule of the kidney. The first two factors listed are, without a doubt, the most potent regulators of mineralocorticoid secretion. Only a slight increase in potassium is required to induce a severalfold increase in aldosterone. Similarly, diminished blood flow to the kidneys activates the renin-angiotensin system, which in turn greatly increases aldosterone secretion. Aldosterone acts on the kidneys to promote potassium excretion and sodium reabsorption, which is accompanied by absorption of water via osmosis. This leads to normalization of blood volume and blood pressure, which is followed by the renin-angiotensin system returning to its normal level of activity. In contrast to potassium and the renin-angiotensin system, sodium and ACTH play comparatively minor roles in controlling aldosterone secretion.

Glucocorticoids

Cortisol is the predominant glucocorticoid secreted by the adrenal cortex. Cortisol is essential for homeostasis and has a significant impact on carbohydrate, protein, and fat metabolism.

Cortisol and Carbohydrate Metabolism
Stimulation of gluconeogenesis by the liver is the most well known metabolic effect of the glucocorticoids. Cortisol increases the activity of enzymes needed to convert amino acids to glucose in the liver. Cortisol also mobilizes amino acids from extrahepatic tissues, predominantly from muscle. More amino acids are therefore available to act as substrates for gluconeogenesis. Finally, cortisol decreases the rate of glucose utilization elsewhere in the body. The cumulative effect of these actions is a rise in serum glucose.

Cortisol and Protein Metabolism
Except in the liver, cortisol reduces protein stores via decreased protein synthesis and increased protein catabolism. Decreased transport of amino acids into extrahepatic cells decreases the intracellular concentration with a consequent reduction in protein synthesis. Proteins already present within the cells are catabolized and amino acids are released into the circulation, leading to a rise in plasma amino acid concentration. Depletion of protein stores elsewhere in the body and an increase in plasma proteins are accompanied by a concomitant increase in hepatic protein. This is due to the differential effect of cortisol on enhancing amino acid transport into hepatic cells, but not into most other cells, as well as to the ability of cortisol to enhance hepatic enzymes needed for protein synthesis.

Cortisol and Fat Metabolism
Just as cortisol promotes mobilization of amino acids from muscle, it also promotes mobilization of fatty acids from adipose tissue, at least in part via diminished transport of glucose into fat cells. The resultant paucity of glucose in fat cells leads to a decrease in α-glycerophosphate, which is derived from glucose and is essential for deposition and maintenance of triglycerides in these cells; in the absence of α-glycerophosphate, cells release fatty acids. This increase of plasma free fatty acids allows for increased utilization of free fatty acids for energy. Oxidation of free fatty acids in cells is also promoted by cortisol.

In times of starvation or other physiological stress, this combination of increased mobilization of fats and increased oxidation of fatty acids helps to shift the metabolism of the cells from utilization of glucose to utilization of fatty acids for energy. Although this cortisol mechanism requires several hours to become fully developed, it is important for long-term conservation of body glucose and glucose stores.

Effects of Stress on Glucocorticoid Secretion
Cortisol is essential for survival during times of physiological stress. The body responds to such stress with a rapid and marked increase in ACTH secretion from the pituitary, which is followed almost immediately by increased secretion of cortisol from the adrenal cortex. Some examples of stressors that result in a glucocorticoid surge are fever, serious infection, trauma, and surgery.

Cardiovascular Effects of Cortisol
Glucocorticoids promote normal cardiovascular function. Cortisol exerts permissive effects on catecholamines, angiotensin II, and arginine vasopressin (AVP), whose vasoconstricting effects maintain adequate cardiac function and vascular tone. In the setting of cortisol deficiency, decreased cardiac contractility and peripheral vascular tone may result in potentially fatal systemic hypotension and cardiovascular collapse. States of cortisol excess, in contrast, are associated with hypertension.

Anti-Inflammatory Effects of Cortisol
Glucocorticoids exert their anti-inflammatory effects both by interfering with the early stages of inflammation and by promoting rapid resolution of established inflammation. The following actions of cortisol prevent inflammation. (1) Through stabilization of lysosomal membranes, cortisol hinders the rupture of intracellular lysosomes. The result is a marked reduction in the quantity of proteolytic enzymes released from damaged cells. (2) Cortisol decreases capillary membrane permeability, thereby preventing leakage of plasma into the tissues. (3) Migration of leukocytes into inflamed areas and phagocytosis of damaged cells are both decreased by glucocorticoids. (4) By suppressing the immune system, cortisol reduces the quantity of circulating T lymphocytes and antibodies, which diminishes tissue reactions that would otherwise exacerbate the inflammatory process.

Specific details about the ability of cortisol to resolve inflammation and promote healing are not completely understood. Regardless of the precise mechanisms, however, the anti-inflammatory properties of glucocorticoids make them extremely useful in the management of diseases such as rheumatoid arthritis and glomerulonephritis, in which local inflammation can be severe and debilitating.

Hematological and Immunological Effects of Cortisol

Cortisol increases red blood cell synthesis and decreases the number of circulating eosinophils and lymphocytes. Hematological abnormalities may therefore be a clue to dysregulated cortisol secretion. Excess cortisol secretion leads to polycythemia, eosinopenia, and lymphocytopenia, whereas decreased cortisol secretion causes anemia.

Excess cortisol causes significant atrophy of lymphoid tissue, which decreases output of T cells and antibodies and reduces immunity against foreign invaders of the body. Organisms that would otherwise be easily destroyed by an intact immune system may result in overwhelming, even lethal, infection. Conversely, this downregulation of immunity makes glucocorticoids highly effective in preventing immunological rejection of transplanted organs.

Regulation of Cortisol Secretion

Recall that mineralocorticoid secretion is mainly controlled by the direct effects of potassium and angiotensin on the zona glomerulosa. In contrast, glucocorticoid secretion is not affected by the direct effects of such stimuli on the inner zones of the adrenal cortex. Rather, cortisol secretion is regulated almost exclusively by ACTH. Hypothalamic secretion of CRH is necessary for the release of ACTH by the anterior pituitary. ACTH then stimulates the formation of cyclic adenosine monophosphate (cAMP) and protein kinase A, which is key for the conversion of cholesterol to pregnenolone in the steroid biosynthetic pathway. This rate-limiting step is of paramount importance in the synthesis and secretion of cortisol.

Baseline cortisol secretion is pulsatile, with the peak release occurring in the early hours of the morning, between 4 AM and 6 AM. As noted earlier, cortisol is also released in response to physiological stress, such as fever, major injury, or surgery, as well as in response to hypoglycemia. In addition, cortisol helps to regulate its own secretion through a direct negative feedback loop by inhibiting continued secretion of CRH from the hypothalamus and ACTH from the pituitary.

Androgens

Regulation of androgen secretion is not as well understood as is that of the other classes of steroid hormones. Androgens are important for normal development of the male genitalia in utero. Newborns have markedly elevated levels of androgens, specifically androstenedione, dehydroepiandrosterone (DHEA), and testosterone. Androgen levels fall within the first few weeks of life and for the most part remain low throughout the prepubertal years. One exception is DHEA, which begins to rise in mid-childhood at approximately age 6 years. In those children with increased end-organ sensitivity, this rise in DHEA can manifest as benign premature adrenarche. In most children, however, adrenarche is associated with the pubertal rise in androgens.

Androstenedione is the most potent adrenal androgen. It is converted outside the adrenal gland to testosterone, an even more potent androgen secreted by the testis. In the target tissue, testosterone is converted to dihydrotestosterone (DHT). Both of these hormones bind to androgen receptors and facilitate the major actions of androgens: gonadotropin regulation, spermatogenesis, and sexual differentiation and maturation. In pubertal and adult males, gonadal steroid synthesis is the major source of androgens. This is in contrast to pubertal and adult females, in whom adrenal androstenedione is the source of more than half of the circulating testosterone.

Disordered secretion of androgens, in and of itself, is not life threatening. Evidence of abnormal androgen secretion may, however, accompany serious disorders caused by dysregulation of the other two classes of steroid hormones and can in fact provide a clue to the possible etiology. For example, excess androgens are responsible for the virilization seen in some forms of salt-losing congenital adrenal hyperplasia (see later). Alternatively, diminished androgen secretion may manifest as sparse pubic and axillary hair in the adolescent with Addison disease.

ADRENAL DEFICIENCY STATES

Adrenal insufficiency ensues when the adrenal gland fails to secrete normal amounts of glucocorticoids and/or mineralocorticoids. Adrenal insufficiency can be primary or secondary. Primary adrenal insufficiency is caused by structural or functional disorders of the adrenal cortex. Malfunction at the level of the hypothalamus or pituitary gland causes central, or secondary, adrenal insufficiency. Patients with primary adrenal insufficiency make inadequate amounts of mineralocorticoids, glucocorticoids, and, in some cases, androgens; those with secondary forms of adrenal insufficiency have only cortisol deficiency.

The list of possible etiologies of adrenal insufficiency is extensive (Box 10-1), but regardless of the cause, inadequate synthesis and/or secretion of glucocorticoids and mineralocorticoids is life threatening. Signs and symptoms of adrenal insufficiency differ depending on the site from which the problem originates. Salt-wasting crisis, the

Box 10-1   Congenital and Acquired Etiologies of Adrenal Insufficiency

Primary adrenal insufficiency (*low* cortisol, *high* adrenocorticotropic hormone [ACTH])

CONGENITAL

Congenital adrenal hyperplasia (CAH)
  (inherited enzymatic deficiencies)

Adrenal hypoplasia congenita (AHC)
  (*DAX-1* gene mutations)

Familial glucocorticoid deficiency (ACTH resistance)

Aldosterone deficiency (true versus pseudo)

Adrenoleukodystrophy (ALD)
Wolman disease

ACQUIRED

Autoimmune
  Isolated
    Polyglandular syndromes (types I, II)
Infectious diseases
  Tuberculosis, histoplasmosis, etc.
  Meningococcemia (Waterhouse-Friderichsen syndrome)
  Associated with human immunodeficiency virus infection
Infiltrative processes
  Sarcoidosis, amyloidosis, etc.
  Neoplasms
Drugs
  Metyrapone, ketoconazole, aminoglutethimide, o,p′-DDD, RU-486

Secondary adrenal insufficiency (*low* cortisol, *low* ACTH)

CONGENITAL

ACTH/CRH deficiency
  Isolated
  Panhypopituitarism
  Associated with structural defects (e.g., septo-optic dysplasia)

ACQUIRED

Lymphocytic hypophysitis
Trauma
Neoplasms*
Exogenous steroids

*ACTH deficiency may be caused by pituitary invasion of the tumor, surgical resection, and/or chemotherapy and radiation.

consequence of both cortisol and aldosterone deficiencies, is a common presentation for patients with primary adrenal insufficiency. In contrast, hypoglycemia due to cortisol deficiency may be the only manifestation of secondary adrenal insufficiency. Except for possibly mild hyponatremia, electrolytes are normal in these individuals because mineralocorticoid function is preserved.

Congenital and Genetic Disorders

Congenital Adrenal Hyperplasia

Primary adrenal insufficiency can be congenital or acquired. The most common inherited etiology for adrenal insufficiency is congenital adrenal hyperplasia (CAH), a group of autosomal recessive disorders in which there is a deficiency of one of the enzymes in the adrenal steroid synthetic pathway. This leads to an inability to synthesize the usual end products of the adrenal cortex (Figure 10-1). Via the feedback pathway between the adrenal cortex and the pituitary gland, inadequate cortisol synthesis promotes the contin-

ued release of ACTH, which leads to chronic stimulation of the adrenal glands. As a result, precursor hormones proximal to the enzyme block accumulate and are shunted to other synthetic pathways. Excessive stimulation of the glands by ACTH leads to the hyperplasia for which the disorder is named. Clinical and biochemical manifestations depend on the specific enzyme deficiency and may include glucocorticoid and mineralocorticoid deficiencies, as well as signs of androgen excess (Table 10-1). Figure 10-2 suggests an approach to making the diagnosis of CAH.

Lipoid Congenital Adrenal Hyperplasia
Lipoid CAH is a severe inborn error of steroid hormone biosynthesis resulting in disrupted synthesis of all adrenal and gonadal steroids. In lipoid CAH, there is a defect in the conversion of cholesterol to pregnenolone, the primary synthetic step in steroid synthesis (see Figure 10-1), due to a deficiency of StAR (steroidogenic acute regulatory) protein. The movement of cholesterol from the outer to the inner mitochondrial membrane where steroid synthesis occurs is an essential first step and is promoted by mechanisms both dependent on, and independent of, StAR protein. In the

Table 10-1   Variants of Congenital Adrenal Hyperplasia (CAH)

Deficiency	Disorder	Ambiguous Genitalia	Salt Metabolism	Excess Hormones	Deficient Hormones	Therapeutic Measures
StAR	Lipoid CAH	Males	Salt-wasting	None	All	Glucocortocoid, mineralocorticoid replacement
3β-OH-steroid dehydrogenase	Classic	Males, females	Salt-wasting	17-OH-pregnenolone, DHEA	Cortisol, aldosterone	Glucocorticoid, mineralocorticoid replacement
	Nonclassic	No	Normal	17-OH-pregnenolone, DHEA	...	Glucocorticoid replacement
11β-hydroxylase	Classic	Females	Hypertension	11-Deoxycortisol, DOC	Cortisol ± aldosterone	Glucocorticoid replacement
	Nonclassic	No	Normal	11-Deoxycortisol ± DOC	...	Glucocorticoid replacement
21-hydroxylase	Classic	Females	Salt-wasting	17-OH-progesterone, androstenedione	Cortisol, aldosterone	Glucocorticoid, mineralocorticoid replacement
	Simple virilizing	Females	Minimally affected	17-OH-progesterone, androstendione	Cortisol	Glucocorticoid replacement
	Nonclassic	No	Normal	17-OH-progesterone, androstenedione	...	Glucocorticoid replacement
17α-hydroxylase	...	Males	Hypertension	DOC, corticosterone	Cortisol	Glucocorticoid replacement

StAR, steroidogenic acute regulatory protein; DHEA, dehydroepiandrosterone; DOC, deoxycorticosterone.

absence of StAR, steroidogenesis does take place but is suboptimal and results in increased ACTH release, which in turn leads to increased production and accumulation of cholesterol within the cell in the form of lipid droplets. In time, lipid droplets engorge the cell, thereby destroying the cytoarchitecture and eliminating all residual steroidogenic capacity. The resultant enlarged appearance of the adrenal glands when viewed on imaging studies is a hallmark of this disorder.

Patients typically present in infancy with salt-wasting crisis. Because of the location of the enzyme deficiency in the synthetic pathway, inadequate androgens are made; genetic males have a female phenotype but lack female internal organs. Genetic females typically do not exhibit signs of virilization. A novel case report of lipoid CAH due to haploinsufficiency of P450 side chain cleavage (P450scc) associated with clitoromegaly has recently been published.

3β-hydroxysteroid Dehydrogenase Deficiency
3β-hydroxysteroid dehydrogenase (3β-HSD) deficiency is responsible for fewer than 5% of cases of CAH. This enzyme converts pregnenolone to progesterone in the mineralocorticoid pathway, 17-OH-pregnenolone to 17-OH-progesterone in the glucocorticoid pathway, and DHEA to androstenedione in the androgen synthetic pathway. Deficiency of 3β-HSD, caused by one of several mutations

in the *HSD3B2* gene on chromosome 1, results in inadequate synthesis of cortisol, aldosterone, and androstenedione. Infants affected with the classic form of this disorder present in salt-wasting crisis. Girls are mildly virilized, whereas boys exhibit signs of incomplete virilization, such as hypospadias or cryptorchidism. Postnatally, females can develop signs of early adrenarche due to excessive secretion of DHEA. Menstrual irregularity, hirsutism, or polycystic ovary syndrome may occur in the adolescent female. Females with the nonclassic form present beyond infancy with premature adrenarche, disordered puberty, and infertility. This form is reported clinically, although no specific genetic mutation has been identified.

11β-hydroxylase Deficiency
11β-hydroxylase deficiency causes 5% to 8% of cases of CAH. This enzyme mediates the conversion of deoxycorticosterone (DOC) to corticosterone in the mineralocorticoid pathway and 11-deoxycortisol to cortisol in the glucocorticoid pathway. Enzyme deficiency, caused by point mutations in the *CPY11B1* gene on chromosome 8, results in inadequate cortisol but excess deoxycorticosterone, 11-deoxycortisol, androstenedione, and testosterone synthesis. In the classic form of this disorder, affected genetic females are severely virilized at birth as a result of the excess androgens in utero. Affected genetic males appear

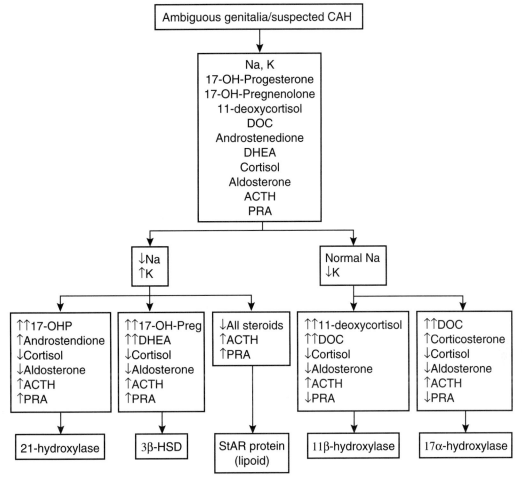

Figure 10-2   Approach to the Infant with Suspected Congenital Adrenal Hyperplasia.
Ambiguous genitalia in genetic females (46,XX) is caused by 21-hydroxylase deficiency, 11β-hydroxylase
deficiency, and 3β-hydroxysteroid dehydrogenase deficiency. Ambiguous genitalia in genetic males (46,XY) is
caused by 3β-hydroxysteroid dehydrogenase deficiency and 17α-hydroxylase deficiency. Males with lipoid
congenital adrenal hyperplasia have a female phenotype.

normal and are not recognized clinically in the newborn
period. Despite the disturbance in the mineralocorticoid
synthetic pathway in this disorder, infants with 11β-
hydroxylase deficiency do not present in salt-wasting crisis.
Deoxycorticosterone has potent mineralocorticoid effects
and leads to sodium retention and potassium excretion. The
resultant volume expansion leads to hypertension, which is
a characteristic feature of this form of CAH. Premature
adrenarche, irregular menses, acne, and/or fertility problems are seen later in life in individuals with the nonclassic
form of this disorder.

21-hydroxylase Deficiency
21-hydroxylase deficiency is the most common cause of
CAH, accounting for more than 90% of cases. The incidence of this disorder is 1:5,000 to 1:15,000. The classic
form of this disorder presents in infancy with ambiguous
genitalia in genetic females and salt-wasting crisis in boys
within the first few weeks of life. 21-hydroxylase converts
17-OH-progesterone to 11-deoxycortisol in the glucocorti-

coid pathway and progesterone to deoxycorticosterone in
the mineralocorticoid pathway. Mutations in the *CYP21B*
gene on chromosome 6 lead to deficiency of the enzyme.
Enzyme deficiency results in inadequate production of
aldosterone and cortisol, which stimulates excessive secretion of ACTH. Precursor hormones before the enzyme
block accumulate and are diverted to the androgen synthetic pathway, resulting in excessive production of
androstenedione and testosterone. These potent male hormones are responsible for the virilization characteristic of
this disorder. Affected 46,XX infants may demonstrate a
range of findings, including clitoromegaly, partial to complete fusion of the labioscrotal folds, and the appearance of
a penile urethra, usually with hypospadias. Internally, they
have normal female reproductive organs.

Nonclassic, or late-onset, CAH due to 21-hydroxylase
deficiency manifests later in childhood or adolescence.
Patients present with premature adrenarche, disordered
puberty, hirsutism, and/or menstrual irregularity. Although

mild salt-wasting, as manifested by elevated plasma renin activity, may occur, neither hyponatremia nor genital ambiguity is a feature of this form.

Newborn Screening

Many states now include 21-hydroxylase deficiency as part of the standard newborn screen, which is performed on the second day of life. The test measures the level of 17-OH-progesterone in a heel stick capillary blood specimen on filter paper. Because premature infants and ill newborns have higher levels of this hormone compared with their well full-term counterparts, abnormal screening values may require clinical interpretation.

17-hydroxylase Deficiency

17-hydroxylase converts pregnenolone and progesterone to 17-OH-pregnenolone and 17-OH-progesterone, respectively. 17,20-lyase then catalyzes the conversion of 17-OH-pregnenolone to DHEA and 17-OH-progesterone to androstenedione. Deficiency of 17-hydroxylase leads to inadequate cortisol synthesis. As in 11β-hydroxylase deficiency, excessive production of deoxycorticosterone causes hypokalemia, hypernatremia, and hypertension. Affected individuals cannot synthesize normal levels of androgens and estrogens. As a result, genetic males appear phenotypically female at birth. Genetic females appear normal but fail to undergo sexual maturation at the expected age for puberty. The lack of sexual development is due to hypergonadotropic hypogonadism.

Treatment

The immediate aim of treatment of CAH is to correct and/or prevent adrenal crisis and its complications. The long-term goals of therapeutic intervention, however, include helping patients to attain normal growth, puberty, sexual function, and fertility. Patients with salt-wasting forms of CAH (lipoid CAH, classic 21-hydroxylase deficiency, classic 3β-HSD deficiency) require both glucocorticoid and mineralocorticoid replacement. Some patients also require sodium supplementation. Those with nonclassic forms of CAH may need to be treated with glucocorticoids. Milder forms of the disorder often require no intervention, but glucocorticoid replacement is indicated if predicted adult height is compromised by a rapidly advancing skeletal age.

Ambiguous Genitalia

Ambiguous genitalia in the neonate requires urgent medical attention. The diagnostic evaluation to determine the underlying disorder should begin promptly in case the infant has a salt-wasting form of congenital adrenal hyperplasia. A multidisciplinary approach that includes evaluations by endocrinology, urology, and psychiatry is useful. Determination of the definitive gender can usually be completed within 48 to 72 hours. Gender assignment can usually be made based on the physical examination, karyotype, and internal pelvic structures while awaiting the results of serum studies. (For a discussion on gender assignment, see Chapter 7.) Females with CAH, even when severely virilized, have good future potential for sexual function and reproduction. For families identified as carriers of CAH mutations, prenatal diagnosis and treatment may limit virilization of the female fetus.

Prenatal Therapy

Prenatal diagnosis of CAH was first reported nearly 30 years ago. Diagnostic modalities include amniotic fluid hormone levels, human leukocyte antigen (HLA) typing of chorionic villus and amniotic fluid cells, and molecular genetic studies of chorionic villus and amniotic fluid cells. Hormonal features of 21-hydroxylase deficiency, for example, include elevated concentrations of 17-OH-progesterone, androstenedione, and testosterone (females only) in amniotic fluid. Testosterone cannot be used to diagnose an affected male fetus because testosterone is normally elevated in males.

Masculinization of fetal external genitalia begins at approximately 8 to 9 weeks of gestation. Suppression of the fetal pituitary-adrenal axis with exogenous steroids (dexamethasone) during this period could then theoretically prevent genital ambiguity in the female fetus with salt-wasting CAH. Later treatment could prevent progressive clitoral enlargement but not fusion of the labioscrotal folds. Attempts at prenatal treatment of CAH, both 21-hydroxylase deficiency and 11β-hydroxylase deficiency, have yielded variable results, from normal to markedly virilized genitalia.

Undesirable events such as spontaneous abortion, late pregnancy fetal death, agenesis of the corpus collosum, hydrocephalus, and hypospadias with cryptorchidism have occurred in pregnant women treated with prenatal steroids, but the events have not been considered to be related to therapy. Most infants treated prenatally have shown normal postnatal growth and development; long-term follow-up, however, is limited. Rare cases of adverse developmental outcomes, such as psychomotor and psychosocial delays and failure to thrive, have been reported. Long-term outcome studies of prenatal steroid therapy are essential.

Potential maternal adverse effects of dexamethasone include hypertension, glucose intolerance, edema, excessive weight gain, severe striae, cushingoid appearance, epigastric discomfort, irritability, anxiety, and facial hair growth. Women with preexisting conditions that may be aggravated by steroid therapy, such as diabetes, gestational diabetes, or hypertension, should be treated only with extreme caution or not at all.

Before initiation of prenatal steroids, the variability of genital outcome and the uncertainty of long-term effects of treatment should be discussed. Treatment should begin by the sixth week of gestation with dexamethasone (20 to 25 μg/kg/day). During the ninth week, women should undergo chorionic villus sampling for karyotyping, HLA typing, and genetic analysis. If the fetus is either a male or an unaffected female, dexamethasone is discontinued. Affected males need not continue to receive prenatal steroids because they develop normal genitalia without any intervention. If the fetus is an affected female, steroids are continued for the duration of the pregnancy. The possibility of physical, hormonal, and metabolic changes in the mother should be monitored closely.

Adrenal Hypoplasia Congenita

Adrenal hypoplasia congenita (AHC) is a rare disorder that presents early in life as salt-wasting crisis due to mineralocorticoid deficiency. There are two forms of the disorder, distinguished by the mode of inheritance and the appearance of the adrenal glands. In the autosomal recessive form, the glands have normal architecture but are hypoplastic. In the X-linked form, the glands are structurally abnormal. The latter form of AHC is caused by abnormalities in the *DAX-1* gene (dosage-sensitive sex reversal–adrenal hypoplasia congenita critical region on the X chromosome). The *DAX-1* gene encodes a member of the nuclear hormone receptor superfamily, which acts as a dominant negative regulator of transcription. More than 40 frameshift, nonsense, and missense mutations in the *DAX-1* gene have been identified, but the disorder can also be caused by gene deletions.

Adrenal insufficiency associated with AHC usually manifests during infancy or early childhood. Affected individuals present with salt-wasting crisis and hyperpigmentation. *DAX-1* mutations also impair gonadotropin synthesis at the levels of the hypothalamus and pituitary. The resultant hypogonadotropic hypogonadism becomes evident during adolescence, when patients fail to manifest signs of puberty.

Familial Glucocorticoid Deficiency (ACTH Unresponsiveness)

Familial glucocorticoid deficiency, or ACTH unresponsiveness, is an autosomal recessive disorder in which adrenal insufficiency results from the inability of the adrenal gland to respond to endogenously secreted ACTH. In some cases, the disorder is caused by missense mutations in the gene that encodes the ACTH receptor, which is also known as the melanocortin-2 receptor (MCR2). Abnormalities distal to the MCR2 have also been suggested as a cause of this entity in patients shown to have normal MCR2 receptors.

Patients with ACTH resistance experience symptoms of cortisol deficiency but without symptoms of mineralocorticoid deficiency. Except for mild hyponatremia, serum electrolytes are normal, and serum glucose may be low. This pattern of electrolytes is characteristic of secondary adrenal insufficiency (due to lack of ACTH), but the combination of very elevated ACTH levels and low cortisol levels is consistent with ACTH resistance. Hyperpigmentation is typical, as ACTH levels are markedly elevated.

When adrenal insufficiency is seen in conjunction with alacrima and achalasia, the triad is referred to as the triple A syndrome, or Allgrove syndrome. As in familial glucocorticoid resistance, adrenal insufficiency is caused by ACTH resistance. Failure of the adrenal glands to respond to ACTH in this disorder, however, has not been shown to be associated with mutations in the ACTH receptor. Mutations in the *AAAS* gene, which encodes the product aladin, on chromosome 12 have been implicated as a cause of this disorder.

Aldosterone Deficiency

True aldosterone deficiency is caused by a deficiency in the enzyme required for synthesis of aldosterone. Patients present with hyponatremia, hyperkalemia, and acidosis. End-organ (kidney) unresponsiveness to aldosterone, also known as pseudohypoaldosteronism, clinically mimics true aldosterone deficiency. These disorders can be distinguished biochemically by measuring levels of aldosterone in blood and urine and plasma renin in blood. In the true form of the disorder, aldosterone is low and renin is high. In pseudohypoaldosteronism, both aldosterone and renin are high. Only true aldosterone deficiency responds to mineralocorticoid replacement; those with pseudohypoaldosteronism require sodium chloride supplementation.

Adrenoleukodystrophy

Adrenoleukodystrophy (ALD) is an X-linked peroxisomal disorder characterized by an inability to degrade very long chain fatty acids (VLCFA) and severe neurological sequelae. Impaired peroxisomal β-oxidation of VLCFA results in progressive demyelination of cerebral white matter and destruction of the adrenal cortex. Elevated VLCFA are found in cultured fibroblasts, plasma, amniotic fluid, and chorionic villi, and prenatal diagnosis is possible.

Multiple phenotypes exist: (1) cerebral ALD, (2) adrenomyeloneuropathy (AMN), (3) adrenal only, (4) asymptomatic, and (5) ALD heterozygotes. Diffuse demyelinating lesions characterize cerebral ALD, which may manifest during childhood (2 to 10 years), adolescence (11 to 21 years), or adulthood (after 21 years). The childhood-onset form of the disease is severe and has a rapidly progressive course; mild behavior changes and deterioration in school performance are followed by blindness, deafness, dementia, and death. Adrenomyeloneuropathy manifests in adulthood, and paraparesis progresses over decades. In 10% to 20% of cases of ALD, adrenal insufficiency is the only presenting manifestation. These patients have a high risk of developing neurological symptoms later in life, as do patients with the asymptomatic form of ALD. There is also a neonatal form of ALD, which manifests during infancy as severe developmental delay, hypotonia, and seizures. Unlike the childhood and adult forms, inheritance is autosomal recessive.

Wolman Disease

Wolman disease is a lysosomal storage disorder caused by lysosomal acid lipase (LIPA) deficiency. Mutations in the *LIPA* gene, which is located on chromosome 10, lead to xanthomatous changes in multiple organs, including liver, spleen, small intestine, lymph nodes, and lungs. This autosomal recessive disorder presents in the neonatal period as a constellation of nonspecific findings such as failure to thrive, emesis, abdominal distension, and organomegaly. Diffuse punctate calcifications of the adrenal glands are typical. Death usually occurs in early infancy.

Acquired Primary Adrenal Insufficiency (Addison Disease)

Etiologies

Autoimmune

Etiologies of acquired primary adrenal insufficiency, or Addison disease, include autoimmune, infectious, infiltrative, traumatic, and drug-induced (see Box 10-1). The majority of cases are caused by an autoimmune process called autoimmune adrenalitis, in which cytotoxic lymphocytes slowly destroy the adrenal cortex. As a result, adrenal cortical function progressively declines until it becomes so severely impaired as to lead to complete metabolic decompensation. In patients with Addison disease, other autoimmune disorders are not uncommon and include, but are not limited to, diabetes mellitus, thyroiditis, Graves disease, hypoparathyroidism, vitiligo, and celiac disease.

Autoimmune Polyglandular Syndromes

Addison disease can be a component of a family of disorders known as the autoimmune polyglandular syndromes (APGs), and making a diagnosis of adrenal insufficiency should prompt an investigation for other autoimmune endocrinopathies. Type I APG consists of adrenal failure and hypoparathyroidism or chronic mucocutaneous candidiasis (CMC). This disorder usually presents in infancy with hypoparathyroidism or candidiasis; adrenal insufficiency follows during childhood. This syndrome is also known as autoimmune polyendocrinopathy candidiasis ectodermal dystrophy (APECED). Vitiligo, alopecia, pernicious anemia, and chronic active hepatitis are among the many nonendocrine autoimmune disorders associated with the APGs.

Type II APG consists of adrenal failure and autoimmune thyroid dysfunction or insulin-dependent diabetes mellitus (IDDM). Hypoparathyroidism and candidiasis are not seen. Presentation of the first endocrinopathy in type II APG may be in the first or second decade. Adrenal insufficiency is not a feature of type III APG, which instead is comprised of autoimmune thyroid dysfunction and one other autoimmune endocrinopathy.

Infectious, Infiltrative, and Traumatic

Several infectious diseases can lead to Addison disease. In fact, tuberculosis was the original etiology of the disorder when first described early in the 20th century. Histoplasmosis and coccidiomycosis may also cause adrenal insufficiency. Meningococcemia can lead to adrenal hemorrhage (Waterhouse-Friderichsen syndrome), and opportunistic human immunodeficiency virus (HIV)-associated infections can interfere with cortisol synthesis. Infiltrative processes such as amyloidosis and sarcoidosis, as well as tumors that destroy the adrenal cortex, can lead to Addison disease. Trauma from birth can cause adrenal hemorrhage, which rarely may precipitate adrenal crisis. More commonly, adrenal calcifications, thought to be remnants of a perinatal adrenal hemorrhage, are discovered incidentally and have no significant clinical sequelae. Surgical trauma and a variety of drugs can also lead to adrenal insufficiency.

Secondary Adrenal Insufficiency

Secondary adrenal insufficiency is caused by a central hormone deficiency in which the hypothalamus or pituitary does not function properly. In such cases, there is deficiency of CRH or ACTH, which results in glucocorticoid deficiency. In contrast to those with primary adrenal insufficiency, patients with secondary adrenal insufficiency do not have mineralocorticoid deficiency because the primary regulator of mineralocorticoid secretion is the renin-angiotensin-aldosterone (RAA) axis, which is preserved in secondary adrenal insufficiency.

Congenital Etiologies

Like primary adrenal insufficiency, secondary adrenal insufficiency can be congenital or acquired. Congenital deficiency of ACTH/CRH can be either isolated or associated with multiple hormonal deficiencies (panhypopituitarism) and often presents with hypoglycemia in infancy. The combination of hypoglycemia and cholestatic jaundice in the newborn is almost always indicative of hypopituitarism. Although the mechanism is still unclear, there is evidence to suggest that pituitary hormones play a role in normal bilirubin metabolism, and jaundice resolves with replacement of the deficient hormones.

Secondary adrenal insufficiency may be caused by anatomic defects of the hypothalamus or pituitary gland or may be idiopathic. Patients with midline defects such as holoprosencephaly and septo-optic dysplasia (SOD) should be evaluated for hypopituitarism. Additional findings on the physical examination that suggest the possibility of pituitary insufficiency include a high arched palate, cleft palate, and micropenis in the male neonate.

Septo-optic Dysplasia
SOD is a disorder characterized by the triad of (1) absence of the septum pellucidum, (2) optic nerve hypoplasia, and (3) hypopituitarism. This disorder can be caused by mutations in the *HESX1* homeobox gene. Pituitary insufficiency may range from isolated deficiency of one specific hormone to complete lack of all pituitary hormones. The adenohypophysis, or anterior pituitary, is more commonly affected than the posterior pituitary. Growth hormone deficiency is the most common abnormality, followed by, in order of decreasing frequency, inadequate thyrotropin-stimulating hormone (TSH), ACTH, luteinizing hormone (LH), and follicle-stimulating hormone (FSH). Prolactin levels may be elevated. When it occurs, involvement of the posterior pituitary results in vasopressin deficiency.

Acquired Causes

Lymphocytic Hypophysitis
Lymphocytic hypophysitis is an autoimmune disorder in which lymphocytic infiltration partially or completely impairs the function of the pituitary. This disorder is most commonly seen in women around the time of childbirth but has been described in children. It may be associated with other autoimmune endocrinopathies, such as thyroiditis. Although the disorder itself tends to resolve, hypopituitarism is permanent.

Trauma
If head trauma results in intracranial hemorrhage or a shear injury to the pituitary stalk, it can lead to secondary adrenal insufficiency. Trauma from surgical resection of a brain tumor, as well as the tumor itself, may also permanently affect ACTH secretion. With the increased number of childhood cancer survivors, it is important to remember that hypopituitarism is a common sequela of chemotherapy and radiation.

Exogenous Glucocorticoids
The most common cause of acquired secondary adrenal insufficiency is the administration of supraphysiological (pharmacological) doses of glucocorticoids as immunosuppressive agents or for the treatment of systemic inflammatory illnesses, such as asthma, juvenile rheumatoid arthritis, and systemic lupus erythematosus. These large doses of glucocorticoids act centrally to inhibit ACTH release. Without ACTH to promote endogenous cortisol release, the adrenal glands are chronically understimulated and may become atrophic. Patients are there-

fore at risk of adrenal crisis if steroids are not adequately tapered to allow for recovery of function of the adrenal glands.

How rapidly steroids can be tapered depends on the following factors: (1) the duration of treatment, (2) the amount and type of steroid used (Box 10-2), and (3) the disease being treated. Steroids should be tapered slowly (e.g., decrease by 10% every 2 weeks) if there is a risk of a flare in the disease when the steroids are reduced. Otherwise, the dose should be reduced by 50% every 2 days until the patient is receiving the equivalent of physiological hydrocortisone replacement (12 to 15 mg/m^2/day). Tapering from physiological dose to complete withdrawal depends on the anticipated degree of adrenal suppression (Figure 10-3). Once the dose is reduced to physiological replacement, the steroid should be changed to a hydrocortisone preparation and the dose reduced by 50% for 2 weeks. At the end of 2 weeks, the patient should withhold the morning dose of hydrocortisone and have a morning cortisol level. If the level is greater that 10 mg/dL, steroid supplementation may be discontinued. If the level is less than 10 mg/dL, steroids must be continued and the test repeated in 1 month. Until full recovery of the adrenal glands is confirmed, stress-dose steroids (50 mg/m^2/day) are indicated during periods of intercurrent illness or surgery.

Clinical Features

History and Physical Findings
Symptoms of adrenal insufficiency are rather nonspecific. Making the diagnosis, therefore, requires a high index of suspicion and can be particularly challenging in the infant or young child who cannot communicate his symptoms. History is remarkable for decreased interest in feeding, vomiting, irritability, and lethargy. Genital ambiguity in the neonate suggests the possibility of a salt-wasting form of

Box 10-2	Relative Potencies of Steroid Preparations	
STEROID	**RELATIVE GLUCO-CORTICOID POTENCY**	**RELATIVE MINERALO-CORTICOID POTENCY**
Hydrocortisone	1	++
Prednisone	3-5	+
Prednisolone	3-5	+
Methylprednisolone	5-6	0
Dexamethasone	25-50	0
Fludrocortisone	15-20	++++

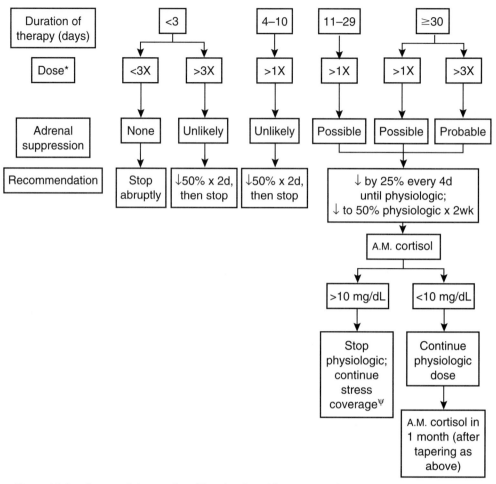

Figure 10-3 **Suggested Approach to Tapering Steroids.** Duration of treatment, amount and type of steroid used, and the disease being treated all influence how quickly steroids can be safely weaned (see text for details). *, Compared with physiological hydrocortisone replacement (12 to 15 mg/m²/day). ψ, Stress coverage is required until adequacy of the pituitary-adrenal response to stress is confirmed with Cortrosyn testing.

CAH. Male neonates with CAH, however, often have normal male genitalia, so the age at presentation, typically at 2 to 3 weeks of life, is an important clue in this age group.

The older child or adolescent with adrenal insufficiency complains of weakness, headache, fever, abdominal pain, and vomiting. More subtle complaints include undue fatigue, myalgias, arthralgias, anorexia, weight loss, and salt-craving. Depending on the age at onset of the disease, pubertal development may be delayed or seem to have an unusually slow progression. Females may report menstrual irregularities or amenorrhea. Patients often appear thin and/or cachetic and, in the setting of adrenal crisis, manifest signs of severe dehydration, including tachycardia, hypotension, and shock.

Hyperpigmentation is the most striking physical finding in Addison disease and is common to all age groups. Areas where hyperpigmentation is typically found include lip borders; buccal mucosa; areolae; skin creases such as axillae, groin, and palms; pressure points; and scarred areas. The heart has a long, thin appearance on chest radiography.

ACTH and melanocyte-stimulating hormone (MSH) are cleaved from the same precursor molecule, pro-opiomelanocortin (POMC), in the pituitary gland so that when the body makes excess ACTH in response to low cortisol, MSH is also released. Both ACTH and MSH are capable of stimulating melanocytes. It is likely the ACTH, however, which is primarily responsible for darkening of the skin because it is produced in such excessive amounts compared to the relatively small amount of MSH. Hyperpigmentation is not a feature of secondary adrenal insufficiency because the defect lies at the level of the hypothalamus or pituitary gland such that the patient is ACTH deficient.

Laboratory Study Abnormalities

Laboratory study findings in adrenal insufficiency depend on whether there is glucocorticoid deficiency, mineralocorticoid deficiency, or both. Cortisol deficiency leads to hypoglycemia and mild hyponatremia due to retention of free water. Patients may also have normochromic anemia and eosinophilia. The hyponatremia of aldosterone deficiency is more profound and is accompanied by hyperkalemia and metabolic acidosis.

Hormonal values that help to distinguish primary from secondary adrenal insufficiency include cortisol, ACTH, aldosterone, and plasma renin. With primary adrenal insufficiency, the ACTH level is markedly elevated in response to a low cortisol level. If there is mineralocorticoid deficiency, the plasma renin level is elevated in response low aldosterone. In secondary adrenal insufficiency, the cortisol level is low, and the ACTH level also is low, indicating that the pituitary gland failed to respond appropriately to an inadequate cortisol level. Because of the nonspecific nature of symptoms of adrenal insufficiency, making a diagnosis requires a high index of suspicion. When adrenal insufficiency is suspected, it is wise to obtain blood for ACTH and cortisol levels and, if possible, to perform provocative testing, before administering steroids. Figure 10-4 provides an approach to differentiating between primary and secondary adrenal insufficiency.

Diagnosis

Primary Adrenal Insufficiency

The definitive test for the diagnosis of Addison disease is the Cortrosyn (cosyntropin) stimulation test. Cortrosyn is a synthetic form of ACTH. After blood is obtained for baseline ACTH and cortisol levels, 250 μg of Cortrosyn is administered intravenously and serial cortisol levels are measured 30 and 60 minutes later. The cortisol level is expected to rise to at least 18 μg/dL in normal individuals. Failure of cortisol level to rise in response to ACTH confirms failure of the adrenal glands.

Additional blood tests that should be ordered in patients presenting with primary adrenal insufficiency include antiadrenal antibodies, which, if present, confirm that an autoimmune process has destroyed the adrenal glands. Plasma renin is elevated, consistent with salt-wasting and mineralocorticoid deficiency. VLCFA is markedly elevated in patients with adrenoleukodystrophy. It is reasonable to screen for thyroid dysfunction by measuring T_4, TSH, and thyroid antibodies. Given the recent resurgence of tuberculosis, a PPD and an anergy panel should be placed.

Secondary Adrenal Insufficiency

If secondary adrenal insufficiency is suspected, a CRH test can be used. Corticorelin (Acthrel) is a synthetic form of CRH and has been shown to be a safe test useful in the evaluation of children with hypopituitarism. After blood for baseline ACTH and cortisol levels is obtained, 1 μg/kg corticorelin is administered intravenously followed by serial measurement of ACTH and cortisol levels at 15, 30, 60, and 90 minutes. Low baseline and low stimulated ACTH and cortisol values are consistent with secondary adrenal insufficiency.

Alternatively, a low-dose (1 μg) Cortrosyn stimulation test can help confirm the diagnosis. The low-dose test is preferable to the standard dose (250 μg) in the setting of ACTH deficiency. Chronically understimulated adrenal glands may have a falsely reassuring response to the standard Cortrosyn dose. On the other hand, chronically understimulated adrenal glands would not be expected to show an adequate response to the lower, more physiological Cortrosyn dose of 1 μg.

Management

Adrenal Crisis

Management of adrenal insufficiency differs in the acute and chronic settings. Emergency measures for the patient who presents in adrenal crisis include aggressive fluid resuscitation with isotonic saline (to restore intravascular volume and renal perfusion), intravenous glucose (3 mL/kg of 10% dextrose) for hypoglycemia, and parenteral hydrocortisone (100 mg/m² as intravenous bolus followed by 100 mg/m²/day in six divided doses). Because this large dose of hydrocortisone has mineralocorticoid activity, additional mineralocorticoid replacement is not needed initially. Measures to correct hyperkalemia may also be required.

Chronic Therapy

Chronic management of adrenal insufficiency requires ongoing replacement of the deficient adrenal hormones. Patients with primary adrenal insufficiency are continued on oral hydrocortisone but at much lower, maintenance doses (12 to 15 mg/m²/day in three divided doses). The actual required physiological replacement dose is 7 to 8 mg/m²/day, but the oral dose is doubled to compensate for the fact that the bioavailability of the oral preparation is only 50%. Patients with mineralocorticoid deficiency must also take oral fludrocortisone (Florinef) 0.1 mg daily, which is usually initiated after diagnosis when the dose of hydrocortisone dose is decreased to maintenance. Patients with secondary adrenal insufficiency require less of a maintenance dose (7 to 8 mg/m²/day) and may take it only once or twice per day. Mineralocorticoid supplementation is not required in these patients.

It is critical that patients with adrenal insufficiency, both primary and secondary, receive "stress doses" of steroids during times of increased physiological stress (e.g., febrile illnesses, surgical procedures) to mimic the body's normal cortisol

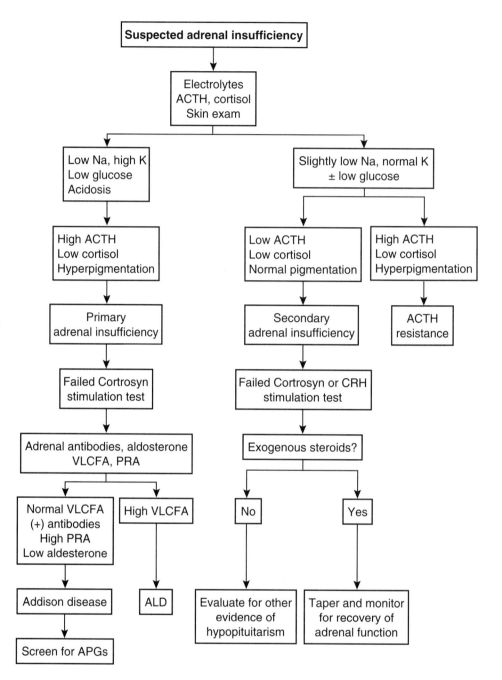

Figure 10-4 **Approach to the Patient with Suspected Adrenal Insufficiency.** Electrolytes, hormonal values, and physical examination findings provide clues for differentiating primary versus secondary adrenal insufficiency. More specific diagnostic tests then help to determine the specific etiology. VLCFA, very long chain fatty acids; ALD, adrenoleukodystrophy; PRA, plasma renin activity; APGs, autoimmune polyglandular syndromes; CRH, corticotropin-releasing hormone.

response to stress. At such times, the maintenance dose of hydrocortisone should be at least tripled (50 mg/m^2/day for minor stress; 100 mg/m^2/day for major stress). Patients should receive the stress dose 3 times daily for 24 hours or for as long as the stress lasts before resuming the maintenance dose. If there is any doubt as to the need for stress dosing, the stress dose should be given since it is dangerous to withhold steroids when the patient is under physiological stress. If unable to tolerate oral fluids, patients should receive parenteral steroids (100 mg/m^2/dose of Solu-Cortef) and seek medical attention as soon as possible, because the duration of action of this for-

mulation is only 4 hours and the parenteral stress dose may need to be continued in a hospital setting.

Prognosis

The prognosis for patients with adrenal insufficiency is generally good if they are compliant with the medication regimen so the disorder is well controlled and if they receive stress-dose steroids when indicated. Sexual function and fertility are normal in Addison disease but may be affected in some forms of CAH, depending on the specific disorder, the genetic sex of the patient, and any anatomical abnormalities of the genitalia. Medic-alert jewelry that identifies the patient as having adrenal insufficiency is highly recommended.

SUGGESTED APPROACH IN CLINICAL PRACTICE

For the patient with suspected *primary* adrenal insufficiency, blood samples should always be sent for ACTH and cortisol levels before steroids are administered. If the stability of the patient's condition allows, it is optimal also to perform a Cortrosyn (250 μg) stimulation test as detailed earlier. High-dose steroids may then be administered while awaiting the results of these studies.

In the infant believed to have adrenal insufficiency caused by CAH, the biochemical investigation should focus on measurement of the steroidogenic precursors, including 17-OH-progesterone, 17-OH-pregnenolone, 11-deoxycortisol, deoxycorticosterone (DOC), androstenedione, and dehydroepiandrosterone (DHEA). Cortisol, aldosterone, ACTH, and plasma renin levels should also be measured. (Figure 10-2 provides interpretation of the results.) For the infant with ambiguous genitalia, a karyotype is needed to determine the genetic sex of the patient. Ultrasonography of the adrenal glands may also be indicated, especially if lipoid CAH is suspected.

In the older child or adolescent with primary adrenal insufficiency, additional diagnostic laboratory studies at the time of presentation should include plasma renin activity, aldosterone, antiadrenal antibodies, and VLCFA. A PPD and an anergy panel should also be placed.

When *secondary* adrenal insufficiency is suspected, blood should be obtained for ACTH and cortisol levels. A CRH test should be done to confirm the diagnosis. A steroid regimen can then be instituted pending the laboratory study results. In the absence of a recent history of exogenous steroid use, the patient should also be evaluated for other pituitary hormone deficiencies.

Long-term Monitoring
Long-term monitoring of children with adrenal insufficiency includes regular monitoring of electrolytes, ACTH, and plasma renin activity. Measurement of specific steroid precursors is part of the routine monitoring in patients with CAH (e.g., 17-OH-progesterone in 21-hydroxylase deficiency). Abnormalities in the electrolytes and the plasma renin value call for an adjustment in the dose of Florinef; an elevated ACTH value or steroid precursor value indicates that the dose of hydrocortisone needs to be adjusted. Clinically, patients should be monitored for adequate growth and pubertal development, as well as changes in pigmentation. After the initiation of treatment, the hyperpig-

mentation resolves. Recurrence of hyperpigmentation can be a clue to the possibility of noncompliance with the medication regimen. Routine screening for other associated disorders that comprise the autoimmune polyglandular syndrome is also important.

ADRENAL EXCESS STATES

Cushing syndrome, or hypercortisolism, refers to the clinical characteristics that result from exposure to excess glucocorticoids, which may be from either an endogenous or exogenous source. When it is an endogenous disorder, hypercortisolism may also be associated with overproduction of other adrenal hormones, mineralocorticoids, and androgens. Hypercortisolism is 10 times more common in adults and is rarely seen among children, but it can occur at any age.

Etiologies

Cushing disease is the name given to the disorder in which an ACTH-producing tumor of the pituitary gland is responsible for cortisol excess. Microadenomas (<10 mm) are most commonly responsible. One other possibility is overstimulation of the corticotroph cells by CRH as a result of an underlying hypothalamic abnormality. In either case, oversecretion of ACTH provides continual stimulation of the adrenal glands, which leads to hyperplasia and the resultant oversecretion of cortisol.

Hypercortisolism that is not central in etiology may by the result of primary oversecretion of cortisol by the adrenal gland itself (hyperplasia), by an adrenal adenoma or carcinoma, or by an ectopic ACTH-secreting tumor.

The patient's age may provide a clue to the etiology of the hypercortisolism. In children older than 7 years, Cushing disease is responsible for the majority of cases of hypercortisolism. Adrenocortical carcinomas, on the other hand, account for the majority of cases of Cushing syndrome in children younger than 7 years. Both disorders are more common in females.

Adrenal neoplasms are rare but can occur at any age from infancy through adolescence. These tumors may secrete one or more classes of steroid hormones and, as such, have various clinical manifestations. Adrenal adenomas are benign tumors of the adrenal cortex that secrete excess glucocorticoids. Affected patients manifest signs and symptoms of Cushing syndrome (see later). Adrenocortical carcinomas are malignant neoplasms, which more commonly secrete excess androgens. Virilization in females and premature adrenarche in males are the predominant clinical manifestations of these tumors. Adrenocortical carcinomas may also secrete glucocorticoids, in which case patients present with signs of both androgen and glucocorticoid excess. Nonadrenal tumors can also lead to Cushing syndrome; examples include neuroblastomas, pheochromocytomas, and islet cell tumors.

Exogenously administered steroids must be considered in the differential diagnosis of an individual being evaluated for possible Cushing syndrome. Prolonged, excessive, or repeated administration of steroids at pharmacological doses can lead to the typical physical features of hypercortisolism (see later). Children with inflammatory disorders such as juvenile rheumatoid arthritis, nephrotic syndrome, and systemic lupus erythematosus, who depend on chronic steroids for control of their disease, have an increased risk of developing Cushing syndrome. Those who have less severe disorders like asthma but receive repeated courses of steroids for intermittent exacerbations are also at risk.

Clinical Features

History and Physical Findings

As in adrenal insufficiency, patients with hypercortisolism report multiple nonspecific symptoms, such as generalized fatigue, weakness, irritability and/or personality changes, and progressive weight gain, usually of gradual onset. The classic description of an individual with hypercortisolism is of someone with centripetal obesity with sparing of the extremities. Fat accumulates predominantly on the trunk, abdomen, face, and neck and gives rise, in part, to the characteristic "cushingoid" appearance. The wasted appearance of the limbs results from increased protein catabolism and loss of muscle mass. In children with hypercortisolism, however, generalized obesity is more typical than truncal obesity.

Cushing syndrome is one of the few endocrine disorders associated with obesity, but obesity itself is not a very helpful finding. Rather, the combination of obesity and short stature suggests the possibility of cortisol excess. In fact, growth failure is the most consistent feature of hypercortisolism in children. It is this feature which best distinguishes hypercortisolism from exogenous obesity, which instead is associated with growth acceleration. One exception is the child with an adrenocortical carcinoma, in whom the excess androgens lead to increased linear growth.

Patients typically have rounded facies, truncal obesity, and an enlarged dorsocervical fat pad, commonly referred to as a "buffalo hump." Hypertension is not a constant finding but when present is due in part to the salt-retaining activity of cortisol. Muscle weakness and generalized fatigue are caused by hypokalemia. Common dermatological findings include ecchymosis and thin skin with violaceous striae on the abdomen and thighs, as well as in the axillae.

Capillary friability leads to easy bruisability and the formation of ecchymoses. Excessive levels of ACTH lead to generalized hyperpigmentation. If there is a concomitant increase in androgen secretion, hirsutism and acne are also seen. Adolescents can have pubertal arrest or disordered menstrual cycles.

Laboratory Study Abnormalities

Sustained hypercortisolism can lead to several undesirable sequelae. As one of the physiological roles of cortisol is to promote gluconeogenesis, hyperglycemia and glycosuria are common. Although adults with this disorder may develop frank diabetes mellitus, children more commonly have impaired glucose tolerance. Hyperlipidemia and hypercholesterolemia may be related to elevated insulin levels, which promote conversion of glucose to lipids. The increased circulating amino acid concentration caused by degradation of extrahepatic protein leads to a negative nitrogen balance.

Despite salt retention, hypernatremia is unusual. Hypokalemia, however, is common. This combination is due to water retention and increased blood volume, which maintain normal sodium but deplete potassium.

Glucocorticoids impair vitamin D–mediated absorption of calcium from the gastrointestinal tract and increase renal excretion of calcium. The resultant decrease in serum calcium stimulates the release of parathyroid hormone (PTH). PTH acts to maintain serum calcium by extracting calcium from the bones, and this process results in osteopenia and/or osteoporosis. The increased activity of PTH usually maintains normal serum calcium but does lead to hypophosphatemia.

Hematological and immune dysfunction is not infrequent with hypercortisolism. The stimulatory effect of cortisol on erythropoiesis leads to polycythemia. Lymphopenia and eosinopenia are common. Impaired immune function, secondary to atrophy of lymphoid tissue and decreased circulating T lymphocytes and antibodies, places patients at increased risk of infection, especially with opportunistic organisms.

Diagnosis

Establishing the Diagnosis

Loss of Diurnal Variation

The physiological diurnal variation of cortisol is not well established until after age 3 years, the age at which differentiation of the adrenal cortex into the mature adult zones is complete. Once diurnal variation is established, however, peak secretion of cortisol normally occurs in the early morning hours. Normal values for 8 AM are within the range of 5 to 25 mg/dL. The level then decreases to less than 50% of the morning value by late evening (11 PM). Loss of this diurnal variation is a hallmark of Cushing syndrome; these patients instead have an elevated mean cortisol level (Figure 10-5).

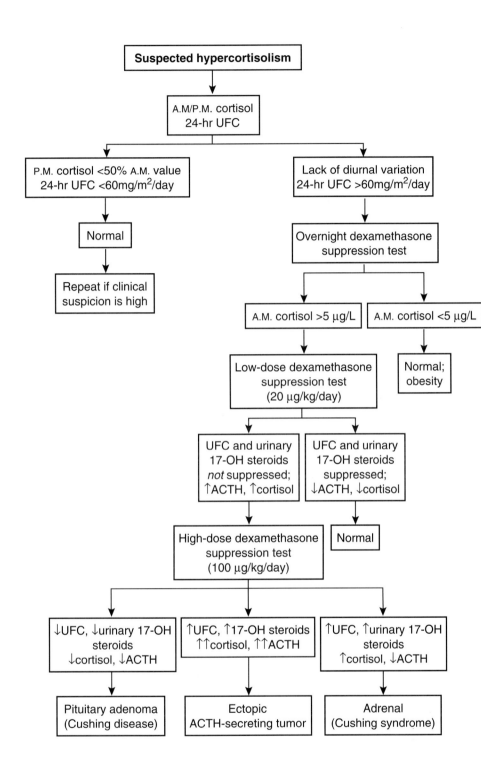

Figure 10-5   Approach to the Patient with Suspected Hypercortisolism. The 24-hour urinary free cortisol (UFC) is a useful test for beginning the evaluation of a patient with suspected hypercortisolism. More specific diagnostic studies, as outlined in the figure algorithm, are usually performed after a formal endocrine evaluation. ACTH, adrenocortricotropic hormone.

Urinary 17-hydroxysteroids

17-hydroxysteroids are cortisol metabolites, representing 25% of the daily cortisol secretion, and so are elevated in the setting of hypercortisolism. The values are also corrected for creatinine and are reported as milligrams per gram of creatinine. A value of greater than 6 mg/g creatinine suggests Cushing syndrome. This test can be affected by obesity and is not as useful as the 24-hour urinary free cortisol (UFC) value (see below).

Twenty-Four-Hour Urinary Free Cortisol

UFC represents a much smaller proportion, only 0.375%, of daily cortisol secretion than do urinary 17-hydroxy-steroids. This value is thought to be a direct reflection of unbound cortisol in blood and therefore to represent biologically active hormone.

The 24-hour UFC is the preferred test for diagnosing hypercortisolism. Patients must collect all urine over a period of 24 hours. On the day the collection begins, the first morning void should be discarded and all subsequent urine, including the first void the next morning, collected. Collection of urine is cumbersome and sometimes difficult to do correctly in both inpatient and outpatient settings. Young children may need to be catheterized for accurate collection of all urine. For older patients and parents, a detailed explanation of the proper method of collection should be provided and the importance of accuracy emphasized.

Urine creatinine must also be determined as the reference values are reported in μg/g creatinine. Normal values differ according to pubertal status and sex, and normal ranges vary according to the type of assay used. Values may be reported based on body surface area. A UFC value of greater than 60 μg/m^2/day is consistent with hypercortisolism. A small percentage of normal individuals can have a UFC value above the normal range at any given time. Conversely, it is possible for an individual with Cushing syndrome to have a normal value. It is therefore preferable to obtain two or three separate collections for determination of UFC.

Overnight Dexamethasone Suppression Test

The overnight dexamethasone suppression test is useful only as a screening tool in the patient suspected of having hypercortisolism, particularly for ruling out hypercortisolism in the patient with exogenous obesity. A single dose of 1 mg (or 0.3 mg/m^2) dexamethasone is administered at 11 PM and an 8 AM fasting cortisol value is obtained the following morning. Suppression of the morning cortisol to less than 5 μg/dL is normal. A value of greater than 5 μg/dL suggests hypercortisolism and warrants additional testing.

Midnight Salivary Cortisol

Measuring a salivary cortisol level at midnight may help obviate the difficulties associated with the aforementioned methods of screening for hypercortisolism. This simple test avoids both the inconvenience of collecting a 24-hour urine specimen and the possibility that a plasma cortisol value may be falsely elevated due to the stress of venipuncture. Like UFC, salivary cortisol is a more accurate index of plasma free cortisol than is total plasma cortisol. Saliva is measured in morning and evening specimens, obtained on 3 consecutive days. As with blood specimens, salivary cortisol reflects the normal diurnal variation of ACTH and plasma cortisol. An elevated salivary cortisol value late in the evening or at midnight indicates loss of this diurnal variation and indicates hypercortisolism.

Determining the Etiology

Corticotropin Levels

Measurement of serum ACTH can be useful in determining if the etiology of the hypercortisolism is central (Cushing disease) or peripheral (Cushing syndrome). If an ACTH-secreting pituitary adenoma is responsible for excess

cortisol production, the ACTH level is expected to be in the upper normal to high range. ACTH is not markedly elevated because the excessive cortisol can still suppress ACTH, albeit only partially, via an intact negative feedback loop. An elevated cortisol level in combination with a mild to moderately elevated normal ACTH level therefore points toward a diagnosis of Cushing disease (Figure 10-5).

Peripheral sources of hypercortisolism include an ectopic ACTH-producing tumor and autonomous hypersecretion of cortisol by the adrenal gland itself. ACTH-secreting neoplasms are very rare among children but, if present, lead to marked elevation of ACTH to a level of greater than 200 pg/mL. If the primary disturbance is with the adrenal gland, the excess cortisol leads to suppression of pituitary ACTH secretion via negative feedback. As a result, the finding of elevated cortisol with suppressed ACTH is consistent with an autonomously functioning adrenal gland.

Androgen Levels

Adrenocortical carcinomas are most commonly virilizing tumors because of the excessive androgens they secrete. As such, the finding of elevated androgen levels suggests the possibility of such a neoplasm. In contrast, benign adrenal adenomas are associated with normal or low levels of androgens.

Dexamethasone Suppression Tests

Dexamethasone is a potent glucocorticoid, approximately 40 times more potent than cortisol. Dexamethasone suppresses secretion of ACTH by the normal pituitary, decreasing the endogenous production of cortisol and therefore of 17-hydroxysteroids. Because so little dexamethasone in needed for suppression of pituitary ACTH, its contribution to urinary 17-hydroxysteroids is relatively small.

Low-Dose Dexamethasone Suppression Test

The low-dose dexamethasone suppression test is used to differentiate patients with hypercortisolism of any etiology from those with a normal HPA axis. For this test, a baseline 24-hour urine specimen for free cortisol and 17-hydroxysteroids must be obtained. Dexamethasone, 20 μg/kg/day, is then administered orally in four divided doses over a period of 48 hours while urine collection is continued. Six hours after the last dose of dexamethasone is administered, the last urine is collected and blood is drawn for cortisol and ACTH. Suppression of UFC and 17-hydroxystreroids to 50% to 90% of baseline values is a normal response and effectively rules out hypercortisolism. Although not required for the test, blood specimens can be confirmatory; ACTH and cortisol are both suppressed. If the low dose fails to show adequate suppression of urinary cortisol metabolites, a high-dose dexamethasone test is indicated.

High-Dose Dexamethasone Suppression Test

The purpose of this test is to differentiate between pituitary and adrenal sources of increased cortisol secretion. The rationale for the high-dose test is that ACTH secretion in Cushing disease is relatively, but not completely, resistant to dexamethasone. Increasing the dose, therefore, can almost always induce suppression of pituitary ACTH secretion. Conversely, nonpituitary tumors that secrete ACTH do not respond to negative feedback by cortisol, and autonomously functioning adrenal tumors in Cushing syndrome secrete cortisol independent of ACTH. In the latter two cases, pituitary ACTH is already suppressed. Therefore, dexamethasone cannot further suppress ACTH and does not affect cortisol secretion regardless of the dose.

To begin this test, a baseline 24-hour urine specimen for free cortisol and 17-hydroxysteroids must be collected. If this test immediately follows the low-dose test, no intervening urine collection is required. Dexamethasone, 100 μg/kg/day, is then administered orally in four divided doses over 48 hours, during which urine collection is continued. Six hours after the final dose of dexamethasone, the last urine is collected and blood is drawn for cortisol and ACTH. Urine is assayed for 17-hydroxysteroids and free cortisol.

A significant decrease in UFC and 17-hydroxysteroids, as well as plasma ACTH and cortisol, suggests a pituitary adenoma (Cushing disease). Lack of suppression of UFC and 17-hydroxysteroids, along with an elevated plasma cortisol level and a low ACTH level, occurs when Cushing syndrome is caused by an adrenal tumor. Most, but not all, ectopic ACTH-secreting tumors also fail to suppress with high-dose dexamethasone. In addition, both plasma ACTH and cortisol remain markedly elevated.

Corticotropin-Releasing Hormone Test
Corticorelin is a synthetic form of CRH. The CRH test involves obtaining a baseline blood sample for ACTH and cortisol levels, administering CRH (1 μg/kg), and obtaining serial ACTH and cortisol levels at 15, 30, 60, and 90 minutes. When administered to patients with a pituitary adenoma, CRH induces an exaggerated rise in ACTH and cortisol. This response pattern indicates an impairment of the negative feedback action of cortisol on the pituitary. In patients with adrenal tumors or ectopic ACTH-secreting tumors, on the other hand, CRH does not significantly affect the already elevated basal levels of ACTH and cortisol.

Challenges in Making the Diagnosis
As with any laboratory test, those described above may yield both false-positive and false-negative results. For example, ACTH fails to suppress in patients experiencing significant physiological stress. Other potential causes of false-positive results are disorders such as clinical depression and anorexia nervosa, both of which are associated with elevated cortisol levels. False-negative results may occur because of erroneous technique, such as incomplete urine collection, or may be the result of individual differences in the metabolism of dexamethasone. If test results contradict a strong clinical suspicion, it is wise to repeat one or more tests to prove or disprove the diagnosis.

Imaging Studies

A radiograph of the skull is almost never useful when diagnosing hypercortisolism. Enlargement of the sella turcica is only rarely seen on a skull radiograph in an individual with a pituitary adenoma once hypercortisolism is documented. Computed tomography (CT) and magnetic resonance imaging (MRI) have therefore replaced plain x-ray films in the diagnosis of hypercortisolism. The radiological study of choice for someone with Cushing disease is MRI with gadolinium, as this yields much more detailed information about the anatomy of the brain and pituitary gland. Due to the small size of most pituitary adenomas, however, MRI accurately localizes the adenoma in only approximately one third of cases. Inferior petrosal sinus sampling combined with CRH is useful in both confirming the presence of a tumor undetected by imaging studies and lateralizing the tumor within the pituitary gland.

Abdominal MRI or CT is indicated in a patient suspected to have an adrenal tumor. CT scanning of the adrenals permits visualization of an adrenal mass measuring 1 cm or greater in diameter. Unilateral enlargement of an adrenal gland is more obvious than bilateral adrenocortical enlargement, which can be difficult to detect.

Management and Treatment Options

Management is primarily determined by the etiology of the hypercortisolism. In Cushing disease, therapy is directed toward the pituitary itself and may include surgery and/or radiation. If the adrenal gland is the etiology of excess cortisol, surgical excision, often in combination with pharmacological intervention, is used.

Surgical Management

Transsphenoidal resection of a pituitary adenoma is potentially curative, but difficulty in localizing the tumor may make this impossible. Success rates of between 70% and 80% have been reported, but recurrence rates of 5% to 25% within 5 years after the initial surgical procedure have been observed. Replacement of glucocorticoids in the perioperative period is essential.

Bilateral adrenalectomy eliminates hypercortisolism because the glands, now absent, no longer respond to trophic stimulation by ACTH and excessive cortisol secretion is quelled. Despite the potential for cure, however, the procedure is associated with both surgical and medical complications. Permanent postoperative glucocorticoid and mineralocorticoid replacement is required for patients undergoing adrenalectomy. Furthermore, patients are at risk of developing an ACTH-producing pituitary tumor that leads to hyperpigmentation (Nelson syndrome).

Radiation Therapy

Radiation directed at the pituitary does not take effect for 6 to 18 months. Radiation induces remission in 45% to 85% of individuals. Efficacy can be enhanced by the addition of medical therapy with o,p'-DDD (mitotane). Partial or complete hypopituitarism that may be caused by radiation is important an potential sequela to keep in mind.

Medical Management

Multiple agents have been used in the medical management of hypercortisolism. Several of these agents interrupt adrenal steroid biosynthesis as follows. Ketoconazole inhibits multiple adrenal enzymes. Aminoglutethamide interrupts steroid production early in the synthetic pathway by inhibiting 20,22-desmolase. Metyrapone inhibits 11β-hydroxylase and trilostane inhibits 3β-HSD. o,p'-DDD (mitotane) and RU486 have different mechanisms of action; the former has adrenolytic effects and the latter is a glucocorticoid receptor antagonist. Using two or more drugs in combination may allow for administration of lower doses of each and therefore induce fewer side effects.

Adrenal Neoplasms

Patients diagnosed with adrenal neoplasms, whether adenomas and carcinomas, require surgical exploration and resection of the mass. The cure rate with surgical excision of an adenoma is virtually 100%. Given the likelihood of atrophy of the contralateral adrenal gland, perioperative glucocorticoid replacement is essential to prevent adrenal crisis after removal of the tumor and affected adrenal gland. Replacement glucocorticoid therapy may need to be continued for several months postoperatively.

Outcome for patients with adrenal carcinomas, on the other hand, is very poor regardless of the size of the tumor. Complete resection of malignant adrenal carcinomas is almost impossible. Even in the absence of radiological and hormonal evidence of residual tumor, micrometastases, most commonly to liver and lung, are very likely. If the pathology report confirms carcinoma, chemotherapy also is required. Potential chemotherapeutic agents include Cytoxan (cyclophosphamide), Adriamycin (doxorubicin), methotrexate, and 5-fluorouracil (5-FU). Persistent hypercortisolism is treated with o,p'-DDD. In patients who have undergone complete tumor resection, high doses of o,p'-DDD may reduce recurrence risk. In those with residual or recurrent disease, it may control hypercortisolism but does not improve survival. Because it is quite difficult to achieve and maintain normal cortisol values, the goal of therapy should be to induce adrenal insufficiency and provide replacement steroids.

Long-Term Monitoring

For those with Cushing disease and benign adrenal neoplasms, maintenance glucocorticoid replacement (12 to 15 mg/m²/day in two or three divided doses) is required until recovery of hypothalamic/pituitary function is confirmed (usually 6 to 12 months). All patients on replacement steroids require increased dosing of hydrocortisone during times of significant physiological stress, such as a febrile illness. The oral dose should be approximately triple that of the maintenance dose (50 mg/m²/day) and should be given in three divided doses. Patients who cannot tolerate oral fluids should receive parenteral hydrocortisone (Solu-Cortef, 100 mg/m²/dose) and should seek medical attention immediately.

During the first week and at 6 weeks after surgery, patients should collect a 24-hour urine specimen for measurement of UFC/ketosteroid secretion. During the week after surgery, if pituitary surgery has been effective, plasma ACTH will be less than 5 pg/mL and cortisol will be undetectable 24 hours after the last dose of hydrocortisone. Stimulation and suppression tests are performed 6 weeks after surgery; hydrocortisone must be withheld before these studies. Close monitoring for recurrence of disease, symptoms of cortisol withdrawal, and hypopituitarism is essential.

Prognosis

The potential for cure in patients with Cushing disease and adrenal adenomas is excellent, as surgical excision is usually curative. Prognosis is poor for those with adrenal carcinomas given the frequency of micrometastases at diagnosis and the high rate of recurrence. Unfortunately, there is no effective therapy for metastatic or recurrent disease. Persistent symptomatic hypercortisolism, however, can be medically controlled.

SUGGESTED APPROACH IN CLINICAL PRACTICE

Evaluation of the patient with suspected hypercortisolism begins with measurement of morning and evening cortisol values and a 24-hour UFC value. If these screening tests yield results suggestive of hypercortisolism, the diagnosis can be established by repeated 24-hour urine collections. Referral to an endocrinologist is then indicated for a more specific diagnostic evaluation aimed at determining the etiology and localizing the source of cortisol excess. In the patient with both virilization and signs of hypercortisolism, serum androgens should also be measured and a CT scan of the adrenal glands obtained.

An intact hypothalamic-pituitary-adrenal axis is required for synthesis of mineralocorticoids, glucocorticoids, and androgens by the adrenal cortex.

The net effect of aldosterone is to promote sodium retention and potassium excretion. Aldosterone secretion is primarily regulated by the extracellular potassium concentration and the renin-angiotensin system.

Because peak cortisol secretion occurs between 4 AM and 6 AM, a first-morning cortisol value above 10 μg/dL indicates normal adrenal function. Due to immaturity of the adrenal glands, this test may not provide a reliable assessment of adrenal function in children under the age of 3 years.

21-hydroxylase deficiency is the most common cause of congenital adrenal hyperplasia (CAH) and is an important cause of ambiguous genitalia in genetic females. Measurement of 17-OH-progesterone to detect this form of CAH is now part of the newborn screening in many states. Unlike most of the other forms of CAH, 11β-hydroxylase deficiency is associated with hypertension and hypokalemia.

Acquired causes of primary adrenal deficiency (Addison disease) include autoimmune, infectious, infiltrative, traumatic, and drug induced. Autoimmune adrenalitis remains the most common cause and may be associated with other autoimmune disorders, both endocrine and nonendocrine.

Secondary adrenal insufficiency is caused by congenital or acquired abnormalities of the hypothalamus or pituitary gland. The most common cause is administration of supraphysiological doses of glucocorticoids used as immunosuppressive agents or for treatment of systemic inflammatory illnesses. Steroids must be tapered carefully (see text for details) to avoid precipitating an adrenal crisis.

Because symptoms of adrenal insufficiency are nonspecific, making the diagnosis requires a high index of suspicion. Symptoms vary with the age of the patient, so physical findings and laboratory study abnormalities are important clues to the diagnosis.

Hyperpigmentation due to increased ACTH and melanocyte-stimulating hormone is consistent with primary adrenal insufficiency. This finding is absent in those with secondary adrenal insufficiency because hypothalamic or pituitary dysfunction leads to ACTH deficiency.

Hyponatremia, hyperkalemia, acidosis, and hypoglycemia are consistent with primary adrenal insufficiency. Patients also have low cortisol levels, along with elevated ACTH and plasma renin activity. Typical laboratory abnormalities in secondary adrenal insufficiency include hypoglycemia and perhaps mild hyponatremia.

It is imperative that patients with both forms of adrenal insufficiency receive "stress-dose" steroids in the setting of increased physiological stress, such as a febrile illness, an infection, or a surgical procedure.

ACTH-producing tumors of the pituitary gland are responsible for the majority of cases of hypercortisolism in children older than 7 years. Adrenocortical carcinomas cause the majority of cases of hypercortisolism in those younger than 7 years. The presence of both virilization and signs of hypercortisolism suggests an adrenal neoplasm.

Growth failure is the most consistent feature of hypercortisolism in children. The combination of obesity and short stature suggests the possibility of cortisol excess and helps distinguish hypercortisolism from exogenous obesity.

Loss of the normal diurnal variation of cortisol secretion is a hallmark of Cushing syndrome. The preferred test for diagnosing this disorder has been the 24-hour urinary free cortisol, but measurement of midnight salivary cortisol values is becoming more popular.

The study of choice for the patient with a suspected ACTH-secreting pituitary adenoma is magnetic resonance imaging with gadolinium. An abdominal magnetic resonance image or computed tomography scan is indicated in the patient suspected to have an adrenal tumor.

SUGGESTED READINGS

American Academy of Pediatrics: Technical report: congenital adrenal hyperplasia, Pediatrics 2000;106:1511.

August GP: Treatment of adrenocortical insufficiency, Pediatr Rev 1997;18:59.

Hughes JM, Whelan MA, Deringer PM: Adrenoleukodystrophy: an important cause of adrenal insufficiency, Endocrinologist 2000;10:271.

Joint LWPES/ESPE CAH Working Group: Consensus statement on 21-hydroxylase deficiency from the Lawson Wilkins Pediatric Endocrine Society and the European Society for Paediatric Endocrinology, J Clin Endocrinol Metab 2002;87:4048.

Magiakou MA, Chrousos GP: Cushing's syndrome in children and adolescents: current diagnostic and therapeutic strategies, J Endocrinol Invest 2002;25:181.

Oelkers W: Adrenal insufficiency, N Engl J Med 1996;335:1206.

Savage MO, Lebrethon MC, Blair JC, et al: Growth abnormalities associated with adrenal disorders and their management, Horm Res 2001;56(suppl 1):19.

Savage MO, Scommegna S, Carroll PV, et al: Growth in disorders of adrenal hyperfunction, Horm Res 2002;58(suppl 1):39.

CALCIUM,
PHOSPHORUS,
AND BONE

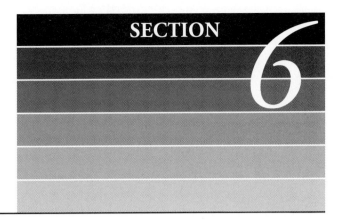

CHAPTER 11

Calcium Regulation and Hypocalcemic Disorders

NEIL CAPLIN

INTRODUCTION

Disorders of calcium, phosphorus, and bone are increasingly common issues for pediatricians. Guidelines in terms of adequate nutritional intake of these minerals and the role of bone health for children are essential knowledge for pediatricians and family physicians. The role of the hormonal, renal, and intestinal regulation of calcium-phosphorus metabolism enables the physician to ascertain those problems that require pharmacological intervention as opposed to nutrient supplementation.

CALCIUM PHYSIOLOGY

The majority of the calcium in the body is contained in the skeleton.

The calcium ion plays a central role in cellular physiology. Despite wide variations in the daily intake and excretion of calcium, the intracellular and extracellular calcium concentrations are maintained within a narrow range. The cytoplasmic calcium concentration is several orders of magnitude lower than the calcium concentration in the extracellular fluid, and this steep gradient is actively maintained. Symptoms occur during both hypocalcemia and hypercalcemia.

About half of the calcium in the serum is bound to protein, predominantly albumin. A small fraction is bound to other chemicals, such as citrate, and the rest is in the free ionized state. Total serum calcium concentration can change with changes in the serum albumin concentration. In contrast, serum ionized calcium concentration is tightly regulated and therefore is the clinically important parameter to measure. The degree of calcium binding to albumin is altered by abnormalities in acid-base status.

The normal serum total calcium concentration is 7.6 (in the newborn) to 10.5 mg/dL (2.1-2.6 mmol/L), and after the neonatal period, it is tightly controlled in the range of 9.0 to 10.5 mg/dL. The normal ionized calcium concentration is 4.4 to 5.2 mg/dL (1.1 to 1.3 mmol/L).

Calcium Intake

Maintenance of optimal bone health depends on an adequate supply of calcium and other essential nutrients. Current dietary intake data indicate that calcium intake is below recommended levels in most individuals. Calcium balance (intake minus the sum of all losses) generally is positive during growth, is essentially zero in the mature adult, and then negative with advancing age. Negative calcium balance can arise from low intake, poor absorption, high obligatory losses, or any combination of these factors and inevitably leads to bone loss if not corrected.

The preferred approach to attaining optimal calcium intake is through dietary sources. For many Americans, dairy products are the major contributors of dietary calcium because of their high calcium content (e.g., approximately 250 to 300 mg in 240 mL of milk) and frequency of consumption. Other good food sources of calcium include some green vegetables (e.g., broccoli, Chinese cabbage), some legumes, canned fish, seeds, nuts, and certain fortified food products. Breads and cereals, although relatively low in calcium, contribute significantly to calcium intake because of their frequency of consumption.

Optimal calcium intake refers to the levels of consumption that are necessary for an individual to maximize peak adult bone mass. Calcium requirements vary throughout an individual's lifetime, with greater needs during the periods of rapid growth in childhood and adolescence, during pregnancy and lactation, and in later adult life. Because 99% of total body calcium is found in bone, the need for calcium is largely determined by skeletal requirements. Body retention of calcium increases with increasing calcium intake up to a threshold, beyond which further calcium intake causes no additional increment in calcium retention.

Calcium intake of exclusively breast-fed infants during the first 6 months of life is in the range of 250 to 330 mg/day, with fractional calcium absorption between 55% and 60%. Cow's milk formulas have a higher calcium content and a lower fractional absorption. There is comparable calcium retention of 150 to 200 mg/day from both formula and breast milk. Net calcium absorption from soy-based formulas is comparable to, or higher than, that of breast milk or cow's milk formulas because of its considerably higher calcium content. The recommended daily allowances for calcium in children are shown in Box 11-1. However, special circumstances such as low birth weight may require higher calcium intake.

For some individuals, calcium supplements may be the preferred way to attain optimal calcium intake. Absorption of calcium supplements is most efficient at individual doses of 500 mg or less and when taken between meals. Ingestion of calcium supplements between meals supports calcium

bioavailability, because food may contain certain compounds that reduce calcium absorption (e.g., oxalates).

Calcium Absorption in the Gastrointestinal Tract

In addition to calcium intake, calcium absorption in the small intestine exerts a major influence on calcium balance. There are a number of factors that influence the absorption of ingested calcium, altering its bioavailability. The efficiency of calcium absorption decreases as intake increases, thereby providing a protective mechanism to lessen the chances of calcium intoxication. This adaptive mechanism can, however, be overcome by a calcium intake of greater than approximately 4 g/day; such excessive calcium intake can result in calcium toxicity, with high blood calcium levels leading to renal damage and ectopic calcium deposition.

There are two mechanisms of calcium absorption from the intestinal tract: (1) a paracellular, unregulated, nonsaturable mechanism that predominates at high calcium intakes and (2) a transcellular, saturable, active-transport mechanism that predominates at low calcium intakes. The paracellular mechanism is responsible for a small proportion of dietary calcium absorption, although at high intakes the absolute amount of absorbed calcium may be large. With the transcellular mechanism, the total amount of calcium that can be absorbed is limited. The active calcium transport system is vitamin D dependent via synthesis of a calcium-binding protein calbindin.

The amount of calcium absorbed in the intestine depends on calcium intake. When intake is low, active transcellular calcium transport in the duodenum is upregulated and becomes the predominant mechanism of calcium absorption. Passive absorption occurs in the jejunum and ileum. Calcium that reaches the large intestine undergoes absorption there via both active and passive processes. Probably no more than 10% of total calcium absorption takes place in the large intestine, whether calcium intake is low or high.

The most important endogenous regulator of calcium absorption is 1,25-dihydroxyvitamin D $[1,25(OH)_2D]$, which stimulates active transport of calcium in the small intestine and colon. Other endogenous cofactors that secondarily enhance net calcium absorption include estrogen, growth hormone, insulin-like growth factor, and parathyroid hormone.

Certain dietary components potentially alter calcium absorption. Foods with high oxalate and phytate content reduce the availability of calcium in these foods. With the exception of large amounts of wheat bran, fiber has not been found to significantly affect calcium absorption. Other dietary components, including fat, phosphate, magnesium, and caffeine, have not been found to significantly

---

Box 11-1	**Recommended Daily Allowances for Calcium**

400 mg/day for infants from birth to 6 months
600 mg/day for infants from 6 months to 12 months
800 mg/day for children 1 to 5 years
800 to 1200 mg/day for children 6 to 10 years
1200 to 1500 mg/day for patients 11 to 24 years

affect calcium absorption or excretion. Glucocorticoids decrease calcium absorption.

Calcium Loss

There are three main avenues of calcium loss: feces, urine, and dermal losses (sweat and sloughed skin cells). At calcium intakes in the range of current recommendations, fecal loss can be as high as 90% of ingested calcium. Fecal losses consist of unabsorbed dietary calcium and calcium from digestive excretions, sloughed intestinal cells, and other endogenous sources. At low calcium intakes, much of the calcium excreted in feces is of endogenous origin. Dermal losses have not been accurately measured but have been estimated to be equivalent to about 30% of normal urinary losses. Urinary loss of calcium is regulated through the actions of the calciotropic hormones, parathyroid hormone (PTH), 1,25(OH)$_2$D, and calcitonin, but is also dependent on protein and sodium intake.

Both active and passive processes mediate calcium absorption in the kidney. Absorption in both proximal tubule and thick ascending limb is mainly coupled indirectly to sodium absorption and is a passive process through the paracellular pathway. In the distal convoluted tubule, calcium absorption is regulated independently of sodium absorption; this is the principal site of action of parathyroid hormone, calcitonin, and 1,25(OH)$_2$D. The fine tuning of calcium ion excretion in the kidney takes place in the distal nephron, which consists of the distal convoluted tubule, connecting tubule, and initial portion of the cortical collecting duct. In these segments, calcium ion is reabsorbed through an active transcellular pathway. Calcium loss can be increased by intake of large amounts of sodium and animal protein, both of which can significantly increase urinary calcium excretion. Aluminum in the form of antacid medication, when taken in excess, may also increase urinary calcium loss.

HORMONAL REGULATION OF CALCIUM BALANCE

Parathyroid Hormone

Parathyroid hormone is a peptide hormone secreted by the parathyroid glands, which are located adjacent to the thyroid gland. Parathyroid hormone alters serum calcium via actions on three target organs: bone, intestinal mucosa, and kidney.

Parathyroid hormone has 84 amino acids and is coded by a gene on chromosome 11. The full biological activity of the hormone is coded by the first 34 amino acids. The actions of PTH are mediated via cell surface PTH receptors in target organs. PTH acts in the kidney on the distal tubule to promote calcium reabsorption and on the proximal tubule to decrease phosphate absorption. The net effect is renal loss of phosphate and conservation of calcium. The actions of PTH on bone are complicated and incompletely understood. PTH increases bone turnover and causes loss of calcium from bone through increases in osteoclast number and activity. PTH also has other effects, including anabolic actions in bone.

The most important stimulus for PTH secretion is hypocalcemia. Parathyroid cells and a number of other cell types sense calcium ion concentrations via a calcium ion sensor (CaSR). The CaSR is a transmembrane, G protein–linked receptor that regulates PTH secretion via intracellular second-messenger systems. The identification of inherited human hypercalcemic and hypocalcemic disorders arising from inactivating and activating mutations of the CaSR, respectively, suggests that the CaSR has an essential, nonredundant role in mineral ion homeostasis. The CaSR also plays numerous roles outside the realm of systemic mineral ion homeostasis. The receptor is involved in the regulation of processes such as cellular proliferation and differentiation, secretion, membrane polarization, and apoptosis in a variety of tissues and cells.

The initial effect of hypocalcemia on the parathyroid gland is the release of preformed PTH from intracellular granules followed by synthesis of the hormone. Parathyroid hormone messenger RNA (mRNA) levels are regulated by calcium, phosphate, and 1,25-dihydroxyvitamin D$_3$. Dietary-induced hypocalcemia increases and hypophosphatemia decreases parathyroid hormone mRNA levels posttranscriptionally.

Circulating PTH has a half-life of 2 to 4 minutes and is predominantly cleared by the liver and kidney. Modern assays for PTH use two-site immunoassays, with one determinant at the amino terminal and the other determinant at the carboxyl terminal. By using the two determinants, the assays are specific for the intact circulating PTH. Measurement of serum concentration of "intact PTH" is generally more useful in evaluating the clinical states of hypercalcemia and hypocalcemia.

Vitamin D

The term *vitamin D* refers to two compounds derived from sterol precursors. Vitamin D$_3$ (cholecalciferol) is produced in the skin after sunlight exposure and is the principal endogenous form of vitamin D. Vitamin D$_2$ (ergocalciferol) is the form derived from plants and is the primary form in food. Vitamin D plays an essential role in maintaining a healthy mineralized skeleton for most land vertebrates including humans. Vitamin D is metabolized in the liver to produce

25-hydroxyvitamin D [25-(OH)D], which is in turn metabolized in the kidney to $1,25(OH)_2D$ is the biologically active form. More polar forms of vitamin D (such as 24,25-dihydroxyvitamin D) are rapidly excreted in urine, not available for conversion to the biologically active form, 1,25-dihydroxyvitamin D. Drugs that increase liver hydroxylases, such as phenobarbital, can reduce the amount of 25-(OH)D available for 1α-hydroxylation to $1,25(OH)_2D$. Such drugs can then cause a form of vitamin D–dependent rickets.

Most foods do not contain any vitamin D. Dietary sources of vitamin D include oily fish, fortified foods, and milk products and multivitamins. Foods fortified with vitamin D have a variable amount present and cannot be depended on as a sole source of vitamin D nutrition. Exposure to sunlight provides most humans with their vitamin D requirement. Factors, including aging and the season, can dramatically affect the cutaneous production of vitamin D_3. Infants receive vitamin D through both sunlight exposure and breast milk and infant formula. The major determinant of the vitamin D concentration of breast milk is maternal vitamin D status. The total vitamin D concentration in human breast milk is 15 to 50 IU/L, an amount insufficient for infants who are completely breast fed, and indicates the need for supplementation with fortified vitamins. The vitamin D concentration of infant formula is higher than that in breast milk.

25-(OH)D is the principal storage form of vitamin D, and its serum concentration is the most useful measure of body stores. Vitamin D and its metabolites are highly protein bound in the circulation. The proteins involved are vitamin D–binding protein and albumin. Vitamin D–binding protein is an α-globulin produced by the liver, the levels of which can be depressed in liver disease.

The major biological function of $1,25-(OH)_2D$ is to keep the serum calcium and phosphorus concentrations within the normal range to maintain essential cellular functions and to promote mineralization of the skeleton. Active vitamin D acts via the vitamin D receptor (VDR), which has a wide tissue distribution. The VDR is a ligand-activated nuclear transcription factor and a member of the steroid-thyroid-retinoid receptor gene superfamily. The vitamin D–VDR complex binds to DNA and acts via gene transcription.

HYPOCALCEMIC DISORDERS

Hypocalcemia is often asymptomatic and is detected incidentally. Hypocalcemia may present acutely with signs of neuromuscular irritability, including perioral paresthesias, tingling of the fingers and toes, and spontaneous or latent tetany. Occasionally, carpopedal spasm and laryngeal spasm producing stridor with grand mal seizures are the present-

ing features. Electrocardiographic abnormalities may be seen, typically prolongation of the QTc interval because of lengthening of the ST segment, which is directly proportional to the degree of hypocalcemia or, otherwise stated, inversely proportional to the serum calcium level. The exact opposite holds true for hypercalcemia. Cardiac arrhythmias are also rarely reported, including torsades de pointes.

Hypocalcemic disorders are traditionally divided into those presenting in the neonatal period and those presenting later. There is some overlap between these presentations. Box 11-2 lists the differential diagnosis of hypocalcemia in the newborn period.

Neonatal Hypocalcemia

Neonatal hypocalcemia is traditionally classified as early and late neonatal hypocalcemia. Early neonatal hypocalcemia occurs in the first 3 days of life and may or may not

---

Box 11-2   Differential Diagnosis of Hypocalcemia

I. Neonatal hypocalcemia
  A. Early neonatal hypocalcemia
    1. Preterm
    2. Asphyxia
    3. Infants of insulin-dependent diabetic mothers
  B. Late neonatal hypocalcemia
    1. Maternal hypercalcemia, vitamin D deficiency
    2. Iatrogenic—bicarbonate or furosemide or phosphate administration, transfusions
    3. Hypoparathyroidism—DiGeorge and other syndromes
    4. Hypomagnesemia
    5. Chronic alkalosis or bicarbonate therapy
II. Childhood hypocalcemia
  A. Hypoparathyroidism
    1. Congenital—late presentation
    2. Iatrogenic—surgery
    3. Resistance to parathyroid hormone—pseudohypoparathyroidism
    4. Component of autoimmune polyglandular syndrome
  B. Vitamin D disorders
    1. Malnutrition—deficiency
    2. Metabolic errors—1α-hydroxylase deficiency, renal tubular phosphate loss
    3. Drugs—anticonvulsants
  C. Hypomagnesemia
  D. Hyperphosphatemia
  E. Drugs—diuretics, phosphate enemas
  F. Critical illness
  G. Other illness—pancreatitis, chronic renal failure, organic acidemia

be symptomatic. Late neonatal hypocalcemia occurs at 5 to 10 days of life and is usually symptomatic.

Normal fetal and neonatal calcium homeostasis is dependent on an adequate supply of calcium from maternal sources. In utero, the fetal serum calcium concentration is higher than maternal serum calcium. Healthy term babies undergo a physiological nadir in serum calcium levels by 24 hours. This fall in serum calcium stimulates PTH secretion, which increases the calcium concentration over the next 24 to 48 hours. The nadir is usually asymptomatic; however, in certain high-risk neonates, symptoms may occur. Early neonatal hypocalcemia is most commonly symptomatic in premature infants, asphyxiated infants, and infants of a diabetic mothers.

Both maternal hypercalcemia and hypocalcemia can cause metabolic bone disease or disorders of calcium homeostasis in neonates. Maternal hypercalcemia can cross the placenta and inhibit PTH secretion by the infant's parathyroid glands, causing neonatal hypocalcemia. Conversely, maternal hypocalcemia can stimulate fetal parathyroid tissue, causing bone demineralization. It is important to assess maternal calcium levels when infants are born with abnormal serum calcium levels or metabolic bone disease.

Hypomagnesemia is an occasional cause of hypocalcemia in the neonate. Occasionally, hypomagnesemia is caused by defects in intestinal or renal magnesium reabsorption. Hypomagnesemia should be corrected in infants found to be hypocalcemic. Autosomal dominant hypocalcemia (ADH) due to gain-of-function mutations in the calcium-sensing receptor gene is a recently described rare cause of neonatal hypocalcemia. Ingestion of formula containing excessive amounts of phosphate was previously a common cause of hypocalcemia in the neonatal period and is still intermittently a cause of late neonatal hypocalcemia, usually presenting at 4 to 6 weeks of age. The associated elevated serum phosphate levels are believed to cause hypocalcemia by increasing bone deposition and inducing PTH resistance.

Neonatal Hypoparathyroidism

Hypoparathyroidism occurring in the neonatal period is most commonly transient, but underlying causes should be sought. It is important to measure plasma magnesium because severe hypomagnesemia can cause hypoparathyroidism. Rarely severe hypomagnesemia is caused by congenital hypomagnesemia, which is a rare genetic disorder characterized by recurrent tetany or convulsions in early infancy. The hypocalcemia is refractory to calcium supplementation but responds to magnesium treatment. In most patients, primary hypomagnesemia is caused by a selective

defect of magnesium absorption in the small intestine. The condition is believed to be an autosomal recessive disease.

Hypoparathyroidism is associated with the DiGeorge syndrome and the Kenny-Caffey syndrome. The DiGeorge syndrome (cardiac defect, abnormal facies, thymic hypoplasia, cleft palate, and hypocalcemia) is caused by a chromosome 22q11.2 microdeletion. The phenotypic features involve many systems ranging from isolated minor findings to multiple, severe anomalies. The neonatal hypocalcemia is frequently transient but may recur in later life. As the abnormal facial appearance is subtle, it is frequently not the presenting feature and often is only appreciated after the discovery of other symptoms such as hypocalcemia but especially cardiac malformations and the absence of thymus. The diagnosis of the syndrome is made by cytogenetic studies, using fluorescent in situ hybridization. If the diagnosis is confirmed, screening for associated renal, immune, cardiac, and central nervous system anomalies is indicated. A suggested evaluation for neonatal hypocalcemia, including historical, physical findings, and laboratory investigations, is listed in Box 11-3.

Childhood Hypocalcemia

Childhood presentation of hypocalcemic disorders is most frequently due to disorders involving vitamin D, including malnutrition, vitamin D resistance, and drugs altering

---

Box 11-3   Evaluation of Neonatal Hypocalcemia

I. History
  A. Gestation history—maternal vitamins, hypercalcemia, diabetes
  B. Symptoms present or absent
  C. Evidence of perinatal "stress"
  D. Medications—bicarbonate, diuretics
  E. Blood transfusion, exchange transfusion
  F. Formula—phosphate content
II. Examination
  A. Signs of tetany—carpopedal spasm, stridor, Chvostek sign
  B. Dysmorphic features
  C. Signs of cardiac disease
III. Investigations
  A. Blood sample—calcium, phosphate, alkaline phosphatase, vitamin D, parathyroid hormone, fluorescent in situ hybridization probe for DiGeorge syndrome
  B. Maternal blood sample—calcium, phosphate, alkaline phosphatase, vitamin D
  C. Chest radiography or other imaging—cardiac and thymic evaluation

86665555556666666666

vitamin metabolism. A differential list of causes of hypocalcemia in the older child is listed in Box 11-2.

Vitamin D Deficiency

Vitamin D deficiency may present as the clinical syndrome of rickets or as hypocalcemia. Surprisingly, vitamin D deficiency probably remains the most common cause of childhood hypocalcemia. The other forms of rickets (i.e., hyperphosphaturic rickets [vitamin D–resistant rickets], vitamin D–dependent [genetic or drug induced], and renal rickets) rarely present with hypocalcemia. The term *rickets* is indicative of defective mineralization of the growth plate and occurs concurrently with osteomalacia (i.e., defective mineralization of the cortical and trabecular bone).

The majority of vitamin D deficiency is secondary to a combination of inadequate exposure to sunlight and inadequate dietary intake of vitamin D. It is most frequently observed in dark-skinned individuals living in northern latitudes and in individuals who, for religious/cultural reasons, shield themselves from sunlight. Exclusively breast-fed infants are at greater risk than are formula-fed infants, with the greatest risk occurring when the mother is vitamin D deficient. There has been a recent increase in the incidence of hypocalcemia secondary to vitamin D deficiency in North America, particularly in African American infants. This has been attributed to an increased prevalence and duration of breastfeeding in this population. Another more recent cause of vitamin D deficiency is vegetarians who ingest only vegetables, abhorring even dairy products. Rarely vitamin D deficiency is due to malabsorption associated with conditions such as cystic fibrosis, short gut, celiac disease, and inflammatory bowel disease.

Infants with gastrointestinal disease and those who are exclusively breast-fed should receive fortified vitamins. There are advocates of breastfeeding who suggest that routine use of fortified vitamins undermines the notion that breast milk provides complete nutrition for the infant. However, just ensuring that mothers in high-risk groups obtain adequate vitamin D does not necessarily prevent vitamin D deficiency in the infant.

When vitamin D deficiency presents as hypocalcemia or rickets, management involves replacement of vitamin D, usually in the form of ergocalciferol in combination with calcium replacement. However, especially in those infants with hypocalcemic tetany or seizures, large amounts of calcium supplementation including intravenous calcium may be necessary as the bones are remineralizing rapidly (the "hungry bones" effect). Once bone healing has occurred, therapy consists of ensuring the patient meets the recommended daily allowances of vitamin D; frequently dietary supplementation is required.

Acute symptomatic hypocalcemia is usually treated with intravenous calcium gluconate. The standard dose is 10% calcium gluconate (9 mg of elemental calcium per ml) at 1 ml/kg body weight. The maximum single dose is 20 ml. Intravenous calcium gluconate is given over 10 to 30 minutes and requires cardiac monitoring throughout the infusion. Care must be taken to avoid extravasation, which can cause subcutaneous tissue necrosis. This dose can be repeated every 6 hours, or given by intravenous infusion (25 to 50 mg/kg of elemental calcium per day).

Hypoparathyroidism

Hypoparathyroidism is characterized by hypocalcemia and hyperphosphatemia. It manifests when parathyroid hormone (PTH) secreted from the parathyroid glands is insufficient to maintain normal extracellular fluid calcium concentrations or, less commonly, when PTH is unable to function optimally in target tissues, despite adequate circulating levels.

The predominant clinical manifestations of hypoparathyroidism are those related to hypocalcemia described earlier. Biochemically, hypoparathyroidism is characterized by low serum calcium and raised serum phosphorus in the presence of normal renal function. Serum concentrations of immunoreactive PTH are low or undetectable, except in the setting of PTH resistance, where levels can be high normal or elevated. Circulating levels of $1,25(OH)_2D$ are usually low or low normal. The 24-hour urinary excretion of calcium is decreased.

Hypoparathyroidism is most commonly due to agenesis or dysgenesis of the parathyroid glands, such as in DiGeorge and other syndromes, or due to autoimmune acquired hypoparathyroidism or due to thyroid surgery. Pseudohypoparathyroidism (PHP) refers to conditions of end-organ resistance to the actions of PTH.

Agenesis or Dysgenesis of the Parathyroid Glands

Congenital developmental defects of the parathyroid glands lead to hypoparathyroidism, which manifests clinically in the neonatal period. These defects can be isolated to parathyroid gland development or be associated with other manifestations as part of a syndrome. Isolated congenital hypoparathyroidism can be either X-linked or autosomal recessive

For the most part, the precise molecular defect or defects in isolated autosomal recessive hypoparathyroidism remain unknown.

Parathyroid gland agenesis or dysgenesis more commonly occurs in association with other developmental abnormalities. In 90% of patients, the etiology is attributed to abnormal development of the third and fourth pharyngeal arches and pouches as a consequence of microdeletions of one copy of the region 22q11.21-q11.23. A small number of patients with a DiGeorge-like phenotype have deletions in other chromosomes. Studies in patients with terminal deletions of chromosome 10p have defined two nonoverlapping regions that contribute to this complex phenotype. These are the DiGeorge critical region II, which is located on 10p13-p14, and the region for the hypoparathyroidism, sensorineural deafness, and renal dysplasia syndrome (HDR syndrome) has a more telomeric location.

Several other complex syndromes have been associated with parathyroid gland agenesis or hypoplasia. In the hypoparathyroidism-retardation-dysmorphism (HRD) syndrome, congenital hypoparathyroidism in association with growth and mental retardation and seizures has been reported in children of consanguineous parents from the Middle East. The locus for this disorder has been mapped to chromosome 1q42-q43. Hypoparathyroidism has also been reported in more than half of the patients with the Kenny-Caffey syndrome, a disorder characterized by growth retardation, craniofacial anomalies, cortical thickening of long bones with medullary stenosis, and basal ganglia calcification. Several of the mitochondrial neuromyopathies, including the Kearns-Sayre syndrome (encephalomyopathy with ophthalmoplegia, pigmentary degeneration of the retina, and cardiomyopathy) and the Pearson marrow pancreas syndrome (neutropenia, sideroblastic anemia, vacuolization of bone marrow cells, and pancreatic exocrine dysfunction), which arise from deletions and duplications of mitochondrial DNA, have been associated with hypoparathyroidism and other endocrinopathies. Hypoparathyroidism as a result of parathyroid agenesis has also been described in a patient with long-chain 3-hydroxyacyl-coenzyme A dehydrogenase deficiency (HADHA; 2p23), an inborn error of fatty acid oxidation.

Destruction of the Parathyroid Glands

Autoimmune-mediated destruction of the parathyroid glands can occur alone or in combination with other disorders in the autoimmune polyglandular syndrome type 1. It is characterized by a variable combination of destructive autoimmune phenomena. In most cases, candidiasis is the first clinical manifestation to appear, usually before the age of 5 years, followed by hypoparathyroidism, before the age of 10 years, and later by primary adrenal insufficiency before the age of 15 years. Overall, these three main components of the syndrome occur in chronological order, but they are present together in only about a third to half of the cases. In the largest reported series of 68 patients from 54 families, hypoparathyroidism was present in 79% of cases, Addison disease in 72%, and candidiasis in 100%.

In adult patients, the most common cause of hypoparathyroidism is surgery, as a result of the removal of all parathyroid tissue or inadvertent interruption of the blood supply to the parathyroid glands. Transient hypoparathyroidism after head and neck surgery can be caused by edema or hemorrhage into the parathyroids. Hypoparathyroidism is a rare complication of radioactive iodine therapy of the thyroid gland for the treatment of Graves disease or after external beam irradiation to the neck region. Finally, the disorder can be the result of infiltrative diseases of the parathyroids such as in hemochromatosis, Wilson disease, and granulomatous diseases. These conditions are rarely seen in the pediatric age group.

Impaired Parathyroid Secretion

Impaired PTH secretion includes maternal hyperparathyroidism suppressing fetal PTH function and hypomagnesemia. Hypomagnesemia, because of losses from either the gastrointestinal tract or from the kidney, can impair PTH secretion and/or action, leading to a state of hypoparathyroidism. Impaired secretion of PTH also arises from gain-of-function mutations in the Ca^{2+}-sensing receptor. Last, primary impaired PTH secretion secondary to various PTH mutations are rare, with only three cases having been described.

The management of hypoparathyroidism is directed at maintaining an adequate serum calcium. Because PTH deficiency impairs renal vitamin D_1 hydroxylation, there usually is an associated 1,25-dihydroxyvitamin D deficiency. Treatment is initiated with calcium and calcitriol supplementation. Once hypocalcemia has been corrected, calcium supplementation may no longer be necessary if there is sufficient calcium in the diet, although generally continued calcium supplementation is necessary. The deficiency of PTH results in an elevated urinary calcium excretion at normal serum calcium levels and places the patient at risk of nephrocalcinosis during treatment. For this reason, clinicians aim to maintain the serum calcium in the low normal range. Monitoring of urinary calcium-to-creatinine ratio and intermittent renal sonography are also used in monitoring therapy.

Pseudohypoparathyroidism

PHP refers collectively to disorders that have the typical biochemical features of hypoparathyroidism (hypocalcemia and hyperphosphatemia) associated with elevated PTH levels. The underlying pathophysiology is end-organ resistance to PTH.

Albright first described an association of PHP with skeletal and developmental abnormalities including a round face, short stature, obesity, brachydactyly, heterotopic calcification, and mental retardation. Originally referred to as Albright's hereditary osteodystrophy (AHO), it is now known as PHP type 1a. A mutation in the gene *(GNAS1)* encoding a stimulatory component of the G protein complex required to activate adenyl cyclase is the cause of PHP type 1. Some patients with PHP1a have additional endocrine abnormalities, such as hypothyroidism and hypogonadism.

Patients with PHP1a have an approximate 50% reduction in expression or activity of the GNAS1 protein. These patients have a reduction in cyclic AMP (cAMP) and phosphate excretion in the urine following infusion of synthetic PTH. *GNAS1* is an imprinted gene with hormone resistance manifesting only in patients who inherit the defective *GNAS1* allele from a female carrier. Paternal transmission of the genetic defect leads to pseudopseudohypoparathyroidism, as described later. This mechanism does not explain the dominant mode of inheritance of the other features of AHO.

Interestingly, there are patients with AHO who exhibit a similar reduction in GNAS1 protein and activity but lack biochemical abnormalities or target-organ resistance to PTH and have a normal urinary cAMP and phosphate response to administration of PTH. Albright described these patients as having pseudopseudohypoparathyroidism, now accepted as being allelic to PHP1a. Therefore, within a given kindred but not within the same generation, some affected individuals have only AHO, whereas others also have PTH resistance, despite equivalent functional deficiency of GNAS1.

Patients with PHP type 1b have biochemical features of PHP, that is, resistance to PTH, hypocalcemia, and hyperphosphatemia, but without the phenotypic features of AHO and with normal Gsα activity. The etiology is presumed to be in the post-PTH receptor pathway.

Patients with PHP type 1c (PHP1c) show phenotypic features similar to those of AHO, in addition to resistance to multiple hormones, but have normal GNAS1 activity, suggesting that another effector of signal transduction, perhaps a defective catalytic unit of adenylate cyclase, accounts for these findings.

Finally, individuals with PHP type 2 (PHP2) lack the phenotypic signs of AHO and are therefore similar to patients with PHP1b. These patients also present with hypocalcemia and hyperphosphatemia with elevated serum PTH. However, in contrast to subjects with PHP1, who fail to show an appropriate increase in urinary excretion of cAMP and phosphate in response to PTH infusion, patients with PHP2 demonstrate a normal increase in urinary cAMP but have an impaired phosphaturic response.

Management of the hypocalcemia in PHP is identical to primary hypoparathyroidism, that is, administration of calcium and calcitriol to maintain low-normal serum calcium concentrations. These patients are at less risk for nephrocalcinosis than are patients with primary hypoparathyroidism. An assessment of the older child presenting with hypocalcemia is shown in Box 11-4.

Hypocalcemia During Critical Illness

Hypocalcemia is often found in critically ill patients, especially those with sepsis, major burns, and pancreatitis. Several factors may be involved, including actions of inflammatory cytokines and chelation of calcium by citrate used in blood products. If the plasma calcium and phosphate return to normal during recovery from such illnesses, further investigation is not indicated.

Box 11-4 Assessment of Childhood Hypocalcemia

I. History
   A. Dietary history—vitamins, ingestion of dairy products
   B. Exposure or lack of exposure to sunlight
   C. Symptoms of other endocrinopathy
   D. Symptoms of renal or gastrointestinal disease
   E. Prior surgery to the neck
   F. Family history of rickets
   G. Family history of endocrine and autoimmune diseases

II. Examination
   A. Growth
   B. Signs of tetany—carpopedal spasm, stridor, Chvostek sign
   C. Dysmorphic features (e.g., short fourth metacarpal)
   D. Cutaneous abnormalities—candidiasis, alopecia, vitiligo
   E. Signs of hypothyroidism and adrenal insufficiency
   F. Signs of rickets—widened metaphyses, rachitic rosary

III. Investigations
   A. Blood for calcium, phosphate, alkaline phosphatase, intact parathyroid hormone, 25-hydroxyvitamin D, and 1,25-dihydroxyvitamin D
   B. Radiographic studies—rickets, osteopenia
   C. Consider other hormone studies—corticotropin, thyroid antibodies
   D. Consider laboratory studies of kidney, liver, pancreas, and intestinal function

MAJOR POINTS

Calcium ion is central to cellular physiology and, despite wide variations in daily intake and excretion, the intracellular and extracellular concentrations are maintained in a very narrow range by a number of physiological mechanisms. These include parathyroid hormone (PTH), hydroxylases, and multiple organs, of which the skeleton, kidneys, and the gastrointestinal tract are key.

Nutrition is an important regulator of calcium physiology as well. The importance of sufficient calcium intake (see Box 11-1) and vitamin D for growing children cannot be underestimated.

The most common cause of hypocalcemia during childhood is still vitamin D deficiency.

Hypocalcemia in the newborn is generally transient, but potential maternal causes should be evaluated.

The most frequent cause of neonatal severe hypocalcemia is most often due to the DiGeorge syndrome (22q11.2 deletion).

Severe hypocalcemia in childhood, if not due to vitamin D deficiency, is generally due to acquired hypoparathyroidism, characterized by low calcium, elevated phosphorus, and low intact PTH.

Pseudohypoparathyroidism, due to an abnormal gain-of-function of the calcium-sensing receptor gene, causes hypocalcemia as a result of essentially target organ resistance to PTH. The classic form is characterized by hypocalcemia with normal to high PTH levels and a phenotype of short stature, rounded facies, and short fourth and fifth metacarpals.

SUGGESTED READINGS

Guise TA, Mundy GR: Clinical review 69: evaluation of hypocalcemia in children and adults, J Clin Endocrinol Metab 1995;80:1473.

Root AW, Diamond FB Jr: Disorders of calcium and phosphorus metabolism in adolescents, Endocrinol Metab Clin North Am 1993;22:573.

Rude RK: Hypocalcemia and hypoparathyroidism, Curr Ther Endocrinol Metab 1997;6:546.

Welch TR, Bergstrom WH, Tsang RC: Vitamin D–deficient rickets: the re-emergence of a once-conquered disease, J Pediatr 2000;137:143.

CHAPTER 12

Hypercalcemic Disorders

WEIZHEN XU

INTRODUCTION AND EPIDEMIOLOGY

Hypercalcemia is defined as total serum calcium level greater than the upper limit of normal range for age and gender. In general, it is above 10.5 to 11 mg/dL but might vary slightly from laboratory to laboratory. The normal serum calcium levels for neonates and older children (9.0 to 10.5 mg/dL) tend to be marginally higher in growing children than in adults by approximately 0.2 mg. The diagnosis of hypercalcemia is often challenging because the clinical presentation is either asymptomatic or too vague and nonspecific to raise the suspicions for testing, with one study suggesting that only 25% of adult patients with biochemical hypercalcemia were not detected. The underdiagnosis of hypercalcemia have significant clinical consequences, even in the mild form of hypercalcemia (calcium levels between 11 and <12 mg/dL), resulting in long-term complications, such as nephrocalcinosis, osteopenia, and pathological fracture. Thus, it is important to recognize, assess, and closely follow children with elevated serum calcium levels.

Calcium is the most abundant mineral in the human body. It is the free diffusible calcium (ionized calcium) that has active and profound biochemical function involving multiple systems and organs. In children, the normal ionized calcium range is 4.4 to 5.2 mg/dL.

Hypercalcemia results from imbalance between fluxes of calcium into and out of extracellular fluid. As iterated in the physiology section, the sources of calcium and target organs for calcium regulation are mainly at bones, renal filtration and reabsorption, and intestinal absorption, under the regulation of parathyroid hormone (PTH) and 1,25-dihydroxyvitamin D [1,25(OH)$_2$D]. Up to 90% of total calcium storage is in skeleton. An increase in net calcium mobilization from the bone is generally the primary cause of hypercalcemia. Although the kidney and gastrointestinal tract are involved in total body calcium homeostasis, and sometimes in maintaining hypercalcemia, there are few hypercalcemic disorders that are thought to be primarily due to calcium hyperabsorption by the intestine or reabsorption by the kidney.

Hypercalcemia in newborn infants differs from older children in respect to etiology, clinical manifestation, and management. Due to various perinatal factors, calcium homeostasis disturbances in neonate have their own characteristics, which make neonatal hypercalcemia a unique disease entity for discussion. In this section, we review the hypercalcemic disorders in newborn infants and in older children, with a focus on their differences.

Epidemiology

Hypercalcemia occurs in children of all ages. The actual incidence of hypercalcemia in children is unknown, although it is clearly less common than in adults. In adults, it is about 0.1% to 1% of the population. Primary hyperparathyroidism is the most common cause of hypercalcemia in the well adult population without malignancy, followed by transient hypercalcemia.

NEONATAL HYPERCALCEMIA

Neonatal hypercalcemia is uncommon but can have potential serious sequelae, including brain damage and bone fractures. The clinical manifestations vary widely, being completely asymptomatic or associated with life-threatening disturbance, coma, or multiple fractures, requiring immediate intervention. The common etiologies are listed in Box 12-1. The most common cause of neonatal hypercalcemia is iatrogenic, due to excessive calcium supplement, usually occurring during intravenous fluid therapy. This form of hypercalcemia is transient and usually mild.

Box 12-1   Etiology of Neonatal Hypercalcemia

I. Maternal hypocalcemia
II. Parathyroid related
  A. Hyperparathyroidism
    1. Neonatal severe hyperparathyroidism
    2. Secondary hyperparathyroidism
  B. Familial hypocalciuric (benign) hypercalcemia
  C. Parathyroid hormone–related protein
  D. Parathyroid receptor mutation—Jansen metaphyseal chondrodysplasia
III. Vitamin D related
  A. Williams syndrome
  B. Idiopathic infantile hypercalcemia
  C. Vitamin D toxicity
  D. Subcutaneous fat necrosis
IV. Miscellaneous
  A. Iatrogenic
  B. Hypophosphatasia
  C. Hypophosphatemia
  D. Blue diaper syndrome

Neonatal Severe Hyperparathyroidism

Neonatal severe hyperparathyroidism (NSHPT) is a rare disorder characterized by marked hypercalcemia (calcium level >16 mg/dL), very high serum concentration of PTH, and skeletal undermineralization. More than 50 cases of NSHPT have been described. Primary hyperparathyroidism in neonates is due to diffuse parathyroid hyperplasia, in contrast to older children and adults, in whom adenoma is more common.

NSHPT is an autosomal recessive disorder that occurs due to mutations of the gene that encodes for the calcium-sensing receptor (CaSR). The affected gene maps to chromosome 3q13.3-q21. CaSR is a plasma membrane G protein–coupled receptor that is expressed in the chief cells of the parathyroid gland and the cells lining the kidney tubule. CaSR senses the extracellular calcium concentration changes and couples this information to intracellular signaling pathways, which include G protein–dependent stimulation of phospholipase C (PLC) activity, accumulation of inositol-1,4,5-triphosphate (IP_3), and the rapid release of calcium ions from intracellular stores, followed by an influx of calcium that ultimately modify PTH secretion or renal cation handling. Loss-of-function mutations at the *CASR* gene are responsible for either NSHPT or familial hypocalciuria hypercalcemia (FHH), whereas gain-of-function mutations at the *CASR* gene leads to hypocalcemia (autosomal dominant/sporadic hypoparathyroidism). NSHPT and FHH are different manifestations of one mutation. The parathyroid cells' "set point" is defined as that calcium concentration at which PTH is 50% of maximal secretion. Both NSHPT and FHH have increased this set point, with the first a greater increase. Homozygous inactivating *CASR* mutations or compound heterozygous mutations have been identified in about two thirds of families described. Autosomal dominant and sporadic cases have also been reported, combined with the reports of other loci linked to FHH (chromosome 19), indicative of genetic heterogeneity.

Hypercalcemia presents as soon as the parathyroid glands, functional in the first trimester of pregnancy, become hyperplastic. This hypercalcemia is associated with significant clinical symptoms. The bony changes of hyperparathyroidism include severe bone deformities due to the generalized demineralization, multiple spontaneous fractures, and subperiosteal resorption. Unexplained anemia, hepatosplenomegaly may be present. Respiratory failure can occur in patients with prominent rib cage bone deformities. In affected babies, serum calcium level is remarkably elevated, so as the urine calcium level. Patients have hypophosphatemia, but hyperphosphaturia. The alkaline phosphate activity may be normal or increased. Serum intact PTH (iPTH) is very high.

Hypercalcemia secondary from NSHPT is often lethal in autosomal recessive patients, unless total parathyroidectomy is performed. Normal saline rehydration and diuresis with furosemide should be delivered urgently, as well as calcitonin in preparation of the surgery. Reimplantation of a small amount of tissue into an ectopic site is often tried, but studies suggest that only total parathyroidectomy is curable in NSHPT. Several reports recently documented less severe forms of NSHPT (generally due to a single heterozygous mutation of the *CASR* gene) but more severe than FHH. They are not associated with FHH kindreds, and they respond well to medical therapy alone.

Familial Hypocalciuric Hypercalcemia

Familial hypocalciuric hypercalcemia (FHH) is also known as familial benign hypercalcemia. Although it is a genetic disorder and hypercalcemia can be detected in the newborn, it is more often detected as a problem of older children and adults, because of its milder clinical picture and later presentation. Occasionally, a calcium level measured for other reasons is a cause for alarm in the newborn. The parents should be assessed for FHH, because urine studies documenting hypocalciuria are more easily performed in the parents.

Secondary Hyperparathyroidism

Neonatal calcium homeostasis is dependent on adequate maternal calcium supplement. Maternal hypocalcemia from diverse etiologies, including hypoparathyroidism or pseudohypoparathyroidism, can stimulate fetal parathyroid hyperplasia that can then result in neonatal disordered calcium homeostasis or bone disease. Studies showed that the PTH itself does not cross the placenta. Regardless the causes, all of these maternal disorders were either undiagnosed or were inadequately treated during the pregnancy. Chronic intrauterine exposure to hypocalcemia results in hyperplasia of fetal parathyroid glands. The affected infants might have, although it is rare, radiographic features of primary hyperparathyroidism and may not have hypercalcemia or may have only hypercalcemia. Management includes an adequate calcium and phosphorus supplement through milk. The condition resolves spontaneously within a few weeks.

Parathyroid Hormone–Related Protein (PTHrP) Hypercalcemia

Hypercalcemia of malignancy in neonate has not been reported. The youngest child previously documented in the literature was a 3-month-old infant with hepatic sarcoma

and elevated parathyroid hormone–related protein (PTHrP) . However, at the 84th Endocrine Society meeting, we presented the case of a 4-day-old Hispanic boy who presented with lethargy, poor oral intake, hyperbilirubinemia, hypercalcemia, elevated PTHrP level, and abdominal mass. He developed marked hypercalcemia with maximal serum calcium concentration of 27 mg/dL. The radiographic findings included rapid progression of diffuse lytic change within 1 month (Figure 12-1). All conventional therapy for hypercalcemia failed until pamidronate was administrated. The tumor was nonresectable, and the pathology was inconclusive. The patient died from a undiagnosed disseminated malignancy in several months.

Jansen Syndrome

Jansen metaphyseal chondrodysplasia is a rare autosomal dominant form of short limb dwarfism characterized by short stature, leg bowing, and a wadding gait, associated with hypercalcemia and normal or low serum concentrations of PTH and PTH-related peptide. These mineral metabolic abnormalities and metaphyseal changes in patients with Jansen disease is caused by an activation mutation in the PTH-PTHrP receptor in kidney, bone, and growth plate chondrocytes, leading to ligand-independent cyclic adenosine monophosphate accumulation. The radiographic and laboratory abnormalities can be detected during the neonatal period, whereas the phenotypic findings become more obvious during early childhood. Radiographic findings include cupped and ragged metaphyses and osteitis fibrosa cystica.

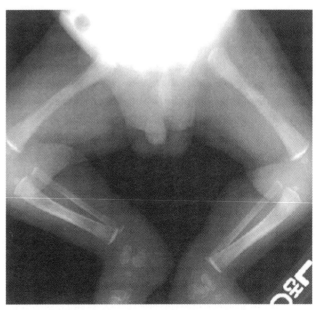

Figure 12-1   Radiograph (anteroposterior) taken 1 month after admission. Baseline film is not shown. Less bone density, with lytic lesions, is seen bilaterally in both femurs.

Laboratory studies show hypercalcemia of serum calcium (13 to 15 mg/dL), hypophosphatemia, hyperphosphatasia, elevated $1,25(OH)_2D$ level, and urine hydroxyproline.

Idiopathic Infantile Hypercalcemia

Idiopathic infantile hypercalcemia (IIH) was originally described in 1950s, after World War II in Britain and Europe, when high-dose vitamin D supplementation was used. Lowering the vitamin D intake has dramatically decreased the incidence of IIH. IIH is a diagnosis of exclusion. The mechanisms responsible for the hypercalcemia vary, indicating that IIH is a heterogeneous disorder. Some of these infants have elevated vitamin D levels, suggesting vitamin D intoxication and/or subtle renal dysregulation of vitamin D metabolism. In others, the vitamin D level was normal, suggesting an increased sensitivity to their vitamin D. Either vitamin D elevation or higher vitamin D sensitivity leads to increased gut absorption.

The disorder was divided into the mild and severe forms. The severe form is now known as Williams syndrome (which is discussed separately). Hypercalcemia in patients with IIH is transient, usually occurring during the first year of life with spontaneous remission. Serum levels of phosphorus and PTH are normal in these patients. Some patients have no clinical symptoms and was detected only when nephrocalcinosis was noted on radiographs. Rarely, others have osteosclerosis or even clinical symptoms of hypercalcemia, such as anorexia, vomiting, constipation, polydipsia, polyuria, and failure to thrive.

Williams Syndrome

Williams syndrome is a multisystem developmental disorder. Williams and coworkers first noticed in 1961 the association of peculiar faces and supravalvular aortic stenosis in children with growth retardation and hypercalcemia. Numerous cases of infantile hypercalcemia had been reported for a decade before Williams' report, and some of the earlier reports described a severe form of IIH that was likely Williams syndrome. With more extensive recognition and reporting, Williams syndrome is now separated from IIH, even the severe subgroup forms, on the basis of clinical, genetic, and pathogenic characteristics.

Williams syndrome occurs due to a contiguous gene deletion at 7q11.23. It composes a 17-gene deletion. The genotype-phenotype correlation is still not clear. There are a variety of physical features associated with Williams syndrome, including elfin facies, a distinctive facial appearance that tend to be more pronounced with age, and with a long philtrum. Cardiac abnormalities occur in 80% of the patients in Williams syndrome, of which the most common is supravalvular aortic stenosis. Hypertension can be seen in 50% of adult patients. Growth and developmental retardation are also characteristics. Two thirds of the infants are small for gestational age at birth, followed by a pattern of growth delay during the first 4 years of life, with catch-up growth in childhood and but low ultimate adult height, frequently remain below the third percentile. Patients also have unique cognitive profile (i.e., a relative sparing of language and facial recognition skills against a background of mental retardation with IQ ranging between 50 and 70). The diagnosis is generally based on the physical and behavioral manifestations.

Hypercalcemia seems to be a variable feature of Williams syndrome. Some patients with Williams syndrome present with hypercalcemia during infancy. However, most with hypercalcemia do not develop symptoms until 3 to 4 months of age, when infants demonstrate irritability (the most frequent symptom) or anorexia, vomiting, constipation, and failure to thrive. The hypercalcemia generally resolves by age 4 years. Therefore, many patients are normocalcemic when they are diagnosed with Williams syndrome. Nephrocalcinosis and other soft tissue calcification in some patients indicate a previous history of hypercalcemia. In still other patients with Williams syndrome, there is neither present nor past evidence of hypercalcemia. Recurrence of hypercalcemia during puberty, on the other hand, has also been reported.

The prognosis is poor in contrast to mild IIH. Approximately 25% die within the first 4 years of life from renal insufficiency, including nephrocalcinosis and renal artery stenosis. Additional sequelae include other renal and cardiac complications and mental retardation.

Subcutaneous Fat Necrosis

Subcutaneous fat necrosis (SFN) of the newborn usually occurs in the first weeks of life associated with perinatal complications surrounding delivery. Fetal distress and direct trauma are noted in the majority of cases. The mechanism of hypercalcemia in SFN is not completely clear. The observations of elevated $1,25(OH)_2D$ and granulomatous infiltration in skin lesion biopsy samples in patients with SFN suggest that unregulated extrarenal $1,25(OH)_2D$ production from involved areas might be responsible for the development of hypercalcemia.

In patients with SFN, erythematous to violaceous, firm, subcutaneous nodules and plaques appear between 1 to 4 weeks postnatally, preceding the development of signs and symptoms of hypercalcemia. The size of the lesions varies from few millimeters to centimeters and can occur as single lesions or generalized lesions. The development of hypercalcemia is during the resolution phase of the fat necrosis;

therefore, the occurrence could be as late as 7 weeks after the onset of SFN, after a period of low or normal serum calcium concentrations. Elevated 1,25(OH)$_2$D levels and suppressed PTH levels are observed in these patients.

In clinical practice, a neonate who develops skin lesions consistent with SFN should be followed for possible onset of hypercalcemia. Fortunately, the hypercalcemia from SFN is transient, lasting about few weeks. Mild cases of hypercalcemia respond to a diet low in calcium and vitamin D; severe hypercalcemia may need to be treated with glucocorticosteroids.

Hypophosphatasia

Hypophosphatasia is a rare inherited metabolic bone disorder associated with deficiency of alkaline phosphatase activity due to the mutation of tissue-nonspecific alkaline phosphatase gene. The defective expression of alkaline phosphatase gene leads to the absence of alkaline phosphatase from bone, an endochondral defect in ossification with severe radiographic bone demineralization, and the elevation of urinary phosphoethanolamine. Hypophosphatasia is inherited as an autosomal recessive disorder, although an autosomal dominant pattern has been reported in a milder form of the disease. The underlying affected gene is in the alkaline phosphatase liver–type gene (*ALPL*, also known as *TNSALP*) and is located on chromosome 1p36.1-34. The accumulation of inorganic pyrophosphate is believed the cause of bone calcification defect in infants and children (rickets) and in adults (osteomalacia).

Severe hypophosphatasia occur in approximately 1:100,000 live births. However, the mild forms are probably more common. About 1:300 individuals in the United States are thought to be carriers for hypophosphatasia. Clinical expression is highly variable, ranging from stillbirth without bone mineralization to pathological fracture that only occurs in adult patients. Hypophosphatasia becomes clinically apparent by 6 months of age. Patients develop hypercalcemia, hypercalciuria, nephrocalcinosis, premature loss of teeth, and severe rickets in the severe form of infantile hypophosphatasia. Some children may have blue sclerae, which resemble osteogenesis imperfecta. Odontohypophosphatasia refers to those who have poor dental formation with no skeletal problems. The disorder may be lethal in utero or shortly after birth because of inadequate bony support of thorax and skull. There is no established medical therapy for this disease.

Hypercalcemia Associated With Phosphate Depletion

Hypophosphatemia is defined as phosphate concentration of less than 4 mg/dL (1.3 mmol/L) in a neonate. It is most often seen in preterm and very low-birth-weight infants (<1500 g) exclusively fed with human milk, which has a relatively low phosphate content. They develop hypercalcemia and "breast milk–induced rickets of prematurity." The low mineral intake and hypophosphatemia decrease bone formation and stimulate 1,25(OH)$_2$D synthesis. The latter, in turn, causes an increase in intestinal calcium absorption. With inadequate low phosphate, calcium deposition in the bone is limited. Hypercalcemia and hypercalciuria eventually result.

Hypophosphatemia may be detected as early as days after birth and persist for months, although mostly infants present after 6 to 8 weeks of life with severe hypophosphatemia and hypercalciuria. Patients usually have normal 25(OH)D and 1,25(OH)$_2$D levels and suppressed serum PTH concentration. With the introduction of commercial available breast milk fortifiers, this condition is now a very rare occurrence.

Blue Diaper Syndrome

Blue diaper syndrome (tryptophan malabsorption), a familial disorder characterized by hypercalcemia, nephrocalcinosis, and indicanuria, is a rare inborn error in which the intestinal transportation of tryptophan is defective. The excessive secretion of indican, an end product of degradation of unabsorbed tryptophan, oxidized to indigo blue on exposure to air, gives the blue stain of the diaper. Clinical symptoms include digestive disturbances, fever, and visual difficulties. Some patients may also develop kidney disease. The disorder is inherited as autosomal recessive but also could be X-linked. Recently, it is proposed that the defect of T-type amino acid transporter-1 (TAT1) gene *SLC16A10* leading to the disruption of aromatic amino acid transport may be the genetic basis of blue diaper syndrome. However, the mechanism of hypercalcemia is yet to be discovered.

Clinical Assessment

Evaluation of neonatal hypercalcemia requires information concerning maternal health, including dietary, potential symptoms and drug history, as well as family history for evidence of calcium disorders or frequent fractures. Anatomical abnormalities (elfin facies), fractures on physical examination, and radiographic examination help differentiate as well as indicate potential severity and diagnosis.

Symptoms and signs of neonatal hypercalcemia are frequently nonspecific. Patients may present with severe dehydration. The dehydration and intravascular depletion trigger an increase in renin-angiotensin activity. Combined with the direct effect of calcium on vasoconstriction and the central nervous system, patients may develop severe hypertension, seizure, lethargy, hypertonia, irritability, and coma. Long-term complications include tissue calcifications, including in particular nephrocalcinosis and renal function impairment. Therefore, unrecognized and untreated hypercalcemia may result in central nervous system and renal damage.

Hypercalcemia is most severe in the patients with parathyroid hyperplasia in this age group. The serum concentration of calcium is commonly in the range of 15 to 20 mg/dL. Serum phosphorus may be as low as 3 mg/dL or even lower. The serum magnesium concentration is also low. However, the alkaline phosphatase is generally normal in this population even if bone involvement is extensive. Both 25(OH)D and 1,25(OH)$_2$D are normal, but PTH is elevated. The urine calcium is elevated, whereas urine phosphorus is low.

Radiological findings include periosteal resorption, best seen along the margins of the phalanges. In advanced cases, there may be generalized rarefaction, cysts, fractures, or deformities. Renal ultrasonography demonstrates the presence of nephrocalcinosis.

Management and Treatment Options

The severity of the hypercalcemia dictates the management. Reduced calcium and vitamin D levels represent the first step in the milder forms of hypercalcemia. For patients who have no response to a low-calcium diet or have life-threatening hypercalcemia, fluid hydration with saline is essential. Calcium-wasting diuretics (e.g., furosemide at a dosage of 1 mg/kg/dose intravenously every 12 hours) should be instituted. In addition, hydrocortisone at a dosage of 1 mg/kg every 6 hours should be used to reduce gut calcium absorption. Calcitonin 10 units/kg intravenously can also be used. Bisphosphonates has been used in adults with hypercalcemia, although they are not approved for use in children. There are reports of successful treatment in children at dose of 0.5 to 1.0 mg/kg/dose of pamidronate intravenously, which could be repeated in 2 to 3 days. In those patients with NSHPT, parathyroidectomy is necessary.

HYPERCALCEMIA IN THE OLDER CHILD

In older children, especially during adolescence, the rate of bone mineralization is dramatically increased under the influence of the sex hormones, growth hormone, and insulin-like growth factor-I. Peak bone mass is achieved by age 18 to 30 years. More than 50% of bone mass is accumulated during puberty, and failure to achieve maximum bone mineralization at this time may lead to osteopenia and

its complications in later adulthood. Therefore, homeostasis of calcium and phosphorus, along with their regulatory hormones and metabolites, is critical in respect to bone health.

Primary Hyperparathyroidism

Primary hyperparathyroidism is generally more common in adult patients and less likely in the pediatric population. It is an uncommonly diagnosed disorder in older children with substantial heterogeneity in regard to the pathology, presenting symptoms, and complications. In adults, especially after the third decade of life, primary hyperparathyroidism is almost always due to a single parathyroid adenoma (75% to 80%). In contrast, in children, it is also almost as frequently due to genetically determined multiple or total parathyroid gland hyperfunction. Loh and coworkers summarized the clinical profile of primary hyperparathyroidism in adolescents and young adults. The study showed that among 22 patients aged 12 to 28 years who were diagnosed with primary hyperparathyroidism, 59% are due to solitary adenoma, 27% to hyperplasia, 9% to multiple adenoma, and 5% to carcinoma.

Solitary parathyroid adenomas account for the majority of primary hyperparathyroidism in older children and adolescents. Most of the parathyroid tumors are monoclonal or oligoclonal, indicating an overgrowth from mutations in parathyroid tumor precursor cells. The underlying gene mutations leading to hyperparathyroidism have been identified in only a minority of tumors. Many of the genes mutated in parathyroid tumors are probably tumor suppressor genes. They contribute to the formation of the tumor through a sequential inactivation of both copies of the gene. *MEN1,* the multiple endocrine neoplasia type 1 gene, is the prototype of known tumor suppressor gene. Parathyroid adenomas have been documented in somatic mutations of both copies of the gene. Inactive tumor suppressor genes may also play an important role in the development of parathyroid tumors. Loss of heterozygosity on chromosome 1p has been reported in 40% of cases of primary hyperparathyroidism. Although the CaSR and vitamin D receptor also inhibit parathyroid gland function, it is noteworthy that no inactivating mutation of either gene has been identified in parathyroid adenoma.

Among the minority of patients with primary hyperparathyroidism caused by hyperfunction of multiple parathyroid glands, only 20% are inherited. These disorders are MEN types 1 and 2, FHH, neonatal severe primary hyperparathyroidism, and jaw tumor syndrome.

Primary hyperparathyroidism is largely asymptomatic. Recent data suggest that the disease is stable in most asymptomatic patients, although there is ample evidence of target organ effects even in those patients. The clinical manifestations of primary hyperparathyroidism are heterogeneous and nonspecific. The most common symptom is fatigue or exhaustion and occurs in 77% of patients, followed by weakness or lethargy and constipation (64% and 41%, respectively). Other symptoms include polyuria, polydipsia, palpitation, hypertension, joint pain, bone pain, pruritis, depression, and poor memory or concentration, occurring in 25% to 33%. Fewer than 20% of patients have anorexia, heartburn, weight loss, headache, fractures, nausea, and vomiting.

With typical hypercalcemia and hypophosphatemia and an elevated PTH level, the diagnosis of hyperparathyroidism is not difficult. Increased bone turnover is the main reason for radiological changes in patients with hyperparathyroidism. These changes include demineralization of bone, osteopenia, pathological fracture, and periosteal "tufting" of the phalanges.

Familial Hypocalciuric Hypercalcemia

FHH is inherited as an autosomal dominant disorder, due to an inactivating gene mutation of *CASR*. The prevalence of FHH is estimated to be 1:78,000. Calcium regulates PTH secretion via the CaSR that is on the surface of parathyroid cells. PTH secretion increases in seconds in response to a low or a falling calcium concentration; in hours through cellular changes in parathyroid messenger RNA level; or in days or months related to parathyroid gland growth. *CASR* loss-of-function mutations lead to complete or partial insensitivity of parathyroid cells to calcium inhibitory effect; therefore, the calcium inhibitory "set point" is shifted, and a higher level of blood calcium is needed to suppress PTH secretion. Furthermore, abnormal calcium-sensor function in the ascending limb of the renal tubule leads to increased calcium reabsorption.

A heterozygous *CASR* mutation usually leads to a mild clinical disorder. The condition is generally asymptomatic in both children and adults. Hypercalcemia is identified incidentally on a chemistry profile, in contrast to homozygous mutations of *CASR* gene, which lead to severe, life-threatening primary hyperparathyroidism at birth and almost always require immediate parathyroid surgery. In older adults with FHH, osteopenia can be a problem, with defective bone mineralization and osteomalacia on bone biopsy. Chondrocalcinosis and pancreatitis have been reported to be associated with FHH.

There are exceptions where a heterozygous *CASR* mutation may lead to more severe problems, although generally not as severe as NSHPT. Specific mutations can lead to a variety and broader spectrum of hypercalcemia and bone problems. There are homozygous *CASR* mutations that result in milder forms with benign elevations of calcium as well as heterozygous mutations that lead to significant hypercalcemia and hypercalciuria, similar to primary hyperparathyroidism. Specific genotyping is necessary, and at the present, such genetic studies are not commercially available.

Biochemical characteristics include mild hypercalcemia with serum calcium levels usually less than 12 mg/dL (3 mmol/L) but occasionally higher. Serum concentration of PTH is inappropriately normal for the degree of hypercalcemia. The serum magnesium concentration is high normal or slightly elevated, instead of the low-normal range in the condition of hyperparathyroidism. There is a positive correlation between the serum total calcium and magnesium concentration in FHH. Hypophosphatemia is mild. Urine calcium is inappropriately low. Therefore, the characteristic finding in FHH is the decreased ratio of urine calcium clearance to that of creatinine as determined by the formula: $U_{Ca} \times S_{Cr}/U_{Cr} \times S_{Ca}$ [(urinary calcium multiplied by serum creatinine) divided by (urinary creatinine multiplied by serum calcium)]. In the majority of the patients with FHH (80%), this ratio is less than 0.01.

In contrast to primary hyperparathyroidism, bone density in patients with FHH usually is normal, although the markers of bone turnover may be slightly elevated.

The treatment of FHH is conservative. There is no evidence of progressive skeletal demineralization or renal injury in the majority of FHH patients. Observation is sufficient in most patients in view of the benign nature, except in the infants with fetal hyperparathyroidism.

Multiple Endocrine Neoplasia

MEN syndromes are not common and consist of type 1 (MEN1, Wermer syndrome) and type 2 (MEN2, Sipple syndrome). About 20 different tumors have been reported in MEN1 but mostly tumors of the parathyroid, enteropancreatic, and anterior pituitary. MEN1 is defined by the presence of two of these primary endocrine-related tumors. *Familial MEN1* is defined as one or more family members diagnosed with MEN1 and one or more first-degree relative with one of the three endocrine-related tumors. The incidence of MEN1 is estimated at 1% to 4% of patients with primary hyperparathyroidism. Hyperparathyroidism is the most common, and generally the earliest endocrinopathy, to present in MEN1. One large sample study in 1996 showed that parathyroid tumors occur in up to 95% of the patients, followed by pancreatic islet tumors (41%) and pituitary tumors (30%). MEN2, on the other hand, has three variants: (1) MEN2A (medullary thyroid carcinoma, pheochromocytoma, and hyperparathyroidism), (2) MEN2B (medullary thyroid carcinoma and pheochromocytoma), and (3) familial medullary thyroid carcinoma only.

MEN1 is inherited as autosomal dominant disorder, although sporadic cases are also reported. The affected gene, mapped to 11q13, is a tumor suppressor gene and codes for a protein product referred as MENIN. More than 80% of the mutations are inactivating and are consistent with the expectation in a tumor suppressor gene. However, there is no clear correlation between the genotype and phenotype documented in MEN1.

MEN2A is also inherited as an autosomal dominant disorder caused by an activating mutation of RET proto-oncogene. The affected gene of MEN2 variants is located on chromosome 10 cen-11.2 and encodes tyrosine kinase receptor. In contrast to the enormous number of various MEN1 mutations, three MEN2 variants have specific mutations at certain locations. Extracellular domain mutations in MEN2A lead to RET homodimerization, whereas the intracellular domain mutations in MEN2B activate the RET kinase catalytic site.

The clinical manifestations of MEN1 depend on the affected tumors and the hormones secreted. Parathyroid disease as the first clinical presentation occurs in about 87% of patients in MEN1, almost never presenting before 5 years of age and always presenting (100%) by the age of 50 years. Compared with primary hyperparathyroidism (HPT) due to adenoma, HPT in MEN1 tends to affect both genders equally and to affect patients earlier (age 20 to 25 years). Usually, multiple parathyroid glands are affected. In addition to the triad of parathyroid, pancreatic, and pituitary tumors, patients may have other tumors, including adrenal cortical tumors (5%) and carcinoid (3.6%). Lipomas, angiofibromas, collagenomas, and other tumors are rare and occur in less than 1% of the patients with MEN1. Among pancreatic tumors, insulinoma is more frequently seen in younger patients (<40 years), but gastrinoma is more common in older patients. Patients with MEN1 associated with the Zöllinger-Ellison syndrome, eventually died from the malignancy with a mortality of 33%.

MEN2A is the more common variant of MEN2, accounting for 75% of cases. In contrast to MEN1, hyperparathyroidism is less common, develops in about 20% to 30% of the patients with MEN2A, and tends to affect patients at an older age. Hyperparathyroidism is milder clinically in MEN2A. Usually, the patients are asymptomatic. Medullary thyroid carcinoma develops in up to 90% of patients with MEN2 and is frequently the cause of death.

Biochemical testing for hyperparathyroidism and gastrin is central in recognizing and for surveillance in MEN1. The MEN1 mutations identified are diverse in type and scatter throughout the coding region, which makes genetic screening more difficult. Germline mutation test by DNA sequencing is the choice for MEN1 mutational analysis. There is an about 10% to 20% failure rate for the detection of mutations in MEN1.

In contrast, RET mutation analysis for MEN2 is more specific and indicates an RET mutation in more than 95% of patients. In families with known MEN2, it is mandatory to test the children because their risk is 50% for having the mutation and the children who are positive for MEN2A are almost 100% likely to develop medullary thyroid carcinoma.

Jaw Tumor Syndrome

Jaw tumor syndrome is a rare disorder characterized by hyperparathyroidism, cemento-ossifying fibromas of the jaw, renal cysts, Wilms tumor, and renal hamartomas. Hyperparathyroidism is commonly caused by single or multiple adenomas. Carcinoma of the parathyroid is less frequently seen; it inherited as an autosomal dominant disease. The gene causing the disease has been mapped to chromosome 1q24.

Hypercalcemia of Malignancy

Parathyroid hormone-related protein (PTHrP) is a tumor product that acts on the PTH receptor, causing hypercalcemia by inducing bone resorption and renal tubular reabsorption of calcium. PTHrP is the predominant factor causing hypercalcemia in cancer patients. Studies showed that at least 80% of adult patients with solid tumors and hypercalcemia have elevated PTHrP level (i.e., hormonal hypercalcemia of malignancy). Although local osteolysis around bone metastases also can induce hypercalcemia, it is the tumor-secreted PTHrP systemic effect on the skeleton that causes hypercalcemia.

PTHrP, structurally homologous with PTH, is found in a variety of tumor types associated with hypercalcemia. Eight of the first 13 amino acids of PTHrP that account for the receptor-activating domain are identical to that of PTH. Thus, PTHrP is considered to mediate effects via the same receptors as PTH, a family of G protein–coupled receptors, in bone and kidney.

Hypercalcemia of malignancy is extremely rare in children and occurs in less than 1% of children with cancer. One retrospective study of 3239 patients with solid tumors and 2816 patients with leukemia or lymphoma over a 29-year period demonstrated a total of only 25 patients with hypercalcemia. Eleven of 25 patients diagnosed with hypercalcemia at the time of their original diagnosis had acute lymphocytic leukemia. The tumors associated with hypercalcemia of malignancy in children are leukemia, lymphoma, rhabdomyosarcoma, and fibrosarcoma, in contrast to adult patients, in whom lung, renal cell, and breast malignancies more commonly produce PTHrP. The clinical picture of hypercalcemia due to PTHrP is very abrupt, acute, and severe, often in the setting of an ill-appearing child who is dehydrated and toxic and may be comatose. Serum calcium levels are markedly elevated. This is extremely different from the hypercalcemia due to HPT, which is milder and more chronic.

Immobilization

Immobility may lead to loss of skeletal mineral and result in hypercalcemia and hypercalciuria. Children and young adults are particular susceptible to rapid bone loss when immobilized. Hypercalcemia can even occur, although rarely so, in growing children and adolescents after single limb fractures. The mechanism of immobilization-induced hypercalcemia is almost entirely attributable to decreased bone mineral accretion, uncoupled integrated action of osteoblasts and osteoclasts, and increased bone reabsorption relative to bone formation. The PTH function and the production of $1,25(OH)_2D$ are suppressed in this primary bone-resorbing process. Calcium reabsorption from distal renal tubules and $1,25(OH)_2D$ synthesis are reduced, and thereby intestinal calcium absorption is decreased. Patients develop hypercalcemia, hypercalciuria, hypertension, acute renal insufficiency, and acute disuse osteoporosis. Clinically, patients with immobilization-induced hypercalcemia may present with nausea, vomiting, obstipation, polyuria, polydipsia, irritability, and emotional instability. Hypercalciuria may lead to calcium oxalate nephrolithiasis and cause abdominal pain mimicking an acute surgical crisis. Laboratory studies indicate that the hypercalcemia is moderate, with plasma calcium concentration elevated but generally less than 18 mg/dL. Early mobilization when possible is the key. Dietary calcium restriction on immobile patients has no effect on urinary calcium excretion. Maintaining a high sodium and water intake in patients with mild hypercalcemia or saline hydration with furosemide administration in moderate to severe hypercalcemic cases should be used to increase urinary calcium excretion and prevent a hypercalcemic crisis.

Granulomatous Diseases

Hypercalcemia is associated with granuloma-forming diseases. The extrarenal overproduction of vitamin D, mainly $1,25(OH)_2D$, from disease-activated macrophages increases intestinal calcium absorption and leads to clinical hypercalcemia. The endogenous synthesized vitamin D metabolite is independent of the usual regulation factors. The granulomatous diseases reported to be associated with hypercal-

cemia include sarcoidosis, tuberculosis, lymphoma, disseminated candidiasis, leprosy, silicone-induced granulomatous disease, Wegener granulomatosis, *Nocardia asteroides* infection, and cat scratch disease (CSD), as well as acquired immune deficiency syndrome and *Pneumocystic carinii*.

The treatment aims at pharmacological inhibition of the abnormal 1-hydroxylation reaction and limitation of substrates for the reaction. The former is best accomplished by the administration of anti-inflammatory concentrations of glucocorticoids and the latter by controlling vitamin D intake and sunlight exposure in susceptible hosts.

Other Causes

Hyperthyroidism. Thyroid hormone stimulates bone resorption. Patients with hyperthyroidism occasionally develop a mild hypercalcemia associated with hypercalciuria.

Adrenal insufficiency. Hemoconcentration may in part account for the hypercalcemia that rarely develops in patients with adrenal insufficiency. Both total calcium and ionized calcium levels are elevated.

Drug-Induced Hypercalcemia

Lithium. Lithium is used in patients with bipolar disorder. Clinical observations showed that after years of therapy, lithium can lead to a mild but persistent serum calcium elevation. It stimulates parathyroid cells, increases the set point for PTH secretion in vitro, and causes parathyroid gland hyperplasia. Hypercalcemia often persists until the therapy is discontinued. Mild hyperparathyroidism occurs in approximately 5% of patients receiving long-term lithium therapy. Withdrawal from lithium therapy and alternative treatment should be considered. Nephrogenic diabetes insipidus, one of the other side effects from lithium treatment, could worsen the hydration status and the severity of hypercalcemia.

Vitamin D intoxication. Excessive vitamin D ingestion may lead to hypercalcemia. It is often seen in patients overtreated for hypoparathyroidism or pseudohypoparathyroidism, hypophosphatemic rickets, or renal osteodystrophy. The mechanism of vitamin D intoxication–induced hypercalcemia is due to increased intestinal absorption and bone resorption. Patients present with weakness nausea, vomiting, mental status change, elevated 25(OH)D levels, and suppressed PTH levels. The serum concentrations of $1,25(OH)_2D$ vary from normal to modestly elevated. Vitamin D is stored in the fat after being absorbed and, as a consequence, hypercalcemia is prolonged and severe. Management for vitamin D toxicity–induced hypercalcemia includes calcium intake restriction, hydration, and corticosteroid administration.

Vitamin A intoxication. The excessive accumulation of vitamin A, either acutely or chronically, results in hypervitaminosis A. Vitamin A intoxication acutely causes clinical symptoms that include nausea, vomiting, drowsiness, and pseudotumor cerebri. Chronic overdosing may lead to anorexia, pruritus, failure to thrive, bone pain and swelling, hypercalcemia, nephrocalcinosis, and osteoporosis. Craniotabes is common. Radiographic findings include periostitis and hyperostosis. The diagnosis can be made on the basis of history of excessive vitamin A intake and elevated vitamin A level.

Clinical Assessment

The clinical features of hypercalcemia are dependent on the nature of the underlying disorder, the age of the child, and the degree of the hypercalcemia. Because of the complex physiological roles of calcium in bone mineralization, enzyme regulation, skeletal and cardiac muscle contraction, cellular secretion, cell growth and division, neural excitation, and light transmission and coagulation, it is no surprise that the clinical findings of hypercalcemia can be both nonspecific and severely morbid. Patients may be completely asymptomatic with mild hypercalcemia or they may present with coma and seizures with severe hypercalcemia. The symptoms of hypercalcemia include polyuria, polydipsia, constipation, hypotonia, poor feeding, vomiting, and failure to thrive (Box 12-2).

Laboratory Investigation

The determination of ionized calcium, as it is the biologically active form, as well as the measurement of total calcium level is important in the biochemical investigation of hypercalcemia. The calcium "set point" for PTH secretion is a serum ionized calcium concentration of 4 mg/dL (1 mmol/dL), where PTH secretion reaches 50% of maximum. Elevation of ionized calcium concentration usually parallels elevation of total calcium level in pathological situations, with some exceptions. A higher protein binding capacity may result in a greater than normal total serum calcium level, yet the ionized calcium is normal. A change in serum albumin of 1 g/dL generally results in a parallel change in total calcium of about 0.2 mmol/L. Conversely, reduced albumin binding of calcium may result in normal serum total calcium in the presence of elevated ionized calcium. Similarly, acidosis decreases the binding coefficient and lowers total calcium and alkalosis increases binding.

Serum intact PTH should be measured at the same time as serum calcium concentration. Common commercial assays for measurement of intact PTH are either an immunochemiluminometric assay (ICMA) or an immunoradiometric assay (IRMA). Both assays are highly sensitive and specific and are highly correlated with PTH secretion.

Box 12-2   Clinical Signs and Symptoms of Hypercalcemia

Cardiovascular
  Hypertension
  Palpitations
  Arrhythmia
  Short QT intervals
Gastrointestinal
  Constipation
  Anorexia
  Nausea or vomiting
  Heartburn
  Peptic ulcer disease
  Pancreatitis
Central nervous system
  Lethargy, drowsiness, fatigue
  Depression
  Psychosis
  Stupor, coma
  Poor memory or concentration
  Headache
Neuromuscular
  Weakness
  Hypotonia
Renal
  Polyuria, nocturia
  Polydipsia
  Nephrocalcinosis
  Nephrolithiasis
Musculoskeletal
  Myalgias, arthralgias
  Osteoporosis
  Pathological fracture
  Osteitis fibrosis cystica
Somatic
  Weight loss
  Failure to thrive
Skin
  Pruritus

Furthermore, there is no cross-reaction between PTH and PTH-related peptide. The assays are two-site immunoassays, detecting both amino-terminal and carboxyl-terminal epitopes of the peptide. Intact PTH is composed of 84 amino acids, with its first 34 amino acids at amino-terminal region containing the full biological activity of the hormone. Intact PTH secreted from parathyroid gland undergoes hepatic metabolism into amino-terminal and carboxyl-terminal fragments. The amino-terminal fragment is further metabolized in the liver, whereas the carboxyl-terminal fragment is excreted from kidney. In renal failure, carboxyl-terminal fragments accumulate and the measurement of carboxyl-terminal PTH is elevated, falsely indicating that secreted PTH is elevated. As a matter of fact, about one-half of intact PTH elevations reported in uremic patients are due to biologically inactive forms of PTH. Therefore, even intact PTH values in patients with chronic renal diseases must be interpreted with caution.

Management of Hypercalcemia

The management of hypercalcemia depends on the underlying mineral metabolic disorders and severity of the high calcium level. Hypercalcemia in some patients may be life-threatening, and it is important to recognize the severity of hypercalcemia and to initiate prompt treatment. Alternatively, with mild hypercalcemia, such as in FHH, no aggressive therapy is necessary.

When the serum calcium reaches 14 mg/dL or greater or the patient demonstrates symptoms of severe hypercalcemia, emergency intervention is imperative. The principles for the management are hydration and correction of volume depletion and electrolyte abnormalities. It is essential to reduce or discontinue any medications that might cause hypercalcemia and to limit dietary calcium and vitamin D. As indicated, the use of diuretics (e.g., furosemide), glucocorticoids, and other medications (as discussed later) may be necessary.

Medical Management

Loop Diuretics and Saline
Urinary calcium excretion is directly proportional to sodium excretion. Calciuric therapy, which includes 0.9% sodium chloride infusion and loop diuretics, is used in the initial management of moderate to severe hypercalcemia. Normal saline given at 2 to 3 times maintenance fluid expands intracellular volume, improves glomerular filtration, and increases renal calcium excretion. Loop diuretics, such as furosemide, not only promote sodium and calcium diuresis but also control fluid overload. The furosemide dosage is 1 to 2 mg/kg/dose every 6 to 12 hours intravenously or intramuscularly. The onset of hydration therapy action usually takes 24 to 48 hours. The reduction of serum calcium in response to this therapy is modest, ranging from 0.5- to 2.0-mg/dL decrements but may ameliorate symptoms to some extent. However, this therapy is generally insufficient to restore normal calcium levels. Furosemide administration should be preceded by the correction of volume depletion and other electrolyte abnormalities. Sodium excretion by furosemide is even more profound than calcium excretion. Uncorrected hyponatremia triggers renal sodium-conserving mechanisms, which in turn decreases both sodium and calcium excretion. Potassium and magnesium losses in the urine are also significant with this regimen. Therefore, careful monitoring of electrolytes and appropriate supplemental therapy are necessary. Severely

hypercalcemic patients should be admitted to the intensive care unit, because electrocardiographic and central venous pressure monitoring are generally required.

Hemodialysis or Peritoneal Dialysis
With calcium-free dialysate, either hemodialysis or peritoneal dialysis can rapidly decrease serum calcium levels. The indications for dialysis are those patients with hypercalcemia due to or associated with severe hypercalcemia of malignancy, congestive heart failure, or significant renal failure. The decrease in serum calcium concentration with dialysis can be extremely rapid, resulting in cardiovascular instability. Cardiac monitoring is necessary with dialysis, and patients may require volume expansion and vasopressor application.

Calcitonin
Calcitonin decreases serum calcium via inhibition of osteoclastic activity and reducing calcium tubular reabsorption. Two forms of pharmacological calcitonin are available: salmon and human. Both are effective in the management of acute hypercalcemia. Calcitonin is characterized by rapid onset of action and the safe and short duration of action. Calcitonin treatment causes a modest reduction in serum calcium levels (i.e., 2- to 3-mg/dL decrease in calcium within 2 to 4 hours after therapy). Therefore, its clinical application is in the treatment of patients with acute hypercalcemia crisis, especially in association with uncorrected dehydration and renal insufficiency. It is particularly useful in the setting of hypercalcemia due to vitamin D intoxication or immobilization. Long-term use of calcitonin for hypercalcemia treatment is limited because of tachyphylaxis. Calcitonin loses its calciuric effect, probably mediated by downregulation of corticosteroid-sensitive receptors, with repetitive dosing beyond 3 to 4 days. This reduction in effectiveness can be partially overcome by the coadministration of corticosteroids, which will sustain the calcium reduction for several weeks.

Calcitonin is given at 1 to 4 IU/kg via continuous infusion or via subcutaneous or intramuscular injections every 6 to 12 hours. Common side effects include nausea, malaise, flushing, or skin rashes.

Bisphosphonates
Bisphosphonates suppress osteoclast-mediated bone resorption and increase bone mineral density. Bisphosphonates are used in adult patients who have increased bone resorption for various pathological reasons, such as Paget disease. Biphosphonates have been used in children with idiopathic juvenile osteoporosis, osteogenesis imperfecta, and corticosteroid-induced osteoporosis, as well as a number of other disorders involving bone.

There have been several reports of the successful use of bisphosphonates to treat acute hypercalcemia or in the long-term management of metabolic bone diseases related to bone resorption. In severe hypercalcemia not responding to conventional hypercalcemia therapy, pamidronate can be given as a single dose of 0.5 to 1.0 mg/kg intravenously over 4 to 6 hours. The effectiveness of treatment usually is seen 2 to 5 days after therapy. The same dose may be repeated as necessary, either in 1 week or at an even shorter interval, as in some studies. Pamidronate should be mixed in normal saline or half-normal saline and administered over a prolonged period (4 hours or longer). Both calcium-containing fluids (e.g., Ringer solution) and coadministration with other drugs should be avoided.

Other Agents Related to Bone Metabolism

Osteoclast Inhibitors. Mithramycin (plicamycin) inhibits RNA synthesis in osteoclasts and belongs to the family of cytotoxic drugs used in anticancer chemotherapy. It is more potent than calcitonin. It decreases calcium level within 12 to 24 hours, and the effects may last as long as 1 to 3 weeks. It has numerous side effects, such as hepatotoxicity, nephrotoxicity, thrombocytopenia, and myelosuppression, that limit its clinical application. The dose is 25 μg/kg via infusion through a central line over 4 to 6 hours. The dose can be repeated in 24 to 48 hours, but should be used with caution because the toxic effects accumulate in a dose-dependent fashion.

Phosphate inhibits osteoclastic activity and increases skeletal mineral accretion. It precipitates renal calcium-phosphate salts and can impair renal function. Phosphate may also result in calcium-phosphorus complex deposits at ectopic soft tissues. Therefore, not only is phosphate contraindicated in patients with renal insufficiency, but also its application in long-term use is limited. Careful monitoring of renal function and radiographs is necessary.

Agents That Decrease Intestinal Calcium Absorption

Glucocorticoids inhibit 1α-hydroxylase and decrease 1,25(OH)$_2$D production and thereby are very effective in reducing intestinal calcium absorption. It is the therapy of choice for 1,25(OH)$_2$D-induced hypercalcemia, such as vitamin D intoxication or ectopic 1,25(OH)$_2$D production or hematological malignancies. The usual dosage is 1 to 2 mg/kg/day of methylprednisolone intravenously every 6 hours. The onset of action is relatively slow, perhaps up to 1 week; the duration of the action is short; and the reduction in calcium is low.

Ketoconazole, an antifungal agent, reduces plasma levels of 1,25(OH)$_2$D in patients with granulomatous disorders. The dosage is 3 to 9 mg/kg/day in three divided doses.

Calcimimetics

Calcimimetics are a new class of pharmacological agents that target the CaSR. Calcimimetics selectively act on the CaSR expressed on parathyroid cells by enhancing the sensitivity of the receptor to extracellular ionized calcium and thereby suppressing PTH secretion. This effect is absent after parathyroidectomy, indicating that the specific effect is on the CaSR of the parathyroid glands. The full molecular mechanism of calcimimetics action has yet to be understood. Two mechanisms via which calcimimetics interfere with PTH secretion have been identified. One mechanism is to act as an agonist of the CaSR, and the second is to act as a positive allosteric modulator to increase the sensitivity of *CASR*. In rats with chronic renal failure, chronic use of calcimimetics prevented the development of parathyroid gland hyperplasia and secondary hyperparathyroidism. In a small clinical study, calcimimetics caused rapid, in a dose-dependent manner, lowering of plasma PTH level in primary hyperparathyroidism. Calcimimetics may provide a novel, potentially very effective approach for treating hypercalcemia due to hyperparathyroidism. Calcimimetics are at the present still under evaluation in clinical trials.

Surgical Management

Parathyroidectomy is the only definitive therapy for hypercalcemia secondary to hyperparathyroidism. It is associated with biochemical normalization and increased bone density. In the hands of an experienced pediatric parathyroid surgeon, the successful rate for parathyroidectomy rate is 90% to 95%, with a complication rate of less than 5%, little morbidity, rare mortality, and brief hospitalization. Depending on the etiology of hyperparathyroidism, partial parathyroidectomy (affected gland) or subtotal parathyroidectomy (3.5 glands) is carried out in patients with parathyroid adenoma and nonfamilial hyperplasia of the parathyroid glands, respectively. Total parathyroidectomy with autotransplantation of one parathyroid gland, cut up in pieces, to the nondominant forearm is the procedure of choice for patients with MEN1.

MAJOR POINTS

Severe hypercalcemia associated with multiple fractures and diffuse osteopenia in a newborn is most often due to homozygous loss of function of the same calcium-sensing receptor gene. The loss of sensing for calcium results in excessive parathyroid hormone (PTH) secretion, that is, neonatal severe hyperparathyroidism.

In older children, mild hypercalcemia is often due to a heterozygous mutation of the calcium-sensing receptor gene, that is, familial hypocalciuric hypercalcemia. This benign disorder is characterized by a decreased ratio (<0.01) of urine calcium clearance to that of creatinine as determined by the formula $U_{Ca} \times S_{Cr}/U_{Cr} \times S_{Ca}$.

Primary hyperparathyroidism is older children is relatively uncommon, and, unlike in adult patients, parathyroid adenoma accounts for only approximately 50% of patients, whereas multiple gland or hyperplasia are as frequent.

Continued

MAJOR POINTS—Cont'd

Vitamin D toxicity is often due to overaggressive treatment for hypoparathyroidism or pseudohypoparathyroidism or immobilization of patients. The treatment is withdrawal of vitamin D and the use of glucocorticosteroids.

Severe hypercalcemia is a medical emergency that can result in coma, irreparable brain damage, and death. The immediate treatment is saline fluid resuscitation and the use of loop diuretics, such as furosemide. Other measures include calcitonin, bisphosphonates, and corticosteroids.

SUGGESTED READINGS

Brandi ML, Gagel RF, Angeli A, et al: Guidelines for diagnosis and therapy of MEN type 1 and type 2, J Clin Endocrinol Metab 2001;86:5658.

Brown EM: Familial hypocalciuric hypercalcemia and other disorders with resistance to extracellular calcium, Endocrinol Metab Clin North Am 2000;29:503.

Loh KC, Duh QY, Shoback D, et al: Clinical profile of primary hyperparathyroidism in adolescents and young adults, Clin Endocrinol (Oxf) 1998;48:435.

Marx SJ: Medical progress: hyperparathyroid and hypoparathyroid disorders, N Engl J Med 2000;343:1863.

Strewler GJ: Medical approaches to primary hyperparathyroidism, Endocrinol Metab Clin North Am 2000;29:523.

CHAPTER 13

Osteoporosis

THOMAS MOSHANG, JR.

INTRODUCTION

The frail old man, stooped over and leaning on a cane, and the well-dressed elderly woman with a "dowager's hump" are not images characteristically part of a pediatrician's practice. These images of outcome effects due to osteoporosis are generally regarded to be a geriatric, not pediatric, problem. The reality is, like much of pediatrics, that such outcomes are often the results of lack of appropriate preventative measures during childhood or iatrogenically induced disease during childhood. There is, however, a growing focus on bone health for the pediatric patients that warrant the practitioner to be well versed in technological advances as well as biochemical advances. This section discusses the regulation of bone growth, techniques used to evaluate bone development, appropriate hormone and chemical studies, the disorders of bone development, and treatment possibilities. It is important to emphasize that the changes in the skeletal system are related to developmental physiological changes occurring during child-

hood. Therefore, it is crucial to understand the age-related and puberty-related changes in bone formation and normative data for bone density in prepubertal, postpubertal, and late adolescent children.

REGULATION OF BONE GROWTH

Primitive mesenchymal tissues are directed during early fetal life to form the bone matrix, organized by a number of factors including those factors regulating calcium-phosphorus metabolism (as outlined in the preceding chapters) and genetic factors, matrix proteins, and collagen. Within weeks after conception, mesenchymal cells form the precursors of bone cells. The fetal skull and clavicle develop from the intramembranous bones. The limbs, ribs, and remaining bones begin to form from endochondral bone. The ossification of the fetal skeleton continues to mature with osteoblasts, and mineralization takes place. The ossification of bone subsequently leads to development of the epiphyseal centers. Remodeling of the skeleton continues with osteoclasts resorbing bone and osteoblasts forming new bone. The fetal skeleton is evident from very early fetal gestation by imaging studies.

During intrauterine life, much of the fetal skeleton is dependent on maternal factors. Calcium, phosphorus and calcitriol (1,25-dihydroxyvitamin D) cross the placental membrane. Inadequate vitamin D intake and decrease calcium absorption by the mother can lead to neonatal rickets and hypocalcemia. Whether this is a direct effect of calcitriol (or a metabolite) on bone mineralization or secondary parathyroid hormone (PTH) excess is not clear. Maternal hyperparathyoidism with increased calcium transport to the infant suppresses fetal parathyroid function, also leading to hypocalcemia in the newborn, albeit transiently.

It is clear that excess parathyroid function can alter bone mineralization in the fetus. In the homozygous form of the genetic disorder of the upregulated calcium sensor, a G protein–linked receptor (benign familial hypercalcemic hypocalcuria), the newborn infant is often born with severe osteoporosis and multiple fractures. Conversely, bone mineralization continues normally due to maternal calcium homeostasis in fetal infants with decreased parathyroid function, such as in the infant with 22q11.2 deletion (DiGeorge syndrome).

After birth, there is gradual continued accruement of new bone with constant remodeling throughout childhood and adolescence and peak bone mass being attained during young adulthood. The bone mineral content (given in g/cm^2) increases in a fairly constant manner with linear growth during childhood and during puberty to reach a peak sometime after maturation. Subsequently, there is a slow decline in bone mineral content because bone resorption outpaces bone formation. The remodeling of bone appears to be related to repairing damage and fatigue and includes replacement of old bone with new bone at the same sites. Bone is composed of osteoblasts and osteoclasts embedded in a matrix of collagen fibers, impregnated with hydroxyapatite, composed from calcium, phosphorus, magnesium, carbonate, and citrate. The osteoclasts are responsible for the removal of old bone, whereas the formation of new bone is regulated by the osteoblasts. The factors regulating the actions of osteoclasts and osteoblasts are multiple and include stress, exercise, nutrition, insulin, growth factors (including growth hormone–dependent growth factors), gonadal steroids, and cytokines.

The origin of the osteoclasts and osteoblasts is bone marrow precursor cells. Mesenchymal stem cells develop into osteoblasts, whereas hematopoietic cells develop into osteoclasts. A number of growth factors have been demonstrated to stimulate osteoblast formation. Similarly, a number of cytokines regulate osteoclast formation. In particular, interleukin (IL)-6 has been studied in some detail. IL-6 increases osteoblasts and bone resorption as well as osteoblast formation. The main hormones regulating osteoclast formation are calcitriol and PTH. As discussed in the section on physiological mechanisms regulating calcium and phosphorus metabolism (Chapter 11), the actions of PTH and calcitriol are interwoven, regulating calcium and phosphorus intestinal absorption, calcium-phosphorus bone formation, and bone resorption. Calcitonin inhibits osteoclast formation and inhibits bone resorption. Gonadal steroids and thyroid hormones alter cytokines but also have direct effects on bone remodeling. The mechanisms by which estrogens and androgens regulate bone remodeling are not clear, but gonadal steroid deficiency is associated with increase in both osteoclast and osteoblast activity. It is believed that estrogen deficiency leads to an imbalance between bone resorption and bone formation because of an increased life span and functional activity of osteoclast; despite the increase in osteoblast activity, there is a decrease in the functional life span of the osteoblast. Glucocorticoid excess causes not only decreased absorption of intestinal calcium and phosphorus but also a secondary hypercalciuria and a secondary hyperparathyoidism. The increase in PTH results in increased bone resorption and decreased bone formation.

Genetic factors regulating bone growth may someday provide a means to evaluate bone disorders. Clearly, the gene mutations of type I collagen lead to various forms of osteogenesis imperfecta (OI). Mutations and deletions within the *SHOX* gene located within the pseudoautosomal region of the short arms of the X and Y chromosomes not only result in the short stature seen in Turner syndrome and Leri-Weil syndrome but also cause limb disproportion and Madelung deformity. Further, the Indian hedgehog gene, parathyroid hormone–related protein (PTHrP) genes, calcium-sensing receptor gene *(CASR),* and others affect bone development and pathology. Some of the proposed genes regulating bone mineral density (BMD) are being mapped using mouse models (e.g., *LRP5* as a potential osteoporosis gene). It is beyond the realm of this book to focus on and discuss the gene abnormalities being discovered, although clearly some of these genetic mutations have been associated with clinical disorders and bone dystrophies. This chapter discusses OI and *CASR* mutations in relation to osteoporosis.

BONE DENSITY DETERMINATION

Techniques to determine bone density are well established for adults but much less so for children. Earlier techniques, such as single-photon and dual-photon absorptiometry or dual-energy X-ray absorptiometry (DEXA), using single beams were useful but technological changes have altered findings so that use in pediatric clinical care (and even in research studies) needs to be continually reevaluated. In adults, DEXA quantification of bone density for adults is based on a comparison of BMD compared with the mean peak BMD, expressed as a T-score. A T-score of –2.5 SDs from the peak bone density is defined as *osteoporosis.* Clearly, osteoporosis in growing children, especially those who are still prepubertal, cannot be assessed against peak bone density, which is not achieved until young adulthood. DEXA also has the disadvantage in children in that normative data (for children) are often based on age and do not factor in height, weight, and pubertal changes. DEXA tends to underestimate bone density in short children. Nevertheless, the best normative data published to date including a significant number of children with equal distribution between male and female children used DEXA with a fan-beam scanning mode. The fan-beam scanning technique is also associated with magnification error. DEXA results are expressed as a Z-score (standard deviations from the mean of a population for children of the same age and gender). More recent techniques used in an effort to overcome the problem of underestimating bone density as a result of small size include quantitative computed tomography (QCT) and quantitative ultrasonography. Normative data still need to be established for children with both of these techniques. One disadvantage of QCT is the cost and the significant amount of irradiation (when evaluating lumbar spine) compared with DEXA. However, for clinical research studies in children, especially those with comorbidities such as growth hormone deficiency or chronic renal failure, this technique may prove to be superior to DEXA once normative data are established.

REQUIREMENTS FOR BONE HEALTH IN CHILDREN

Peak bone mass is achieved subsequent to puberty and is achieved sometime in young adulthood. Peak bone mass is the maximum level of bone mineral content attained and is recognized as the major association for risk of osteoporosis or lack thereof in later life. The achievement of peak bone mass can be altered to some degree by lifestyle interventions. Poor nutrition, especially the inadequate intake of calcium and vitamin D, and lack of physical activity can substantially reduce bone density. There are genetic factors influencing the attainment of adequate bone densities, but comorbidities and treatment of disease states probably account for significant reduction of bone density in children.

A number of studies evaluating calcium intake in children, including double-blind placebo-control studies, have all indicated in general that calcium supplementation enhances bone density to a significant degree. However, studies also indicate that after discontinuation of calcium supplementation, differences in achieved bone density did not persist, indicative that continuing calcium supplementation is warranted. Dietary studies indicate that calcium intake declines as children grow older, especially when the need is greatest during adolescence. The current recommendation is that children should receive at least 800 mg of elemental calcium before puberty and increase their intake to 1200 and 1500 mg through puberty and postpuberty, respectively.

Vitamin D intake also is reduced when children decrease their milk intake and ingestion of routine vitamins, being almost completely dependent on sunlight as a source. Fish and fish oils, another potential source of vitamin D, are not a frequent dietary staple in the United States. In Asian Americans and African Americans, the incidence of lactose intolerance is high, further reducing the likelihood of these two ethnic groups to ingest milk and milk products for any length of time. The suggested intake for vitamin D is 100 to 200 IU/day, but the need increases after puberty and in the adult, with recommendations being 400 to 800 IU/day.

Physical activity, as related to mechanical stresses, is important for bone remodeling. A number of studies indicated that severe immobilization results in osteopenia and is a known cause of hypercalcemia. Conversely, even in normally active children, increased activity will further increase BMD.

DIFFERENTIAL DIAGNOSIS OF DISORDERS RESULTING IN OSTEOPOROSIS

The frequency or incidence of osteoporosis during childhood is not known. It is only during the past decade that interest in osteoporosis has led to evaluation of BMD during childhood and late adolescence. The normative data for BMD and BMC are still being established, as discussed earlier, with some of the difficulties compounded by improving technology and changing software, which makes data obtained by one type of bone densitometer no longer valid with newer models. Nevertheless, it is clear that osteoporosis is a major pediatric issue, above and beyond the genetic forms of OI, especially because the most frequent causes of osteoporosis are probably iatrogenic.

Infants and Newborns

Other than in the neonate, fractures during infancy are by and large due to child abuse. Nevertheless, pediatricians have to be aware that there are some conditions predisposing to osteoporosis and easier fractures. The most common problem still is vitamin D deficiency, which occurs most frequently in black children in urban areas. Less common disorders include vitamin D dependency (1α–hydroxylase deficiency) and hypophosphatemic rickets (as discussed in Chapter 11). Congenital renal disease and renal rickets predispose the infant to osteopenia. Rare conditions resulting in severe fractures in the newborn include the homozygous inactivating mutation of the *CASR* gene and mutations of type I collagen genes leading to OI.

Mutations of Calcium-Sensing Receptor Gene

In the newborn, homozygous inactivating mutations of the *CASR* gene lead to insensitivity to calcium concentrations with a resultant hyperparathyroid state. The heterozygous condition causes benign familial hypocalciuric hypercalcemia (FHH), a disorder characterized by slightly elevated calcium levels but no associated pathology. Conversely, the homozygous state leads to neonatal severe hyperparathyroidism (NSHPT), with fractures at birth associated with very poorly formed and osteoporotic bones. There also are less common mutations of *CASR* that have a dominant negative inactivation. These heterozygous mutations result in a clinical state that is more severe than FHH, with the newborn often having poorly developed bones, some fractures, and hypercalcemia, but generally the condition is less clinically severe than NSHPT. Equally as rare in the newborn are the severe forms of OI (types II and III), as discussed later.

Osteogenesis Imperfecta

OI is an inherited disorder that occurs due to gene mutations (at least 200 gene mutations) of type I collagen genes. The disorder is inherited in general in an autosomal dominant mode. However, there are significant numbers of children born with new gene mutations that are then transmitted in a dominant mode of inheritance, as well as the relatively uncommon patients with OI due to autosomal recessive gene inheritance. In the past, OI was classified as osteogenesis imperfecta congenita and tarda, distinguishing those children with clinical presentations early, including the severely affected infant who often died in utero, and those with more mild forms presenting later in life with fractures. During the past 30 years, with genetic discoveries, the classification of OI was divided into four types, as summarized in Box 13-1, originally so classified by Sillence in 1973. Because there is considerable overlap with genotype and phenotype expression, it is at times difficult to actually separate the four types clinically. As well, the variable expression makes the incidence

difficult to ascertain, including the fact that perhaps some have been diagnosed as having juvenile idiopathic osteoporosis.

Clinical manifestations of OI vary from the most severe perinatal lethal variety (type II) to a mild form, with some nondeforming fractures and normal stature (type I). A summary of the different clinical manifestations is included in Box 13-1. Type I, which is most mild form of OI, which may also be the most common. This form is manifested by frequent fractures, sometimes as early as in the perinatal period. In addition, these children have blue sclera, a high incidence of hearing loss, and dental abnormalities, but the fractures heal relatively well with good callus formation. The fracture rate may be very high or only a small number of fractures. The lack of bony deformities and normal stature is most consistent with type I. The fracture rate appears to decrease after puberty, suggestive that the gonadal hormones aid in improving the bone density in this type of OI. The various types clinically overlap, although the most severe form demonstrates marked bony deformities at birth and the infant may die in utero. The infants are born with very dark sclera, soft calvaria, beaked nose, thin beaded ribs, and fractures in the long bones and often die soon after birth. Most characteristically, the infants have telescoped femurs and bowed tibias. The diagnosis is recognizable by most pediatric radiologists. Most genetic studies, despite the presence of a few families with multiple siblings born with this form (which is believed to be a germline mutation), appear to be new autosomal dominant gene mutations. The other intermediate types (types III and IV) overlap types I and II. Type III is similar initially to type II at birth, with thin calvaria and in utero fractures. The sclerae are, however, light blue (not dark) and may become blue-gray in time. If there are no fractures at birth, fractures occur in life and the healing is poor. The bones appear to be soft and bowing occurs.

TYPE	INHERITANCE	PRESENTATION
I	Autosomal dominant	Fractures, decreased bone mineral density, blue sclerae, and hearing loss but normal height, and scoliosis uncommon. (Mildest form)
II	Autosomal dominant (new mutations) Rare autosomal recessive	Lethal in utero and neonatal period. Very dark sclerae. Severe osteoporosis with severe deformities of skull, clavicles, femur, and ribs noted at birth.
III	Autosomal dominant Rare autosomal recessive	May have fractures at birth but progressive fractures, bone deformities, markedly short stature, dental abnormalities, and hearing loss. Sclerae are blue-gray.
IV	Autosomal dominant	Mild but deforming, sclerae are normal to light blue-gray. Mild short stature, fractures with mild bone deformities. Also have hearing loss and dental abnormalities.

Box 13-1   Major Classifications of Osteogenesis Imperfecta

These children often have poor healing, microfractures, and cyst-like lesions in the epiphyses. These poorly healing and frequent fractures result in marked short stature. Many of the children develop marked kyphoscoliosis, which is virtually impossible to treat because of the poor bone formation. Type IV is often similar to type I, the mild form, but patients usually have fractures at birth or early in life. By age 2 years, short stature may become apparent. The sclerae are light gray to normal. The fractures are generally frequent, the healing is not normal, and bowing occurs. Scoliosis is common in this form and adult stature is generally less than the 25th percentile of the adult population. The fracture rate, like type I, decreases after puberty but is greater than expected with aging, especially in postmenopausal women.

Management and Treatment Options

Infants born with severe fractures and clinical findings consistent with OI types II and III and variations of NSHPT require expert guidance. Consultations must be obtained with surgeons, geneticists, orthopedic surgeons, and endocrinologists. The first order is to distinguish infants with neonatal fractures as to etiology, because therapy may be very different, such as metabolic disorders causing poorly formed bones (I cell disease and other storage disorders). Patients with more severe forms of OI have been treated with a number of bone formation therapies, including calcitonin injections and even bone marrow transplantation. More recently, there are increasing positive reports using bisphosphonate therapy for OI patients. Bisphosponates are antiresorptive drugs that interfere with osteoclast activity. The fractures in the more severe form are very difficult to deal with and generally treated conservatively. The neonates with NSHPT and the severe forms of calcium-sensing receptor–inactivating gene mutations are severely hyperparathyroid and require parathyroidectomy as a life-saving procedure. These infants die of respiratory problems due to the lack of skeletal development of their ribs. Temporizing therapies include intravenous saline, furosemide, and injections of calcitonin. These patients require subsequent treatment of the hypoparathyroid state. A more complete discussion of therapy and the antihypercalcemic agents, including the bisphosphonates, is provided in Chapter 12.

Children and Adolescents

The finding of osteoporosis in older children and adolescents who have been relatively well is often serendipitous, seen on a radiograph taken after a fracture that suggests osteopenia. There are no incidence data available regarding the number of fractures that are normal for the pediatric age group. Certainly an "unusual" number of fractures occurring after minor injury should raise the suspicion of the cli-

nician as to the possibility of a bone disorder. There are known iatrogenic causes of osteoporosis, such as treatment for malignancy with radiation and chemotherapy or chronic glucocorticoid therapy. There are conditions that are associated with fractures, such as the McCune-Albright syndrome with polyostotic fibrous dysplasia. Box 13-2 lists the primary endocrine and other disorders associated with osteoporosis. The endocrine disorders, other than hypogonadism, cause osteopenia by mobilizing calcium from bone. The osteoporosis due to rickets, malabsorption syndrome, and acquired immune deficiency syndrome is related to vitamin D deficieny and malnutrition. Renal disease can cause tubular phosphate loss, inherited as an X-linked dominant disorder (vitamin D–resistant rickets), or phosphate retention in chronic renal failure with resultant renal rickets and secondary hyperparathyoidism.

Box 13-2 Differential Diagnosis of Osteoporosis

NEWBORNS AND INFANTS
Homozygous familial hypercalcemic hypocalciuria
Neonatal primary hyperparathyroidism
Maternal vitamin D deficiency
Renal disease
Vitamin D deficiency
Vitamin D dependency
Hypophosphatemic rickets
Osteogenesis imperfecta

CHILDREN AND ADOLESCENTS
Hyperparathyroidism
Hyperthyroidism
Hypogonadism
Cushing syndrome
Rickets
Malabsorption syndromes
Acquired immune deficiency sysndrome
Renal disease
Malignancies—leukemia or parathyroid hormone–related proteins
Medications
 Anticonvulsants
 Antimalignancy chemotherapy, radiation
 Immunosuppressive agents
 Glucocorticoids
Behavioral
 Immobilization
 Anorexia nervosa
 Drug abuse
Primary bone disorders
 Polyostotic fibrous dysplasia
 Osteogenesis imperfecta
 Juvenile idiopathic osteoporosis

Malignancies

Malignant conditions can involve bone, such as sarcomas or metastatic lesions. However, certain malignancies, especially of the reticuloendothelial system, often cause a generalized osteoporosis. This can occur in leukemias and lymphomas in children but is especially likely in adults with multiple myeloma. Certain malignancies seem to produce a parathyroid-like humoral substance or PTHrP that causes phosphate loss and hypercalcemia. In general, these latter patients have severe life-threatening hypercalcemia that is of greater concern than for bone disease.

In terms of osteoporosis, it is more likely that it is the primary oncology treatments, both radiation and chemotherapy, including glucocorticoids, that are the primary causes of osteopenia in children surviving malignancy. The successes over the past several decades in terms of treatment of malignant disease in children have led to a greater need to evaluate the late effects of oncologic therapies. These children who survive cancer often develop primary endocrine dysfunctions that contribute to osteopenia, including growth hormone deficiency and hypogonadism. As well, there is clear evidence of osteoporosis in young adults treated with radiation and chemotherapy who have osteoporosis without endocrine or nutritional deficiency.

Iatrogenic Osteoporosis

A number of medications can affect bone modeling, resulting in osteopenia. Anticonvulsants, such as phenytoin, alter vitamin D metabolism by increasing hydrolysis of vitamin D. The resultant polar metabolites of 25-hydroxyvitamin D (e.g., 24,25-dihydroxyvitamin D) are rapidly excreted and not available for conversion to the active form of vitamin D (i.e., 1,25-dihydroxyvitamin D). Thus, the patients on anticonvulsant therapy have a lack of active 1,25-dihydroxyvitamin D, essentially resulting in vitamin D–deficient osteopenia.

The most common iatrogenic cause of osteoporosis during childhood is related to chronic glucocorticoid use. Glucocorticoids are prescribed (albeit less frequently now) for severe asthma but remain a mainstay for the treatment of inflammatory bowel disease, nephrotic syndrome, and other autoimmune inflammatory diseases (e.g., lupus, rheumatoid arthritis). Glucocorticoids cause both bone resorption and decreased bone formation. The decreased bone formation is due to inhibition of the osteoblasts. As well, glucocorticoids inhibit calcium gastrointestinal absorption of calcium and phosphorus. In turn, there is a secondary rise in PTH with a resultant hypercalciuria and hypophosphaturia. The osteoporosis in chronic glucocorticoid use is often so severe that the children fail to grow, have markedly delayed bone age, and develop vertebral and hip fractures.

Juvenile Idiopathic Osteoporosis

Juvenile idiopathic osteoporosis (JIO) is clearly a diagnosis of exclusion. Box 13-2 lists the disorders that must be excluded, some of which are more clearly identifiable than other conditions. JIO occurs in the peripubertal or younger child, especially during periods of rapid growth. It is reported that a sudden loss of bone mass appears to be discovered because of a recent onslaught of frequent fractures and bone pain. Evaluation finds relatively severe osteoporosis without a discernible cause. The age of onset varies from 5 years to 16 years, and the problem often remits within several years, especially with puberty. Frequently, the earliest symptom is a gradual onset of pain in the lower extremities with subsequent fractures occurring. There can be physical sequelae, including kyphosis, bowed legs, and loss of height and bone deformities. The most important consideration is to rule out possible treatable disorders and then embark on a program of treatment and rehabilitation in an effort to prevent physical sequelae. It is possible that JIO may be forms of yet undiscovered variants of OI or other genetic bone disorders.

Management and Treatment Options

In older children and adolescents, a history of fractures to a degree that the clinician becomes concerned about the possibility of osteoporosis requires, first, a careful assessment of lifestyle, nutritional history, and past medical history as well as examination. The possibility of previous therapies, such as chronic glucocorticoid exposure or immobilization, raises the real possibility of osteoporosis. The history of known medical disorders associated with loss of bone, such as hypogonadal disorders, growth hormone deficiency, and brain tumor survival, raises further clinical concern of osteoporosis. The physical findings of blue sclerae or limb disproportion, scoliosis, kyphosis, or rachitic changes are of equal clinical significance.

If the clinician is concerned that there is a significant risk for osteopenia, the child should have an evaluation of bone density with a DEXA scan (recognizing that DEXA scans overestimate osteopenia in short children, such as glucocorticoid-induced growth failure and osteoporosis). Furthermore, the DEXA scan should be performed in an institution with appropriate standards for children (as discussed earlier). Children with a BMD standard deviation score (Z-score) of −1 to −2.5 SDs is defined as being *osteopenic*. Children with a BMD Z-score of less than −2.5 SDs is defined as having *osteoporosis*. If the concern was raised by the frequency of fractures, then the subsequent finding abnormal bone density by DEXA indicates the need for diagnostic as well as therapeutic measures.

The clinician can at least maximize nutritional intake of calcium and vitamin D. Biochemical studies should include a complete blood cell count to evaluate for anemia and a biochemical panel that includes liver function tests, renal function, calcium, phosphorus, and alkaline phosphatase. Measurements of 25-hydroxyvitamin D and 1,25-dihydroxyvitamin D and intact PTH should be made. Referral to a geneticist to rule out the possibility of OI may be necessary because the more mild forms of OI, unless blue sclerae are present, may be difficult to distinguish from juvenile idiopathic osteoporosis without genetic studies. In severe osteoporosis, whether due to OI, JIO, or a known iatrogenic cause, such as glucocorticoid-induced osteoporosis, therapies may need to be more aggressive. As an example, in older children, if fractures are extremely frequent and mobility is limited, orthopedic surgeons have used rods during treatment to stabilize the spine or limbs. Similarly, if osteoporosis is severe and fractures frequent, injections of calcitonin have been tried but the bisphosphonates may be the drug of choice. There was (and still is) some concern that these drugs, which interfere with osteoclast activity and bone resorption, may also cause premature fusion of growth epiphyses. However, recent reports, especially in children with OI, have been very positive, and the use of these drugs is expanding into other areas of osteoporosis in childhood and adolescence. If the osteoporosis is severe with multiple fractures and calcitonin therapy is inadequate, bisphosphonates can be used chronically either intravenously or orally. For chronic therapy, pamidronate can be given as 0.5 to 1.0 mg/kg/dose for 3 days every 4 to 6 months or as a single administration every 3 to 4 weeks. In addition, oral forms of bisphosphonates are available as a daily dose or a weekly dose.

The common adverse effects of bisphosphonates include fever, flu-like symptoms, nausea, dyspepsia, esophagitis, abdominal pain, diarrhea, gastrointestinal bleeding, abnormal taste, iritis, conjunctivitis, scleritis, hypocalcemia, and hypophosphatemia. Therefore, bisphosphonates are contraindicated in patients with achalasia and esophageal stricture and relatively contraindicated in patients with gastroesophageal reflux.

CONCLUSIONS

Bone health in pediatrics is still a developing science. Despite the technological advances such as DEXA and quantitative CT in assessing bone density and bone mineral content, normative data based upon variations in height, weight, and pubertal development for children have not yet been established. What is considered a "normal" number of fractures for active children to distinguish those children with an "abnormal" number of fractures in

order for the clinician to decide that bone health assessment is necessary is not yet defined. However, it is clear that bone health of children is within the purview of the pediatricians, and progress in this area must be of major interest for pediatricians.

The differential diagnosis of the cause of osteoporosis is age dependent. Osteoporosis in children and adolescents is most frequently due to iatrogenic causes, such as the chronic use of corticosteroids and chemotherapy for treatment of pediatric cancers. In the younger child, child abuse must be suspected as a cause of frequent fractures. Nutritional deficiencies, occasionally due to changes in dietary fashions, can result in lack of appropriate vitamins and minerals leading to decreased bone density and osteoporosis. Genetic causes, such a osteogenesis imperfecta and mutations of the calcium-sensor gene, must be entertained in the newborn with multiple fractures and in children with severe osteoporosis.

Therapy should be directed to the root cause if possible, such as appropriate vitamin needs. Parathyroidectomy may be necessary in those infants with a mutation of the calcium sensor gene. Newer medical therapies, including calcitonin, bisphosphonates, and parathyroid hormone are still being evaluated in pediatric use.

MAJOR POINTS

Osteoporosis is a concern for pediatricians because helping children to achieve an appropriate peak bone density can reduce a major health risk in the future.

A major problem is the ascertainment of decreased bone density because normative data for children are not available in many institutions. The dual-energy X-ray absorptiometry (DEXA) scan is appropriate only if normative data are available for children; the DEXA scan overestimates the degree of osteopenia in short children.

Puberty or the lack of puberty also can result in misinterpretation of bone density determinations even if normative data for age are available. There are almost no normative data for bone density relating to stages of pubertal development.

Osteoporosis in childhood is most often due to iatrogenic causes, such as glucocorticosteroid therapy or radiation and chemotherapy.

In severe osteoporosis, if not due to medical treatments, osteogenesis inperfecta syndromes and juvenile idiopathic osteoporosis are diagnoses to be considered.

In severe osteoporosis associated with frequent fractures, first-line treatment is to increase calcium and vitamin D supplementation. If inadequate, the use of calcitonin and bisphosphonates may be necessary.

SUGGESTED READINGS

Brumsen C: Long-term effects of bisphosphonates on the growing skeleton, Medicine 1997;76:266.

Leonard MB, Zemel BS: Current concepts in pediatric bone disease, Pediatr Clin North Am 2002;49:143.

Paterson CR: Osteogenesis imperfecta and other heritable disorders of bone, Baillieres Clin Endocrinol Metab 1997;11:195.

Smith R: Idiopathic juvenile osteoporosis: experience of twenty-one patients, Br J Rheumatol 1995;34:68.

Srivastava T: Bisphosphonates: from grandparents to grandchildren, Clin Pediatr 1999;38:687.

VASOPRESSIN AND DISORDERS OF FLUIDS AND ELECTROLYTES

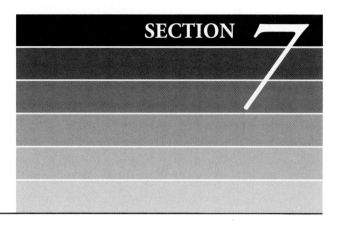

SECTION 7

CHAPTER 14

Hormonal Control of Fluid and Electrolytes

ROBERT J. FERRY, JR.

INTRODUCTION

Electrolyte homeostasis is essential for normal growth and development. Four endocrine subsystems exert continuous control over fluid and electrolytes: the renin-angiotensin-aldosterone axis, the neurohypophyseal antidiuretic hormone arginine-vasopressin (AVP), thirst, and atrial natriuretic peptide (ANP). Chapter 10 discusses adrenal mineralocorticoid physiology, so this chapter primarily considers the contributions of the other three subsystems. Thyroid hormone and adrenal glucocorticoids also regulate fluid homeostasis but are not the primary focus of this discussion.

OSMORECEPTOR-MEDIATED AND NONOSMOTIC ENDOCRINE RESPONSES TO DEHYDRATION

The most common fluid disturbance occurring in the pediatric population is acute volume depletion, usually as a result of increased sensible losses (diarrhea), increased insensible losses (tachypnea, fever, sweating), or inadequate intake (anorexia, inanition). The author assumes that the reader has conducted a history and physical examination of

the patient and is now deciding the etiology of dehydration or hypervolemia based on this information. Consideration of osmolality is a useful approach to understanding fluid disorders related to posterior pituitary physiology, because osmolality serves both as a stimulus and as a clinical outcome in fluid homeostasis. By definition, osmolality is the ratio of solute content per liter of water (mOsm/L, or mOsm/kg because 1 L of water weighs 1 kg). Sodium, urea, and glucose comprise the primary solutes determining extracellular fluid (ECF) volume. Serum osmolality can be estimated by calculating the sum of their relative contributions as follows:

$$2 \cdot [\text{serum Na (mEq/L)}] + [\text{serum glucose (mg/dL)}/18] + [\text{blood urea nitrogen (mg/dL)}/2.8]$$

(Although seldom of clinical relevance in pediatric patients, one should add the terms $2 \cdot [\text{serum K (mEq/L)}]$ or $[\text{ethanol (mg/dL)}/4.6]$ in the appropriate circumstance.) Calculated serum osmolality should be compared to the actual measured serum osmolality. The difference between the calculated and the measured serum osmolality normally ranges between -3 and $+3$. If the value exceeds $+3$, the clinician should ascertain the identity of the additional osmolyte(s). The usual suspects in this search are ethanol, ethylene glycol, methyl alcohol, and isopropyl alcohol.

A 2% rise in ECF osmolality stimulates independent osmoreceptors of the hypothalamus regulating AVP release and thirst. AVP increases water resorption at the renal collecting duct (Figure 14-1). Hypervolemia stimulates high-pressure baroreceptors of the carotid sinus, aortic arch, and heart ventricles, leading to release of brain and atrial natriuretic peptides. In human serum, α-ANP is the predominant natriuretic peptide and constitutes a major feedback loop that inhibits several distinct endocrine effects. Among effects inhibited by α-ANP are AVP-induced antidiuresis, aldosterone-induced sodium reabsorption, and vasoconstriction by diverse hormones (see Figure 14-1). The oropharyngeal reflex is another potent inhibitor of AVP release. Ingestion of any fluid (hypotonic, isotonic, or hypertonic), cold water above all, inhibits AVP release even before absorption of the water from the gut. Ingestion of solids does not appear to stimulate the oropharyngeal reflex.

A drop in ECF volume stimulates low-pressure baroreceptors of the pulmonary capillaries, cardiac atria, and right ventricle as well as the renal juxtaglomerular mechanism. The juxtaglomerular apparatus induces aldosterone release from the adrenal cortex (zona glomerulosa), which increases renal reabsorption of sodium (see Figure 14-1). Angiotensin II action also stimulates aldosterone release, potentiating mineralocorticoid effects.

RENAL HANDLING OF SODIUM

Aldosterone physiology is detailed in Chapter 10. Briefly, renal reabsorption of sodium occurs via the sodium-potassium (Na^+/K^+) transporter, an ion channel driven by

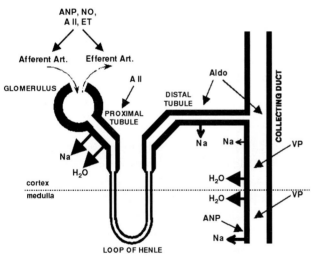

Figure 14-1   Renal actions of atrial natriuretic peptide (ANP), arginine vasopressin (AVP), aldosterone (aldo), nitric oxide (NO), and angiotensin II (A II). ANP vasodilates afferent arterioles, vasoconstricts efferent arterioles, and inhibits sodium reabsorption in the medullary collecting tubule. AVP inhibits water excretion in the cortical and medullary portions of the collecting duct. ANP overrides the antidiuretic action of AVP at the distal collecting tubule. Aldosterone stimulates sodium reabsorption in the distal tubule and cortical section of the collecting duct, and aldosterone also stimulates potassium loss at the distal tubule (not shown). Nitric oxide vasodilates both afferent and efferent arterioles, while increasing interstitial pressure by inhibiting sodium and water reabsorption in the proximal tubule. Renal autonomic nerves and angiotensin II vasoconstrict both afferent and efferent arterioles while enhancing sodium and water reabsorption in the proximal tubule. Endothelin vasoconstricts both afferent and efferent arterioles. (Adapted with permission from Martin P-Y, Schrier RW: Renal sodium excretion and edematous disorders, Endocrinol Metab Clin North Am 1995;24:459 © WB Saunders Co.)

ATP hydrolysis. To maintain electroneutrality across the cell membrane, one potassium cation and two chloride anions are exchanged with each sodium cation. Hyperaldosteronism is rare in childhood; Box 14-1 summarizes the most frequent etiologies of hyperaldosteronism. Paradoxically, chronic hyperaldosteronism does not cause hypernatremia or edema. The first reported patient with hyperaldosteronism, who was reported by Conn in 1955, displayed a single adrenal adenoma with hypokalemia and asymptomatic hypertension. This classic presentation probably represents downregulation of the receptor(s) for the sodium-retaining action of the mineralocorticoid combined with the activation of the atrial natriuretic peptide as a "pop-off" valve. The hallmark of chronic hyperaldosteronism is potassium depletion that presents as muscle cramps, weakness, tetany, or periodic paralysis.

The more common fluid disturbance in infants related to aldosterone physiology is salt wasting, most often in the setting of adrenal enzymatic defects (classically, 21-α-hydroxylase deficiency). Cortisol potentiates the mineralocorticoid action of aldosterone. In the combined absence of mineralocorticoids and glucocorticoids, tremendous natriuresis can occur with consequent diuresis. The physician should remember that the classic presentation of salt wasting due to 21-α-hydroxylase deficiency (one form of congenital adrenal hyperplasia) is hyponatremic dehydration, with hyperkalemia secondary to metabolic acidosis, that presents as dehydration toward the end of the first week of life. The delayed presentation of this congenital disorder is due to transplacental import of maternal steroids protecting the fetus, an effect that disappears over the first few days of life.

In normal physiology, renal sodium excretion is offset by 60% reabsorption at the proximal tubule and an additional 20% at the loop of Henle and distal convoluted tubule respectively (see Figure 14-1). Falling sodium delivery to the distal tubule or a drop in renal perfusion pressure induces the juxtaglomerular cells to secrete renin. Renin induces angiotensin II production, which increases vascular

---

Box 14-1   Endocrine Etiologies of Hypertension due to Sodium Retention

Exogenous glucocorticoid excess
Primary hyperaldosteronism
    Cortical adenoma (Conn syndrome)
    Bilateral adrenal cortical hyperplasia
Hypercortisolism
    Cushing disease
    Cushing syndrome
17α-hydroxylase deficiency
11-hydroxylase deficiency

tone and aldosterone release (see Figure 14-1). The resultant sodium retention draws water to the intravascular space. If overcompensation to hypo-osmolality occurs, such as excessive water intake, ANP is released.

ANP release occurs primarily when hypervolemia stretches the atrial muscle. ANP directly counteracts the antidiuretic effect of vasopressin at the renal collecting duct by increasing sodium excretion (natriuresis), which forces obligate water excretion (diuresis) (see Figure 14-1). The intracellular action of ANP occurs proximal to the antidiuretic effect of vasopressin, which stimulates adenylate cyclase (as demonstrated by the lack of ANP effect on cAMP- or forskolin-stimulated water flow in isolated rabbit cortical collecting tubules). In the syndrome of inappropriate ADH secretion (SIADH), hypervolemia stimulates ANP release, which serves as a pop-off valve preventing hypertension. In addition to hypervolemia, a drop in ECF osmolality induces ANP release via the autonomic nervous system. Thus, a hypotonic fluid challenge stimulates ANP release, leading to natriuresis and diuresis of the free water load. Clinical disorders of the natriuretic peptides are discussed in further detail at the end of this chapter.

SODIUM INTAKE AND REPLACEMENT

Daily sodium requirements in infants and young children typically range between 3 and 6 mEq/kg of body weight. Sodium requirements increase most dramatically with salt wasting, hemorrhage, or diarrhea and, to a lesser degree, with fever or emesis. As discussed in detail at the end of this chapter, salt wasting in children resulting from abnormal release of ANP can increase daily sodium requirements in excess of 20 mEq/kg body weight! Close, serial monitoring of serum sodium level, the hydration status, and select serum electrolyte levels guides clinical management. Salt replacement should include maintenance requirements as well as ongoing losses. Ongoing losses can be estimated from the initial urinary sodium excretion rate. Unfortunately, in many clinical settings the urinary sodium excretion rate is reported too slowly to guide management of the patient. The rate of restoration of serum sodium level to the normal range should occur no faster than 10 mEq/L in each 24-hour period. To illustrate this critical point, a serum sodium level of 195 mEq/L would be corrected over no less than 5 days.

Salt may be administered orally to chronic salt wasters who lack definitive treatment, if the dose of sodium required to maintain eunatremia is known. A rounded tablespoon of standard household salt weighs about 6 g and contains approximately 250 mEq of sodium. (Although not the preferred course, the author has used this home remedy

to treat a child with cerebral salt wasting who was terminally ill under a "do not resuscitate" order, when the mother requested the least invasive intervention.)

Daily urinary potassium excretion in excess of 20 mEq in the presence of hypokalemia (serum potassium level <3.5 mEq/L) suggests inappropriate potassium wasting. A thorough evaluation to identify the underlying etiology is similar to the evaluation for hyponatremia as discussed in Chapter 10. In the event of renal potassium wasting, potassium chloride, which tastes uncomfortably bitter, can be administered orally in three or four divided doses daily, as needed to maintain eukalemia.

COUNTERREGULATORY RESPONSE TO VOLUME EXPANSION OR HYPEROSMOLALITY: THIRST AND ATRIAL NATRIURETIC PEPTIDE

Two primary mechanisms counteract the renin-aldosterone axis: thirst mediated by hypothalamic osmoreceptors and the release of ANP (previously called atrial natriuretic factor, atrial natriuretic hormone, cardionatrin, atriopeptin, auriculin, or cardiodilantin). A rise in serum osmolality is the primary stimulus for thirst. The presence of hypothalamic osmoreceptors for thirst was first demonstrated more than 50 years ago by Andersson, and clinical disorders of thirst first described in adults in 1976 were reported in children by 1986. The primary disorder of thirst is hypothalamic adipsia, which has also been called a *reset osmostat*. Hypothalamic lesions are the most common cause of reset osmostat in the pediatric population (Box 14-2). Reset osmostat can cause hyponatremia or hypernatremia. Hyponatremia results in more symptomatic dehydration than the same excursion of serum sodium level toward

---

Box 14-2 Etiologies of Disorders of Thirst (Reset Osmostat)

Hypothalamic tumor
Midline facial defects
  Holoprosencephaly [sonic hedgehog (*SHH*) mutation]—
    higher threshold to induce thirst results in
    hypernatremia
Cerebral palsy
Thyrotoxicosis—increased water ingestion due to stimulated
  thirst
Drugs
  Venlafaxine
  Ethanol—downset osmostat
Tuberculosis—downset osmostat

hypernatremia. Unless suspected by the astute clinician, reset osmostat resulting in hypernatremia often goes undetected, because affected children are typically neurologically compromised or institutionalized. Children most likely to possess a reset osmostat are those with congenital malformations of the midline central nervous system, and serum sodium level should be assessed during the initial, routine health maintenance visits and during any evaluation of growth failure. Chronic hypernatremia is associated with poor growth.

CLINICAL ASSESSMENT OF THIRST

The assessment of thirst is crucial to the management of fluid disorders. Intact thirst is confirmed by the history and is suggested if the infant's cry is soothed by fluid intake. Absent thirst, or hypothalamic adipsia, is apparent when the patient is not thirsty despite hypernatremia and should be suspected in patients with recurrent episodes of hypernatremic dehydration. Provocative testing may be required to assess thirst in patients unable to express their thirst adequately. Measurement of the urinary AVP level and plasma osmolality in response to 3% saline or volume challenge can distinguish reset osmostat from other disorders (Table 14-1).

The safest treatment for hypernatremia due to absent thirst is simply replacement of water to meet daily needs. The water dose should be administered enterally, because gastrointestinal absorption is efficient and regulated.

Daily water requirements vary dramatically with age and clinical status. Among several methods developed to estimate daily water requirements, in the early 1960s Holliday developed a method based on body surface area. A comparison with other methods is beyond the scope of this chapter; moreover, the author generally prefers the Holliday method for its practical utility on a busy clinical service. One convenient formula for determining body surface area is:

$$BSA\ (m^2) = \sqrt{\frac{Weight\ (kg) \times Height\ (cm)}{3600}}$$

Children generally require 1500 mL water/m^2 daily. The reader is referred elsewhere for discussion of the clinical investigations since the 1970s that developed adjustments for common clinical states, such as burns, diarrhea, fever, and so on.

ENDOCRINE LABORATORY ASSESSMENT OF DEHYDRATION AND HYPERVOLEMIA

The most useful, initial laboratory assessment for the differential diagnosis of fluid and electrolyte disorders is the common chemistry panel, which typically measures serum levels of sodium, potassium, chloride, bicarbonate, urea, glucose, and creatinine. Uric acid is also a useful test. Azotemia and hyperuricemia are reliable markers of ECF volume contraction. Specialized endocrine tests are indi-

---

Table 14-1 Tests to Distinguish Primary Disorders of Fluid Balance

Etiology	Plasma Osmolality (mOsm/kg)	Urinary Osmolality (mOsm/kg)	Δ[Plasma AVP] (pg/mL) After Volume or 3% Saline Challenge
Normal	285-295	50-1200, depending on hydration	Rise by at least 10
Primary hyperaldosteronism	285-295	100-1200	Rise by at least 10, but failure to suppress PAC*
Reset osmostat (hypernatremia)	295-320	>350 until rehydrated	No rise until plasma osmolality exceeds the reset threshold
Central diabetes insipidus (complete)	>295	<100	Below 1 at baseline and no rise
Central diabetes insipidus (partial)	>295	Not more than 800, even when hypernatremic	Below 5 at baseline and rise <10 from baseline
Essential hypertension	285-295	50-1000 depending on hydration	Normal
Nephrogenic diabetes insipidus	>295	<100	Normal
Psychogenic polydipsia	285-295	<100	Normal

AVP, arginine-vasopressin; PAC, plasma aldosterone concentration. An accepted protocol for volume challenge in children (with stable cardiac function) weighing between 10 and 50 kg body weight is administration of 30 mL/kg body weight of a 0.9% NaCl solution over 2 hours. Children weighing at least 50 kg may receive 2000 mL of 0.9% saline over 2 hours or 10 g NaCl daily for 3 days. Alternatively, 3% saline challenge can be used to raise serum sodium level to between 145 and 150 mEq/L.
*Volume challenge should not be administered to patients with a compromised cardiovascular system.

cated when this primary survey suggests an endocrine disorder. The most commonly considered tests are plasma renin activity and plasma aldosterone concentration. Figure 14-2 contrasts these laboratory values in disorders of aldosterone physiology.

Intense pediatric studies over the past decade have established ranges for plasma ANP levels across several conditions and gestational ages, but this result is seldom available in time to guide clinical management. In practice, plasma ANP levels do not distinguish the hyponatremic disorders of cerebral salt wasting and SIADH. Moreover, the conditions most often associated with elevated ANP levels (Box 14-3) are apparent clinically without this test. Due to its inhibitory role in fluid physiology, ANP deficiency could theoretically lead to uncontrolled hypertension, but no such disorder of primary ANP deficiency or resistance has been reported to date. When ANP deficiency occurs (as in low cardiac output with low atrial pressure), the lack of inhibition is probably compensated by other regulators of vascular tone, such as nitric oxide (NO). Nevertheless, valuable physiological insights from this research have been gained.

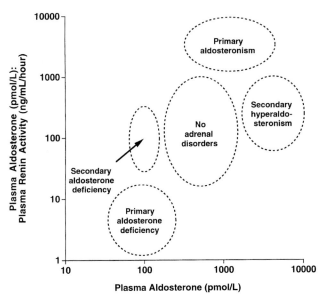

Figure 14-2 Laboratory findings that distinguish disorders of aldosterone action. The proper method for collection of the plasma to determine renin activity and aldosterone is to draw blood at 7 to 8 AM before the patient rises. The task is to keep the patient supine after sleep overnight. Properly collected in this manner, the plasma renin activity and plasma aldosterone concentration can be used to distinguish the disorders of aldosterone action, as noted in the figure. (Adapted with permission from White PC: Disorders of aldosterone biosynthesis and action, N Engl J Med 1994;331:253, as adapted from McKenna TJ, Sequeira SJ, Heffernan A, et al: Diagnosis under random conditions of all disorders of the renin-angiotensin-aldosterone axis, including primary hyperaldosteronism, J Clin Endocrinol Metab 1991;73:952, © The Endocrine Society.)

Box 14-3 Conditions Associated With Elevated Atrial Natriuretic Peptide Levels (in Peripheral or Umbilical Plasma)

Central hypervolemia
Respiratory distress
Prematurity
Hydrocephalus
Patent ductus arteriosus
Acute cardiac failure (unless atrial pressures are low)
Primary hyperaldosteronism
Chronic renal failure
Pregnancy (mild elevation)
Cirrhosis with ascites
Acute pulmonary embolus
Fetal distress
Systolic cardiac dysfunction due to doxorubicin

Although the renal threshold for sodium reabsorption at the proximal tubule rises over the second and third trimesters of gestation, the premature infant's ability to conserve sodium is significantly impaired. Postnatal salt loss is related to ANP release. Postnatal growth of premature infants improves significantly with sodium supplementation, and not simply as a result of water retention. Providing 4 to 5 mmol (or mEq) of sodium/kg daily to infants born under 34 weeks' gestational age for the first two postnatal weeks safely improves growth and electrolyte balance but should be delayed until 5% to 6% of the birth weight has been lost. ANP levels of infants are lower in the cerebrospinal fluid than in plasma, and plasma levels of brain natriuretic peptide are highest immediately after birth.

Undetectable plasma AVP levels in the setting of hypernatremia and dilute polyuria reliably confirm the diagnosis of diabetes insipidus. Plasma AVP levels can be elevated in both SIADH and nephrogenic diabetes insipidus, so these conditions are distinguished clinically by the history and clinical course. Further discussion of the endocrine laboratory evaluation of the posterior pituitary disorders was provided earlier.

CONCLUSIONS

The clinical approach to the management of fluid and electrolyte abnormalities in infancy and childhood begins with a careful history and a thorough physical examination to assess hydration status. Routine serum electrolyte and serum osmolality determinations guide the differential diagnosis. Serial assessment of serum electrolytes is indicated in conditions requiring salt administration. Chapters 15 and 16 detail the pathophysiology and management of diabetes insipidus, thirst disorders, SIADH, and salt wasting.

MAJOR POINTS

Renal, adrenal, cardiac, and hypothalamic endocrine mechanisms interface to regulate sodium and free water balance.

Outpatient screening for central diabetes insipidus begins with assessment of 24-hour urinary volume.

Water deprivation is the definitive diagnostic test for diabetes insipidus.

SUGGESTED READINGS

Al-Dahhan J, Haycock GB, Nichol B, et al: Sodium homeostasis in term and preterm neonates. III. Effect of salt supplementation, Arch Dis Child 1984;59:945.

Assadi FK, Agrawal R, Jocher C, et al: Hyponatremia secondary to reset osmostat, J Pediatr 1986;108:262.

Chevalier RL: The moth and the aspen tree: sodium in early postnatal development, Kidney Int 2001;59:1617.

Conn JW: Primary aldosteronism, a new clinical entity, J Lab Clin Med 1955;45:6.

de Bold AJ, Borenstein HB, Veress AT, et al: A rapid and potent natriuretic response to intravenous injection of atrial myocardial extract in rats, Life Sci 1981;28:89.

DeFronzo RA, Goldberg M, Agus ZS: Normal diluting capacity in hyponatremic patients, Reset osmostat or a variant of the syndrome of inappropriate antidiuretic hormone secretion, Ann Intern Med 1976;84:538.

Dillingham MA, Anderson RJ: Inhibition of vasopressin action by atrial natriuretic factor, Science 1986;231:1572.

Fitzsimons JT: Bengt Andersson's pioneering demonstration of the hypothalamic "drinking area" and the subsequent osmoreceptor/sodium receptor controversy, Acta Physiol Scand 1989;583:15.

Fleming SM, O'Gorman T, O'Byrne L, et al: Cardiac troponin I and N-terminal pro-brain natriuretic peptide in umbilical artery blood in relation to fetal heart rate abnormalities during labor, Pediatr Cardiol 2001;22:393.

Glasser L, Sternglanz PD, Combie J, et al: Serum osmolality and its applicability to drug overdose, Am J Clin Pathol 1973;60:695.

Hartnoll G, Betremieux P, Modi N: Randomised controlled trial of postnatal sodium supplementation on oxygen dependency and body weight in 25-30 week gestational age infants, Arch Dis Child Fetal Neonatal Ed 2000;82:F19 (comment in Arch Dis Child Fetal Neonatal Ed 2000;83:F160).

Hayakawa H, Komada Y, Hirayama M, et al: Plasma levels of natriuretic peptides in relation to doxorubicin-induced cardiotoxicity and cardiac function in children with cancer, Med Pediatr Oncol 2001;37:4.

Hill AR, Uribarri J, Mann J, et al: Altered water metabolism in tuberculosis: role of vasopressin, Am J Med 1990;88:357 (comment in Am J Med 1991;90:407).

Holliday MA, Potter D, Jarrah A, et al: The relation of metabolic rate to body weight and organ size, Pediatr Res 1967;1:185.

Holmstrom H, Hall C, Stokke TO, et al: Plasma levels of N-terminal proatrial natriuretic peptide in children are dependent on renal function and age, Scand J Clin Lab Invest 2000;60:149.

Modi N, Betremieux P, Midgley J, et al: Postnatal weight loss and contraction of the extracellular compartment is triggered by atrial natriuretic peptide, Early Hum Dev 2000;59:201.

Siberry G, Iannone R, eds: Harriet Lane Handbook, ed 15, Philadelphia, 2000, Harcourt Health Sciences.

Tulassay T, Khoor A, Bald M, et al: Cerebrospinal fluid concentrations of atrial natriuretic peptide in children, Acta Paediatr Hung 1990;30:201.

Yoshibayashi M, Kamiya T, Saito Y, et al: Plasma brain natriuretic peptide concentrations in healthy children from birth to adolescence: marked and rapid increase after birth, Eur J Endocrinol 1995;133:207.

Diabetes Insipidus

SARASWATI KACHE

ROBERT J. FERRY, JR.

INTRODUCTION

In his 1947 Croonian lecture at Cambridge University, Ernest Basil Verney summarized his work of over three decades to identify and characterize arginine-vasopressin (AVP) as the primary antidiuretic hormone (ADH). *Diabetes insipidus* (DI) is defined by large volumes of dilute urine and polydipsia that occur in the absence of intrinsic renal or adrenal disease. DI results from inadequate release of AVP by the posterior pituitary gland or from unresponsiveness of the renal collecting duct to AVP. Understanding this straightforward pathophysiology of DI facilitates both diagnosis and treatment.

PHYSIOLOGY

AVP is synthesized in the supraoptic and paraventricular nuclei of the hypothalamus and then transported within axons of the pituitary stalk to be stored in the posterior pituitary (pars distalis). Elevated serum osmolality is the prime stimulus for AVP release. *Osmolality* is defined as the ratio of solute content to water volume (expressed as mOsm/L or mOsm/kg for most fluids of biological relevance). Normal serum osmolality in humans is maintained within the narrow range of 280 to 295 mOsm/kg. Aquaporins, which are

water-specific channels in the distal renal collecting duct, play a pivotal role in maintaining normal serum osmolality by reabsorbing free water from the collecting ducts. AVP binds V_2 receptors on the basal epithelium of the distal renal collecting duct cells. These receptors are coupled to a G protein signal transduction system, which increases intracellular cyclic adenosine monophosphate (cAMP) levels. The elevated cAMP triggers protein kinase A (PKA), which induces translocation of aquaporin-2 channels to the luminal membrane of these ductal cells. To decrease serum osmolality, aquaporins transport water across the membrane, reabsorbing 10% to 20% of the water in the glomerular filtrate (water arriving at the collecting ducts has not been reabsorbed in the proximal nephron). Dehydration due to water losses in sweat, emesis, stools, or urine directly raises serum osmolality. It has been postulated that increased serum osmolality in the hypothalamus leads to water egress from the hypothalamic neurons and that the consequent physical changes in cellular volume trigger AVP release from the posterior pituitary.

THIRST

Thirst is a critical regulator of AVP release and therefore must be assessed by the clinician. The thirst center is located within the organum vasculosum of the lamina terminalis along the anterior wall of the third ventricle, close to the sites of AVP synthesis. Bengt Andersson of Stockholm, who worked extensively with goats from the 1940s on, first proposed "the drinking area" of the brain. Thirst receptors are distinct from the osmoreceptors, which regulate AVP secretion and respond at a higher threshold, specifically when serum osmolality rises above 295 mOsm/kg. The normal relationship between the increase in serum osmolality and thirst is linear; however, the set point for the osmoreception regulating AVP release is lower than that for thirst. Thus, the initial physiological response by the body to dehydration (or to increased serum osmolality) is to release AVP; thirst is a later adaptation to dehydration. Humans can maximize renal concentrating capacity to achieve urinary osmolality approaching 1200 mOsm/kg. (Incidentally, the most concentrated urine in the animal kingdom occurs in the Australian hopping mouse, which can achieve urinary osmolality in excess of 2000 mOsm/kg!) When serum osmolality rises despite maximal resorption of free water by the kidneys under the action of AVP, thirst is activated. Thirst is best satisfied by cold water, which triggers the oropharyngeal reflex. Indeed, the suppression of AVP release by this reflex occurs even before the absorption of ingested liquid across the bowel lumen, because contact of the oropharyngeal mucous membranes with liquid activates this reflex. Patients with DI who lack an intact thirst are at the highest risk of the development of hypernatremia.

DIFFERENTIAL DIAGNOSIS

Because DI is a rare cause of polyuria, screening should be performed to exclude more common etiologies of polyuria. The differential diagnosis of polyuria is considered in Table 15-1. Screening tests to be performed in the initial outpatient evaluation include serum electrolyte concentrations

Table 15-1   Differential Diagnosis of Polyuria

Diabetes mellitus	The most common cause of pathologic polyuria in the outpatient setting, hyperglycemia and glucosuria are the hallmarks of diabetes mellitus. Polyuria results from the increased solute load presented to the kidney.
Renal tubular acidosis (RTA)	Four types of RTAs exist, with types I and II being the most common. Patients with type I or type II RTA manifest hypokalemic, hyperchloremic, metabolic acidosis. Type III is normokalemic, hyperchloremic acidosis. Relative hypoaldosteronism constitutes type IV RTA, characterized by hyperkalemia, hyperchloremia, and hypernatremia. All forms of RTA result in nongap metabolic acidosis.
Fanconi syndrome	Impaired proximal tubular dysfunction causes polyuria, with impaired resorption of amino acids, glucose, phosphate, citrate, urate, and bicarbonate. Patients typically present with rickets.
Chronic renal failure	Intrinsic loss of urinary concentrating mechanism. Common signs and symptoms include elevated blood urea nitrogen, elevated serum creatinine level, anemia, renal osteodystrophy, and hypertension.
Urinary tract infections	Urine culture is positive for the infective organism or organisms.
Acute tubular necrosis	Signs of acute renal failure are present, e.g., elevated blood urea nitrogen level or elevated serum creatinine level. Polyuria usually develops as renal function improves. Common causes include ischemia, nephrotoxins, disseminated intravascular coagulation, and trauma.
Renal tubulointerstitial disease	Chronic tubulointerstitial disease may present as polyuria due to either vasopressin insensitivity or inability to concentrate the urine. Common causes include vesicoureteral reflux, chronic analgesic ingestion (particularly nonsteroidal anti-inflammatory drugs), and obstructive uropathy.
Cushing syndrome	Polyuria results from increased free water clearance. Classic findings of hypercortisolism include central obesity, moon facies, buffalo hump, protuberant abdomen, thin extremities, and hypertension. Other common signs are hyperglycemia, glucosuria, and hypokalemia. The most appropriate screening test is a 24-hour urinary excretion of free cortisol, which should be normalized to body surface area and repeated if the initial results are equivocal. A single, normal 24-hour urinary free cortisol value does not exclude hypercortisolism (Cushing syndrome); however, serial normal values exclude this disease. Hypercortisolism (Cushing syndrome) may occur from excess endogenous cortisol production or from exogenous steroid administration.
Primary hyperaldosteronism	Hypernatremia, hypokalemia, metabolic alkalosis, low plasma renin activity, and diastolic hypertension. The most common etiology is aldosterone-hypersecreting adrenal adenoma (Conn syndrome). Bilateral cortical nodular hyperplasia is another common etiology.
Primary polydipsia	The primary problem of inappropriate fluid intake is caused by dipsogenic diabetes insipidus (an abnormal thirst mechanism) or psychogenic polydipsia. This diagnosis can be distinguished from diabetes insipidus by the desmopressin challenge as described in the text. Psychogenic etiologies include schizophrenia and mania. Dipsogenic causes include granulomatous disease (e.g., sarcoid), vasculitis, and multiple sclerosis.
Adrenal insufficiency	This is caused by combined or isolated mineralocorticoid (e.g., aldosterone) and/or glucocorticoid (e.g., cortisol) deficiencies.
Cerebral salt wasting	Inappropriate release of natriuretic peptides induces natriuresis and obligate diuresis, resulting in hyponatremic dehydration. Occurs most commonly after neurosurgery and has been reported with various central nervous system injuries or chemotherapies. Inappropriate administration of exogenous antidiuretic hormone to salt wasters aggravates the hyponatremia.

(specifically, glucose, sodium, potassium, calcium, urea nitrogen, creatinine, and osmolality) and complete urinalysis (with urinary specific gravity and urinary osmolality). Classic findings for DI are elevations of serum sodium, blood urea nitrogen, creatinine, and calcium levels. With uncontrolled DI, urinary specific gravity is typically below 1.005, urinary osmolality below 300 mOsm/kg, and urinary-to-serum osmolality ratio below 1.

Clinicians distinguish two primary forms of DI: central (neurogenic) and nephrogenic. Central diabetes insipidus (CDI) results from inadequate production or release of vasopressin. Brain tumors and their treatment comprise the most common recognizable etiologies of CDI (Box 15-1). The most common causes of permanent nephrogenic DI (NDI) include congenital defects of the vasopressin receptors and aquaporins. Adverse effects of commonly administered medications are the most frequent causes of transient NDI. Other etiologies of NDI are summarized in Box 15-2. Partial NDI is defined as inadequate AVP release (i.e., inability to maximally concentrate the urine despite an appropriate stimulus [rising serum osmolality]). Patients with partial NDI demonstrate some response to AVP but do not maximally concentrate their urine in response to ADH.

The clinician should recognize the triphasic presentation of DI, which can develop after trauma or neurosurgery. During the initial phase, the patient develops polyuria lasting 4 to 8 days due to loss of regulation of AVP release after neuronal damage. The second phase is a pseudo-remission with antidiuresis lasting 1 to 14 days as a result of uncontrolled AVP release by dying neurons that produce the hormone. The final phase is permanent DI due to complete AVP deficiency from neuronal death.

DIAGNOSIS

A thorough history and physical examination should be acquired at initial consultation, although the diagnosis of DI is confirmed only by appropriate laboratory testing. The primary complaints include polyuria and polydipsia and, in children, enuresis. The clinician should pose questions about possible head trauma, previous neurosurgical procedures, endocrine deficiencies, current medications, congenital abnormalities, systemic disease processes (particularly those in Table 15-1), and family history of similar symptoms. Symptoms of hypernatremia include restlessness, irritability, lethargy, muscular twitching, seizures, nausea, and vomiting. At least 50% of patients with CDI have one or more anterior pituitary hormone deficiencies, with the most common being isolated growth hormone deficiency. Deficiencies of thyrotropin, corticotropin, follicle-stimulating hormone, and luteinizing hormone should be excluded by a complete eval-

Box 15-1   Etiologies of Central Diabetes Insipidus

Idiopathic
Head trauma
Postneurosurgery
Neoplasm
  Craniopharyngioma
  Meningioma
  Pituitary tumor
  Leukemia/lymphoma
  Metastatic tumor
  Pineal tumor
  Germinoma
  Glioma
  Benign cysts
Ischemia
  Brain death
  Sheehan syndrome
Infiltration
  Histiocytosis X (formerly called Letterer-Siwe disease)
  Sarcoidosis
  Wegener granulomatosis
  Bronchocentric granulomatosis
Infection
  Viral encephalitis
  Bacterial meningitis
  Tuberculosis
  Syphilis
  Blastomycosis
  Toxoplasmosis
Autoimmune (also called hypophysitis)
Congenital
  Familial (autosomal dominant)
  Prepro-arginine-vasopressin-neurophysin II mutation, http://www3.ncbi.nlm.nih.gov/htbin-post/Omim/dispmim?125700
  Septo-optic dysplasia (de Morsier syndrome): *HESX1* mutation, http://www3.ncbi.nlm.nih.gov/htbin-post/Omim/dispmim?182230
  DIDMOAD (Wolfram syndrome): diabetes insipidus with diabetes mellitus, optic atrophy, and deafness (WFS1 mutation), http://www3.ncbi.nlm.nih.gov/htbin-post/Omim/dispmim?606201#CLONING
  Hypopituitarism
  PIT1 mutation
  PROP1 mutation, http://www3.ncbi.nlm.nih.gov/htbin-post/Omim/dispmim?601538
Cytomegalovirus infection

uation. Begin with a careful assessment of the prior growth pattern and ascertain growth failure, anorexia, weakness, cold intolerance, behavioral changes, signs of hypotension, and pubertal development. Consult the endocrinologist if linear growth is below the third percentile, has dropped more than two curves on the standard growth chart, or is more than 2 SDs below the mid-parental height.

Box 15-2   Etiologies of Nephrogenic Diabetes Insipidus

Electrolyte disturbances
  Hypokalemia
  Hypercalcemia (resulting in hypercalciuria)
  Hypermagnesemia
Genetic (familial)
  X-linked dominant
    Vasopressin V_2 receptor (*AVP2R* mutation),
      http://www3.ncbi.nlm.nih.gov/omim/
  Autosomal recessive or autosomal dominant
    Aquaporin-2 water channel (*AQP2* mutation), OMIM
      222000427
Psychogenic polydipsia with loss of the medullary
  concentrating gradient
Cerebral salt wasting
  Neurosurgery
  Irradiation
  Head trauma
  Tumor-related: usually hypothalamic or pituitary
    neoplasms
  Fever
  Autonomic failure
Adrenal insufficiency
  Glucocorticoid deficiency
  Mineralocorticoid deficiency
Drugs
  Loop diuretics (e.g., furosemide)
  Diphenylhydantoin
  Reserpine
  Cisplatin
  Rifampin
  Ethanol
  Lithium: may become permanent
  Demeclocycline
  Chlorpromazine
  Volatile anesthetics
  Foscarnet
  Amphotericin B
  α-Interferon
  Mannitol
Chronic tubulointerstitial diseases
  Nephropathy of analgesic abuse
  Sickle cell nephropathy
  Multiple myeloma
  Amyloidosis
  Sarcoidosis
  Sjögren syndrome
  Autoimmune/lupus
  Renal medullary cystic disease
  Polycystic kidney disease

Physical examination should focus on the state of perfusion. Patients at the highest risk of developing severe dehydration are those with inadequate access to water (such as infants) and patients without an intact thirst mechanism (typically, patients with central neurological deficits). The

practitioner should identify any neurological deficits. Patients with hypernatremic dehydration classically have hyperreflexia, spasticity, seizures, or labored breathing. Masses or lesions of the central nervous system may cause specific focal deficits, including visual field deficits. The classic physical finding for a mass of the optic chiasm is bitemporal hemianopsia. Midline facial deformities, such as single central incisor, cleft lip or palate, or bifid uvula (which is associated with submucosal cleft palate), are frequently associated with abnormal pituitary function. Patients with CDI should be evaluated for anterior pituitary hormone deficiencies. Signs of panhypopituitarism include growth failure, precocious puberty, hypoactive deep tendon reflexes, dry skin, pallor, and myxedema.

LABORATORY EVALUATION

If the patient is hemodynamically stable and eunatremic and possesses an intact thirst, then urinary volume assessment can be performed at home. Instruct the patient (or parent) to collect all urine voided over a 24-hour period as follows. The patient should use the toilet immediately after waking in the morning and discard this specimen. The patient should measure and log the volume of each void produced over the subsequent 24 hours. If any sample is missed, the patient should abort the test and begin a new collection the next morning. Fluid intake must be unrestricted during this evaluation. Never restrict water intake unless the patient is hospitalized under close surveillance. Adjunct tests to be performed include early morning urinary osmolality with simultaneous serum sodium level and serum osmolality. If urine osmolality is at least 2 times higher than in serum, the patient does not have complete DI. If the patient's 24-hour urinary output exceeds 4 L/day in an adult or 2 L/m² in a child, then DI is likely. A convenient formula for estimating body surface area is

$$\text{BSA (m}^2) = \sqrt{\frac{\text{Height (cm)} \times \text{Weight (kg)}}{3600}}$$

In the absence of classic history such as surgical transsection of the pituitary stalk, the definitive diagnosis of DI entails a formal water deprivation test. Although it is the most sensitive and most specific test, the water deprivation test requires admission to the hospital for controlled sampling under the close supervision of the endocrinologist. The test should be performed when the clinical presentation is equivocal or when the clinician cannot distinguish partial CDI from an abnormal osmostat (abnormal thirst). Box 15-3 illustrates one accepted protocol for the water deprivation test and desmopressin challenge. Figures 15-1, 15-2, and 15-3 illustrate the correct interpretation of the water deprivation test.

Box 15-3 Provocative Tests to Distinguish Causes of Polyuria

FLUID (WATER) DEPRIVATION TEST

Allow access to fluid ad libitum the night before test.

Start fluid deprivation for 7 or 8 hours at 8 AM.

Measure serum osmolality, urine osmolality, urinary volume, and patient weight at the start of the test, every 2 hours during the test, and at completion of the test.

Also collect plasma antidiuretic hormone level at completion of test.

Test should be aborted if patient has greater than 5% weight loss or develops hemodynamic compromise.

DESMOPRESSIN CHALLENGE (IMMEDIATELY AFTER THE WATER DEPRIVATION TEST)

Administer desmopressin: 0.3 μg intramuscularly, intravenously, or subcutaneously or 10 μg intranasally.

Allow patient free access to fluids.

Determine urinary osmolality and volume 4 hours after administration.

Results are interpreted as follows.

| | AT THE END OF WATER DEPRIVATION | | AFTER DESMOPRESSIN CHALLENGE |
	Urine:Serum Osmolality	Plasma Arginine-Vasopressin (pg/mL)	Urine Osmolality (mOsm/kg)
Normal	>1	1-5	Over 800 mOsm/kg
Central DI	<1	<1	>50% rise
Nephrogenic DI	<1	>5	<50% rise
Primary polydipsia	>1	1-5	<10% rise
Partial DI	>1	1-5	<10% rise

DIFFERENTIATING PARTIAL DIABETES INSIPIDUS (DI) FROM PRIMARY POLYDIPSIA

Administer arginine-vasopressin daily for 4 days: 1 to 2 μg subcutaneously every 12 hours.

Monitor daily weight, plasma sodium, urinary volume, urinary osmolality, and intake of fluids.

Interpretation of results

 Resolution of polyuria and polydipsia indicates central DI.

 No effect indicates nephrogenic DI.

 Progressive thirst with hyponatremia indicates primary polydipsia (avoid hypo-osmolemia and hyponatremia).

Figure 15-4 presents the algorithm for the evaluation of suspected DI. Once the patient has been diagnosed with DI, it is imperative to determine the primary etiology. Patients with "idiopathic" CDI must undergo magnetic resonance imaging (MRI) to evaluate the hypothalamus, hypothalamic stalk, and pituitary. Loss of the normal, hyperintense signal of the posterior pituitary on T1-weighted MRI is noted in 94% of pediatric patients. On a scale from 1 to 9, appropriateness criteria developed in 1999 by the American College of Radiology rank MRI without contrast as an 8 and with contrast as 6 for imaging the brain when the diagnosis of DI is considered. The most concerning MRI findings include: (1) thickened pituitary stalk, suggestive of an infiltrative lesion such as histiocytosis; (2) ectopic posterior pituitary tissue, which is only noted in patients with neurohypophyseal pathology and not in normal subjects; and (3) hypoplastic anterior pituitary, which has frequently been associated with at least one anterior pituitary hormone deficiency.

Patients with any of these abnormal findings should undergo thorough endocrine evaluation, including provocative testing for deficiencies of anterior pituitary hormones as indicated by screening tests. Initial screening tests should include serum levels of insulin-like growth factor (IGF)-I (formerly called somatomedin C), IGF binding protein-3 (IGFBP-3), free serum thyroxine (T_4) level by equilibrium dialysis, and luteinizing hormone by a third-generation assay (such as immunochemiluminometric assay). Cerebrospinal fluid (CSF) sampling and biopsy are occasionally indicated to obtain informative cytology during the evaluation of a central nervous system mass and should be supervised by the neurologist or neurosurgeon. Detection of human chorionic gonadotropin in the CSF suggests a germinoma. Lumbar puncture to obtain CSF should not be performed if elevated intracranial pressure is suspected on the basis of the physical examination or radiographic studies. It is essential to remember that anterior pituitary hormone deficiencies, in particular, growth hormone deficiency, may present several years after the presentation of DI. Thus, ongoing visits for MRI of the brain and growth assessments should occur every 6 months for the first 3 years after the diagnosis of "idiopathic" CDI and annually thereafter for the life of the patient.

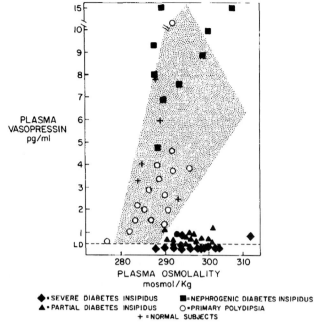

PLASMA VASOPRESSIN pg/ml

PLASMA OSMOLALITY mosmol/Kg

◆=SEVERE DIABETES INSIPIDUS   ■=NEPHROGENIC DIABETES INSIPIDUS
▲=PARTIAL DIABETES INSIPIDUS   ○=PRIMARY POLYDIPSIA
+ = NORMAL SUBJECTS

Figure 15-1 Plasma arginine-vasopressin (AVP) levels in relation to plasma osmolality during fluid deprivation. Patients with neurogenic diabetes insipidus (DI) or partial neurogenic DI display AVP levels below 1 pg/mL in the face of elevated serum osmolality. Patients with nephrogenic DI or dipsogenic DI have AVP levels greater than or equal to normal levels. Patients with partial DI partially concentrate their urine but cannot maximally concentrate their urine. Reset osmostat does not change the rate of rise in urinary osmolality but shifts the threshold for concentration to the right (parallel to the normal response). (With permission from Robertson GL: Differential diagnosis of polyuria, Annu Rev Med 1988;39:425.)

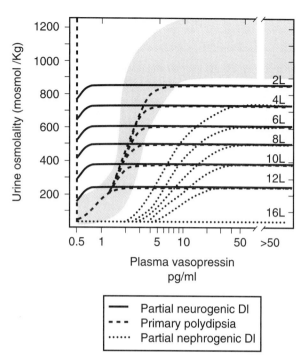

Urine osmolality (mosmol /Kg)

Plasma vasopressin pg/ml

—— Partial neurogenic DI
- - - Primary polydipsia
····· Partial nephrogenic DI

Figure 15-3 Relation of urinary osmolality to rising plasma vasopressin level in patients with partial diabetes insipidus (DI) and primary polydipsia. The vertical axis reflects daily urine output (2 to 12 L). The shaded area encompasses normal responses. Impaired urinary concentrating ability is directly proportional to the degree of polyuria. The rate of response of urinary concentration to rising plasma vasopressin level distinguishes partial central DI, partial nephrogenic DI, and primary polydipsia. (With permission from Robertson GL: Differential diagnosis of polyuria, Annu Rev Med 1988;39:425.)

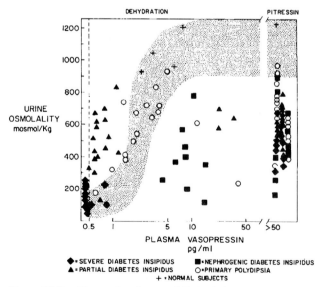

DEHYDRATION   PITRESSIN

URINE OSMOLALITY mosmol/Kg

PLASMA VASOPRESSIN pg/ml

◆=SEVERE DIABETES INSIPIDUS   ■=NEPHROGENIC DIABETES INSIPIDUS
▲=PARTIAL DIABETES INSIPIDUS   ○=PRIMARY POLYDIPSIA
+ = NORMAL SUBJECTS

Figure 15-2 Changes in urine osmolality and plasma vasopressin with fluid deprivation. The shaded area indicates the normal response. Patients with complete central diabetes insipidus (DI) show low plasma arginine-vasopressin (AVP) levels and low urinary osmolality. Patients with nephrogenic DI show inappropriately high AVP levels without a concomitant rise in urine osmolality. (With permission from Robertson GL: Differential diagnosis of polyuria, Annu Rev Med 1988;39:425.)

NDI is usually acquired rather than congenital. Medications commonly cause NDI. All patients with non-pharmacological NDI should undergo renal ultrasonography to exclude anatomic abnormalities, such as polycystic disease. Consultation by the nephrologist should be considered for any patient with NDI to evaluate underlying renal pathology and to exclude X-linked or autosomal recessive NDI. More than 90% of congenital DI is X-linked, caused by mutations of AVP receptor subtype 2. The autosomal recessive form is caused by mutations of the aquaporin-2 gene. Patients with congenital DI typically present as neonates with polyuria, irritability, and frequent vomiting. They have symptoms of constipation, unexplained fevers, poor skin turgor, and perhaps seizures if they develop hypernatremia. The infant may be treated for hypernatremic dehydration on multiple occasions before there is suspicion of NDI by an astute clinician. The long-term complications of untreated congenital DI include lower urinary tract dilation and obstruction, growth retardation, and poor development. Production of large volumes of urine is the most likely cause of urinary tract dilation. Consumption of noncaloric fluids to maintain adequate

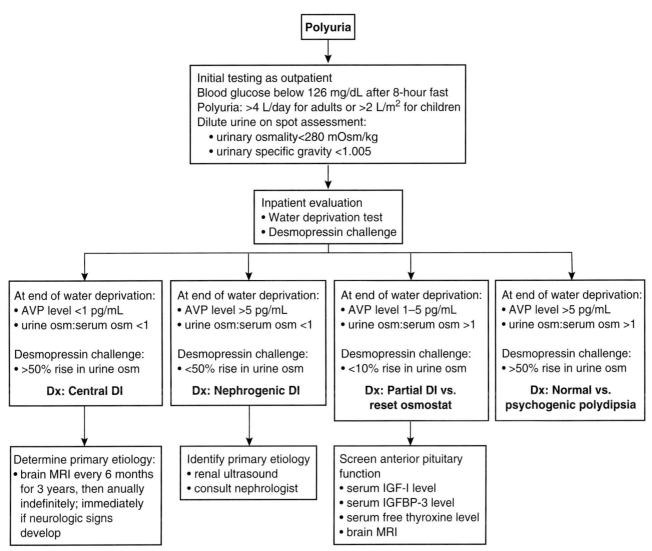

Figure 15-4   Algorithm for the evaluation of suspected diabetes insipidus.

hydration leads to growth retardation. Poor nutritional status in combination with intermittent hypernatremia may also lead to developmental delay. As expected, a delay in diagnosis in treatment increases the severity of developmental delay.

MANAGEMENT AND TREATMENT OPTIONS

Both pharmacological and nonpharmacological therapies are available to treat DI. The patient with an intact thirst and adequate access to water who develops DI maintains normal serum osmolality and eunatremia simply by drinking water. Drug therapy for patients with intact thirst improves quality of life by decreasing polyuria and polydipsia. Although inconvenient, simple fluid administration

always remains the safest and most effective method of managing DI in infants and in patients with dipsogenic DI (discussed later). Management of CDI in infants generally should not include exogenous ADH administration because infants receive their nutrition in liquid form (milk or formula). Consequently, antidiuresis can interfere with adequate caloric intake. These young patients with DI are best managed with dilute formula (one-tenth strength) provided ad libitum. Despite the attendant inconvenience of uncontrolled polyuria, simple fluid replacement therapy is safest with respect to growth and prevention of adverse events related to pharmacological therapy. Such management is usually best undertaken by the endocrinologist.

The approach to managing the critically ill patient focuses on restoring hemodynamic homeostasis. The patient presenting with shock (secondary to dehydration) should receive 20 mL isotonic fluid/kg body weight as initial resuscitation given as rapidly as possible. After initial resuscitation, the urinary output should be replaced with hypotonic fluid consisting of 2.5% dextrose in 0.22% saline to gradually restore eunatremia. If the urinary output is replaced with 5% dextrose in water, patients with large volume of urine will develop hyperglycemia and resultant glucosuria will aggravate polyuria. Dynamic DI (especially after neurosurgery) increases the risk of hyponatremia. A vasopressin infusion under management of an experienced physician provides rapid control and is easily titrated. The initial dose of a vasopressin drip is 0.25 to 1.0 mU/kg/hr and should be titrated as required to achieve eunatremia with urine output ranging from 2 to 3 mL/kg body weight each hour. Urinary output should be assessed hourly. Serum sodium level, serum osmolality, and urinary specific gravity should be checked every 4 to 6 hours whenever the patient receives a vasopressin infusion. Changes in urine specific gravity closely reflect the changes in vasopressin action, and this simple bedside test in conjunction with the serum sodium level represents the most effective and convenient assays for titrating the vasopressin infusion. The most significant adverse effect of vasopressin is potent vasoconstriction, which may aggravate existing central nervous system injury or cause myocardial compromise. This severe vasoconstriction can induce lactic acidosis by impairing tissue perfusion. Permanent DI is easily managed in the outpatient setting by analogues such as 1-deamino-8-D-argininevasopressin (desmopressin or DDAVP), which lack significant vasoconstrictive actions.

Because patients with DI are at risk of developing hypernatremia, proper management of this electrolyte disturbance is briefly discussed. Box 15-4 lists the differential diagnosis of hypernatremia. Hypernatremia can lead to dehydration along with tissue injury. The brain adapts to chronic hypernatremia by slowly accumulating intracellular osmolytes. Overly rapid correction of hypernatremia places the patient at risk of developing cerebral edema because these endogenous osmolytes cannot be eliminated quickly and they retain intraneuronal water. Hypernatremia is treated by providing sufficient water to replace the deficit, as estimated by the following equation:

$$\text{Free water deficit} = 0.6 \cdot \text{body weight (kg)} \cdot [(\text{plasma sodium level (in mEq/L)}/140) - 1]$$

The fluids used for replacement can either be enteral free water ad libitum, or the intravenous administration of hypotonic saline or 5% dextrose in water. The patient's ongoing fluid losses should also be replaced in addition to the original free water deficit. Hypernatremia should not be corrected any faster than 2 mM/hr nor faster than 10 mM over a 24-hour period. More rapid correction places the patient at high risk of developing cerebral edema and her-

---

Box 15-4   Etiologies of Hypernatremia

Free water loss
    Fever
    Hyperventilation
    Diabetes insipidus
Hypotonic fluid loss
    Gastrointestinal losses (e.g., vomiting or diarrhea)
    Renal losses (e.g., renal tubular acidosis)
    Loop diuretics
    Osmotic diuresis (e.g., hyperglycemia)
    Burns
Sodium overload
    Infusion of hypertonic solutions (e.g., 3% NaCl solution)
    Tube feedings with hypertonic solution
Decreased free water intake
    Inadequate access to free water
    Altered sensorium (e.g., intubated or sedated)
    Reset osmostat (hypothalamic adipsia)

---

niation. The nurse or physician should frequently assess the patient's neurological status during correction of the hypernatremia to monitor for symptoms of cerebral edema (e.g., headache, altered sensorium). The serum sodium level should be determined every 2 to 4 hours during correction to ensure that eunatremia is restored gently and slowly.

In the nonacute setting, the drug of choice for the treatment of CDI is DDAVP. DDAVP is a synthetic AVP analogue with a longer half-life, 10 to 100 times the native antidiuretic effect, but no vasopressor activity. (A unique side effect of DDAVP is release of coagulation factor VIIIc and von Willebrand factor. Thus, DDAVP has been used for coagulopathic patients with these factor deficiencies.) DDAVP is administered intranasally at a dose between 2.5 and 40 μg (10 μg/0.1 mL or per puff), daily or twice daily as needed to control polyuria. The absorption of intranasal DDAVP is highly variable depending on mucosal atrophy, scarring, nasal discharge, or congestion. DDAVP can also be administered subcutaneously at doses of 2 to 4 μg, either daily or twice as a day, with more reliable absorption than intranasal administration. The dose of oral DDAVP ranges from 0.05 to 0.8 mg, administered 2 or 3 times through the day as needed, reflecting the lower bioavailability of enteral dosing. DDAVP can be administered as a crushed or chewable tablet, or as an oral solution. All formulations are equally efficacious.

Patients receiving DDAVP should be allowed to have breakthrough polyuria at least once each day, and no less frequently than once each week. Such episodes of polyuria reduce the risk of water intoxication. Hyponatremia increases the risk of cerebral edema, and overly rapid correction of hyponatremia can result in central pontine myelinolysis. Breakthrough polyuria also allows monitoring for possible disease remission. Patients with DI after trauma or neurosurgery have been reported to recover AVP function as late as 10 years after the initial insult.

NDI is more challenging to treat than CDI, and the former patients typically require multiple medications to achieve adequate control. The mainstay of medical therapy is hydrochlorothiazide (or other thiazide diuretics) administered at a dose of 50 to 100 mg, 1 or 2 times each day. The thiazide diuretics induce natriuresis at the convoluted portion of the distal tubule, and the patient must be maintained on salt restriction to achieve this desired effect. Hypokalemia is the most concerning adverse effect of thiazide therapy, and patients may be switched to a potassium-sparing agent (e.g., amiloride). Amiloride, given daily or twice daily in 5- to 20-mg doses, is considered the drug of choice in patients with lithium-induced NDI. Prostaglandin prevents reabsorption of solutes in the medulla and antagonizes AVP action. Inhibitors of prostaglandin synthesis, such as indomethacin, at daily doses of 1.5 to 3.0 mg/kg body weight, have proved to be effective, particularly in conjunction with thiazide diuretics and desmopressin.

Partial DI should be treated according to its primary cause. Partial CDI may be treated with DDAVP alone or with chlorpropamide at doses of 100 to 500 mg, 1 or 2 times per day. Chlorpropamide stimulates AVP release from the hypothalamus and potentiates its renal effects. The primary adverse effect of chlorpropamide is hypoglycemia, which is of particular concern in children. Clofibrate and carbamazepine exert similar actions to chlorpropamide but are not favored due to more significant adverse effects. Adequate control of partial NDI usually requires a combination of DDAVP and diuretic (Table 15-2).

Patients with dipsogenic DI lack intact thirst. These patients should be prescribed a daily amount of water intake with or without DDAVP. The water prescribed for each day should be tailored to the individual patient and appropriately increased during periods of increased requirement (e.g., exercise). These patients or their caretakers should be vigilant for signs of dehydration, hyponatremia, and hypernatremia. The daily weight log guides fluid replacement.

The patient and/or parent should be educated about DI after the diagnosis is confirmed. Education includes understanding the treatment, proper administration of medications, and their potential side effects. Intranasal DDAVP is correctly administered by spray applied to the midportion of the nose to prevent runoff at the nare, with delivery beyond the turbinates. Patients should be supervised on the proper technique. Conditions affecting the absorption of DDAVP, such as nasal congestion or discharge, should be identified by the patient to prompt monitoring for symptoms of underdosing.

COMPLICATIONS AND MONITORING

Patients with DI are at risk of developing severe, symptomatic dehydration if they lack intact thirst. It is imperative,

---

Table 15-2   Pharmacological Management of Diabetes Insipidus

Medication	Primary Use	Mechanism of Action	Dosing	Side Effects
DDAVP (desmopressin, 1-desamino-8-D-arginine-vasopressin)	Chronic treatment of central DI	Antidiuretic hormone analog	10-40 µg, every 12-24 hours, intranasally	Irritation to mucous membranes
Vasopressin	Central DI in the ICU	Short-acting vasopressin	0.5-1.0 mU/kg/hr as continuous IV infusion*	Potent vasoconstrictor
Chlorpropamide	Partial central DI	Release of AVP from the hypothalamus and increase its renal effects	100-500 mg, every 12-24 hours, PO	Hypoglycemia
Thiazide diuretics	Nephrogenic DI	Increase sodium excretion by the kidney	50-100 mg, every 12-24 hours, PO	Hypokalemia
Amiloride	Lithium-induced nephrogenic DI	Block lithium action on collecting ducts in the kidney	5-20 mg, every 12-24 hours, PO	Antikaliuretic
Nonsteroidal anti-inflammatory drugs (indomethacin)	Nephrogenic DI	Block prostaglandin synthesis and decrease solute reabsorption	1.5-3.0 mg/kg, every 8-12 hours, PO	Gastrointestinal hemorrhage

*Note the unusual unit dose, because this is a frequent source of iatrogenic error.

therefore, that patients always have free access to water. As mentioned, patients with dipsogenic DI in particular should be encouraged to maintain their daily prescription of water. An intercurrent illness should prompt immediate attention to forestall dehydration. The patient can be admitted for management to prevent severe electrolyte disturbances during the intercurrent illness. The physician should evaluate any patient who becomes unresponsive to treatment. These points should be reinforced during outpatient evaluations. Patients should wear a medical identification bracelet or necklace that states "diabetes insipidus" and the name and contact telephone number of the physician. This promotes immediate identification of the disease process if the patient becomes obtunded.

Initial outpatient follow-up of children with DI occurs in 2 to 4 weeks after initiation of therapy to ascertain fluid status. Subsequent follow-up at 3-month intervals for infants and 6-month intervals for older children and adolescents permits longitudinal assessments of growth and development. At follow-up, patients and caretakers should report polyuria, nocturia, polydipsia, change in mental status from baseline, neurological deficits, adverse effects of medications, and convenience of the treatment regimen. The clinician should inquire about symptoms suggesting deficiencies of anterior pituitary hormones, including weakness, cold intolerance, lethargy, or gastrointestinal disturbance. Physical examination should include thorough neurological assessment for interim changes in cognitive function, focal deficits, or visual fields. Serum electrolyte monitoring and urinalysis are not routinely indicated.

Patients with idiopathic CDI must undergo brain MRI every 6 months for the initial 3 years, then annually thereafter for life, because occult brain lesions may present radiographically many years after the diagnosis of DI. Patients who develop anterior pituitary hormone deficiencies should be followed closely for MRI changes. The most common occult lesions reported as etiologies for "idiopathic" DI include histiocytosis X, intracranial tumors, skull fractures, autoimmune polyendocrinopathy, and familial DI. Cerebrospinal fluid evaluation is indicated in cases of suspected malignancy or infection.

Primary care physicians should consult a specialist in particular circumstances. The endocrinologist or nephrologist should assist the intensive management of severe electrolyte derangements. The endocrinologist must be consulted for water deprivation testing or desmopressin challenge. The pediatric endocrinologist should co-manage DI in infants or patients lacking intact thirst to ensure proper growth and development. The endocrinologist should be consulted for the evaluation of anterior pituitary hormone deficiencies. The nephrologist should evaluate patients with NDI for underlying renal pathology such as polycystic kidney disease. Neurosurgeons and oncologists should be consulted to evaluate and manage central nervous system lesions. Patients and parents of patients with inheritable forms of DI should receive genetic counseling. The Hormone Foundation is a superb resource for patients and families (http://www.hormone.org).

DI is a disease with a straightforward pathophysiology, managed easily once the diagnosis is established. The etiology must be determined to ensure normal growth and development. Outpatient management can be handled by the primary care physician. Consultations should be obtained during initial diagnosis and treatment, during any inpatient admission, and to treat the underlying cause. Educating the patient and caretaker about the disease and its management helps prevent adverse sequelae.

MAJOR POINTS

The two major categories of diabetes insipidus (DI) are central and nephrogenic.

Assessment of the thirst mechanism is critical to selection of appropriate therapy.

It is nearly impossible to overdose 1-deamino-8-D-arginine-vasopressin (desmopressin or DDAVP), due to its lack of vasogenic action.

The most significant iatrogenic complications during therapy for DI relate to inappropriate fluid administration during antidiuresis (water intoxication) and overly rapid correction of hypernatremia.

Annual magnetic resonance imaging of the brain is indicated to monitor patients with acquired, idiopathic central DI.

Germinoma is a tumor commonly associated with central DI.

Education resources should be available to families to reduce apprehension.

SUGGESTED READINGS

American College of Radiology: Appropriateness criteria 2000, Radiology 2000;215:1.

Baylis PH, Cheetham T: Diabetes insipidus, Arch Dis Child 1998;79:84.

Bichet DG: Nephrogenic diabetes insipidus, Am J Med 1998;105:431.

Buonocore CM, Robinson AG: The diagnosis and management of diabetes insipidus during medical emergencies, Endocrinol Metab Clin North Am 1993;22:411, 1993.

Dreifus LS, Frank MN, Bellet S: Determination of osmotic pressure in diabetes insipidus: a new diagnostic test, N Engl J Med 1954;251:1091.

Frasier SD, Kutnik LA, Schmidt RT, et al: A water deprivation test for the diagnosis of diabetes insipidus in children, Am J Dis Child 1967;114:157.

Fried LF, Palevsky PM: Hyponatremia and hypernatremia, Med Clin North Am 1997;81:585.

King LS, Agre P: Pathophysiology of the aquaporin water channels, Annu Rev Physiol 1996;58:619.

Knoers N, Monnens L: Nephrogenic diabetes insipidus, Semin Nephrol 1999;19:344.

Lugo N, Silver P, Nimkoff L, et al: Diagnosis and management algorithm of acute onset of central diabetes insipidus in critically ill children, J Pediatr Endocrinol Metab 1997;10:633.

Maghnie M, Cosi G, Genovese E, et al: Central diabetes insipidus in children and young adults, N Engl J Med 2000;343:998.

Mootha SL, Barkovich AJ, Grumbach MM, et al: Idiopathic hypothalamic diabetes insipidus, pituitary stalk thickening, and the occult intracranial germinoma in children and adolescents, J Clin Endocrinol Metab 1997;82:1362.

Robertson GL: Diabetes insipidus, Endocrinol Metab Clin North Am 1995;24:549.

Robertson GL: Differential diagnosis of polyuria, Annu Rev Med 1988;39:425.

Rogers MC, Helfaer MA, editors: Handbook of Pediatric Intensive Care, ed 3, Baltimore, 1999, Williams & Wilkins.

Seckl JR, Dunger DB: Diabetes insipidus: current treatment recommendations, Drugs 1992;44:216.

Singer I, Oster JR, Fishman LM: The management of diabetes insipidus in adults, Arch Intern Med 1997;157:1293.

Thrasher TN, Keil LC: Regulation of drinking and vasopressin secretion: role of organum vasculosum laminae terminalis, Am J Physiol 1987;253:R108.

Zimmerman EA, Nilaver G, Hou-yu A, et al: Vasopressinergic and oxytocinergic pathways in the central nervous system, Fed Proc 1984;43:91.

CHAPTER 16

Salt Wasting and the Syndrome of Inappropriate Antidiuretic Hormone

ROBERT J. FERRY, JR.

INTRODUCTION

In 1950, Peters and colleagues first described three patients with intracranial disorders (specifically, intracranial hemorrhage, bulbar poliomyelitis, and meningitis) who developed hyponatremia with high urinary output, high urinary specific gravity (indicating concentrated urine), and extracellular hypovolemia. They coined the term *cerebral salt wasting* (CSW) to describe this syndrome, and additional reports of similar patients soon followed. In 1954 Cort reported a patient with astrocytoma who developed hyponatremia and manifested negative sodium balance despite low sodium intake over 9 days; the patient recovered with liberal salt administration. Cort's patient had no demonstrable defect in anterior pituitary or adrenal function and had intact antinatriuretic and antikaliuretic responses to deoxycorticosterone acetate, suggesting that CSW was not primarily due to defective action of the antidiuretic hormone (ADH) arginine-vasopressin nor adrenal dysfunction. During the 1980s and 1990s, the molecular pathophysiology of CSW was established by several investigators who discovered and characterized a family of natriuretic peptides, which are released from human atrial muscle in response to atrial distension induced by hypervolemia. Atrial natriuretic peptide (ANP) also inhibits ADH release through feedback inhibition.

In 1957, Schwartz and colleagues reported a series of hyponatremic patients with low urinary output despite natriuresis, which they established as the syndrome of inappropriate secretion of antidiuretic hormone (SIADH). Verney's earlier discovery of ADH set the stage for insight into the mechanism underlying the new syndrome. The clear pathophysiology of SIADH combined with the clinical difficulty of quantifying hypovolemia (to support the diagnosis of CSW) made SIADH the more attractive diagnosis for clinicians from the 1950s through the 1990s. Unfortunately, many clinicians still debate the existence of CSW as a diagnostic entity, and even busy neurosurgeons claim they have not encountered salt wasters in practice. How is this possible? Two reasons are most likely.

First, natriuresis, although a convenient clinical marker, occurs in both SIADH and CSW, although to a markedly higher degree in salt wasters. Second, fluid restriction reduces renal perfusion and thereby decreases salt delivery to the distal tubule, which may temporarily exert a salutary effect on salt wasting. For both reasons, clinicians usually fluid restrict the hyponatremic patient, unless profound dehydration is noted. The number of salt wasters who deteriorate with fluid restriction is probably smaller than the number of patients with SIADH who inappropriately receive excessive fluid resuscitation. Unfortunately, misdiagnosis leading to inappropriate management, morbidity, and fatality has been reported with both CSW and SIADH. Hyponatremia commands close attention because it remains the most common electrolyte disorder in hospitalized patients, and the distinction of SIADH from CSW is particularly crucial, because optimal therapeutic interventions differ dramatically for these disorders. This chapter describes the author's clinical approach to these disorders of sodium and water homeostasis. We begin by asking, "What should prompt the clinician to consider dysnatremia at the initial clinical presentation?"

HISTORY

Patients with SIADH or CSW present with unusually low or high fluid intake and urinary output, respectively. The clinician should ask about previous hospitalizations for dehydration or fluid resuscitation. Useful historical information to obtain includes review of intake and output of hospitalized patients, anorexia, lethargy, changes in urine output, weight loss, weight gain, intrinsic renal disease, diarrhea, vomiting, burns, liver or heart disease, use of diuretics, and brain injuries, such as trauma, surgery, hypoxia, or toxic ingestion.

Essential historical data for management are whether the patient possesses an intact thirst mechanism. To assess the status of thirst, determine what times of day and night, how much, and what kind of liquids the patient drinks. The classic patient with central diabetes insipidus (DI) prefers cold water over other liquids, consistently wakes from sleep in order to drink, and urinates more than 4 L daily (or in a child, more than 75 mL/kg body weight). Salt wasters may crave salt, but in our experience, these patients have typically complained of extreme thirst, which is improved by salt intake as well as water. Patients with SIADH generally are not thirsty. Patients who sleep through the night without drinking or without enuresis do not have DI or CSW, because these conditions are associated with extremely high urinary flow rates. CSW has occurred in patients with pre-existing central DI (ADH deficiency). The key historical feature that must prompt consideration of CSW as a contributor to polyuria is the occurrence of ADH-unresponsive polyuria in a patient whose DI previously responded to exogenous ADH.

PHYSICAL EXAMINATION

The key physical sign to distinguish SIADH and CSW is the patient's hydration status. Euvolemia to hypervolemia characterizes SIADH, whereas salt wasting results in extracellular hypovolemia. Classic signs of dehydration include tachycardia (heart rate more than 2 SDs above the mean for age), tenting or decreased skin turgor, cool skin, and prolonged capillary refill time (>3 seconds). Either orthostatic hypotension in the absence of autonomic failure or acute weight loss supports the diagnosis of hypovolemia. Although most clinicians rapidly identify the dehydrated patient by these bedside methods, precise quantification of the extracellular volume requires invasive procedures (Box

16-1). Even these invasive techniques only approximate the extracellular fluid volume, and fortunately, these values are not routinely required to either initiate or guide clinical management. Finally, signs of hypervolemia, which can occur with SIADH, include headache, pulmonary edema, or signs of congestive heart failure.

It is critical to exclude adrenal insufficiency as a cause of salt wasting. Physical signs suggesting primary adrenal insufficiency (Addison disease) include hyperpigmented skin or mucous membranes (e.g., crura, oral membranes, and areolae). Hypotension unresponsive to aggressive fluid administration should also raise the suspicion of cortisol deficiency.

LABORATORY EVALUATION

Indications for prompt assessment of serum electrolyte levels include (1) idiopathic dehydration; (2) extreme dehydration, even when the etiology is certain; (3) previously well-controlled central DI that has become acutely unresponsive to medical therapy (i.e., exogenous ADH); (4) abnormal thirst mechanism; (5) hospitalized patients receiving intravenous fluid therapy simultaneously with medications known to disturb electrolyte balance or impair ADH action; (6) new-onset incontinence; (7) recent cranial irradiation; and (8) disorders associated with impaired ADH action (see Chapter 15), particularly head trauma or neurosurgery, or increased ADH or ADH-like action (Box 16-2). Box 16-3 lists other conditions in the differential diagnosis of the dysnatremic patient.

Hyponatremia is easily confirmed with commonly available laboratory tests, originally flame photometry in the early 1940s and, more recently, indirect potentiometry, also called the ion-selective electrode (ISE) method. Bedside techniques have become widely available and provide rapid, accurate determinations of serum electrolyte composition. Contemporary assays quantify free sodium ion concentrations in any body fluid with great accuracy and precision across low to high values. An important caveat to remember is that high glucose concentrations lower the apparent reading of sodium concentration. The following formula corrects this pseudohyponatremia:

Box 16-1 Assessments of Extracellular Volume

Capillary wedge pressure
Central venous pressure (normal range is 3-6 mm Hg at the
   right atrium in supine patients)
Isotope hemodilution

Box 16-2 Causes of Syndrome of Inappropriate Antidiuretic Hormone

Idiopathic
Central nervous system (CNS) pathology causing increased
 secretion of antidiuretic hormone (ADH) or ADH-like
 peptides

Subarachnoid hemorrhage	Cerebral venous thrombosis
Brain tumor	Neurosurgery
Retinoblastoma	Meningitis
Craniopharyngioma	Guillain-Barré syndrome
Hypothalamic glioma	Meningitis
Head trauma	Encephalitis
Brain abscess	Hydrocephalus
Hypoxia	

Non-CNS tumor with independent secretion of ADH or
 ADH-like peptides

Bronchogenic carcinoma	Pancreatic carcinoma

Pulmonary disease (leading to secondary elevation in ADH
 secretion or ADH-like peptides)

Pneumonia	Asthma
Cystic fibrosis	Positive-pressure ventilation

Oat cell carcinoma (rarely occurs in pediatric population)
Tuberculosis
Hypothyroidism
Cortisol deficiency (adrenal insufficiency)
Drugs (which mimic ADH or stimulate its release)

Carbamazepine (Dilantin)	Vincristine
Cyclophosphamide (Cytoxan)	Chlorpropamide
Phenothiazines	(Glyburide)
Nicotine	Clofibrate
Sertraline	Fluoxetine (Prozac)

Anorexia nervosa
Schizophrenia

Box 16-3 Differential Diagnosis of Dysnatremia

Hyponatremic dehydration (diarrhea)
Congestive heart failure
Adrenal insufficiency
Nephrotic syndrome
Renal failure
Severe potassium depletion
Cerebral salt wasting
Cirrhosis
Hypothyroidism
Water intoxication
Reset hypothalamic osmostat

$$\text{True serum [Na] (mM)} = \text{measured [Na]} + 1.6 \cdot \{\text{measured [glucose]} - 200 \text{ mg/dL}\}/100$$

Several tests can be used to distinguish CSW and SIADH (Table 16-1). Blood urea nitrogen and serum creatinine concentrations are most helpful to establish the diagnosis of prerenal azotemia characteristic of CSW. Plasma atrial natriuretic peptide (α-ANP) can be quantified by a commercial radioimmunoassay available at Mayo Reference Laboratories (Rochester, MN), and several reference laboratories provide reliable ADH assays. However, the diagnosis of SIADH or CSW does *not* require an assessment of urinary sodium excretion, plasma α-ANP, or ADH concentrations. First, these results are usually not available in time to guide clinical management, and, second, the range of values may overlap in mild forms of each disorder. Notwithstanding these limitations, these tests are useful for retrospective confirmation of the diagnosis in the context of the clinical course. Recognition and delineation of CSW in patients at risk permit anticipatory management during subsequent medical and surgical interventions to militate morbidity.

Hypervolemia and hypernatremia are the most potent stimuli for ANP release. Low α-ANP concentration is consistent with hypovolemia, and the normal range for plasma α-ANP concentrations in adults with normal cardiac filling pressures (with or without cardiovascular disease) was

Table 16-1 Laboratory Values Distinguishing Common Causes of Dysnatremia

Diagnosis	Serum [Na] (mM)	Urinary Specific Gravity	FE_{Na}	Plasma [ADH]	Plasma [ANP]	Plasma [Aldosterone]
SIADH*	<130	>1.025	<1%	High	High	Low
Central DI	>145	<1.005	<1%	Very low	Normal	High
CSW	<130	>1.015	>1%	Normal-high	High	High
CAH	<130	>1.015	>1%	Normal-high	Low-normal	Low

FE_{Na}, fractional excretion of sodium; ADH, antidiuretic hormone; ANP, atrial natriuretic peptide; DI, diabetes insipidus; CAH, congenital adrenal hyperplasia. Note that the blood urea nitrogen (BUN) is the most convenient test to distinguish syndrome of inappropriate antidiuretic hormone (SIADH) (low BUN level, <22 mg/dL) from cerebral salt wasting (CSW) (high BUN level, >22 mg/dL).
*Obtain simultaneous urinary osmolality, urinary sodium, serum osmolality, serum sodium, and uric acid; typically, the serum sodium is <125 mM, serum osmolality <260 mOsm/kg, and serum uric acid <2.4 mg/dL, whereas simultaneous urinary osmolality exceeds 100 mOsm/kg.

reported as 22 to 104 pg/mL. Studies to define thresholds in the pediatric population are warranted. Plasma α-ANP concentration may be elevated in both CSW and SIADH; thus, elevated α-ANP levels do not always distinguish these two conditions. Basal assessment of plasma renin activity and plasma aldosterone level can aid differential diagnosis of SIADH from CSW (see Table 16-1). Salt wasting that results in dehydration stimulates renin and aldosterone release, whereas in SIADH, these hormones tend to be suppressed or near the lower limit of the normal range due to attendant hypervolemia. The fractional excretion of sodium (FE_{Na}) exceeds 1% at the time of salt wasting but often tops 3%. It must be remembered that with severe dehydration, after prolonged salt wasting, decreased renal perfusion may reduce salt excretion despite the ongoing natriuretic stimulus of elevated α-ANP. Such patients demonstrate massive salt loss as fluid resuscitation restores intravascular volume and improves renal perfusion. (As an aside, most clinicians have observed this phenomenon more commonly in the dehydrated, hyperglycemic, diabetic patient whose blood glucose level drops precipitously with the initial diuresis during fluid resuscitation.) With SIADH, FE_{Na} is typically below 1%, although the attendant hypervolemia can stimulate significant natriuresis. The following formula yields FE_{Na}:

$$FE_{Na} = 100 \cdot (U_{Na} \cdot P_{Cr})/(P_{Na} \cdot U_{Cr})$$

where U indicates the urinary and P, the plasma concentrations of sodium or creatinine, respectively.

MANAGEMENT AND TREATMENT OPTIONS

The safest, most effective treatment for CSW is replacement of ongoing salt and water losses. The natriuresis associated with CSW can be tremendous, exceeding normal physiological requirements by 20-fold. Moreover, the triggers for CSW may be sudden (Box 16-4), resulting in abrupt onset and/or abrupt resolution of the natriuresis. The author proposes a simple delivery system that permits rapid, independent titration of saline and water to match the clinical status (Figure 16-1). This method allows the clinician to titrate water and salt doses immediately during dynamic care, reducing delays for preparation time by the pharmacy as well as hospital costs associated with the preparation of multiple infusion sets during the hospitalization. Fluid and salt delivery is calculated using conventional formulas. The following formula conveniently estimates the total sodium deficit:

Total Na deficit (mM or mEq/L) = 0.6 · body weight (kg) · {135−actual serum [Na]}

Box 16-4   Conditions Associated with Salt Wasting

Renal medullary cystic disease
Neurosurgery
Cranial irradiation
Head trauma
Tumor related, usually hypothalamic or pituitary neoplasms
Fever
Autonomic failure
Adrenal insufficiency
Drugs
   Loop diuretics (e.g., furosemide)
   Diphenylhydantoin
   Cisplatin
   Foscarnet
   Amphotericin B
   α-Interferon
   Mannitol

Initial administration of hypertonic saline (3% NaCl solution) should be limited to that required to halt clinical seizure activity. Raising the serum sodium level above 115 mM often ceases generalized seizure activity. If the child is not demonstrating an active seizure, there is no need to aggressively raise the serum sodium level above 115 mM.

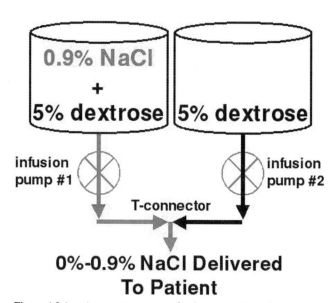

Figure 16-1   A convenient system for dynamic, independent control of salt and water administration. Only to simplify the illustration, potassium, phosphate, and other salts have been excluded from the diagram. Two bags of nearly identical electrolyte composition, differing only in sodium content, are infused via separate pumps. The clinician controls flow on each individual pump to permit independent, immediate adjustment of sodium and total fluid administration to the clinical condition. For extremely high rates of natriuresis, the author has successfully used a 3% saline solution for bag 1.

Indeed, overly rapid correction of hyponatremia dramatically increases the risk of central pontine myelinolysis. The author recommends correction of hyponatremia no more rapidly than 2 mM/hr, up to 10 mM over each 24-hour period. Close monitoring (every 1 to 4 hours) of serum sodium levels during initial resuscitation and subsequent management should guide titration of the sodium infusion. Typical sodium infusion rates required by cerebral salt wasters range from 6 to 20 mEq Na daily per kg body weight. It is essential to quantify urinary volumes to guide replacement of free water in salt wasters. Monitoring urinary sodium excretion may be helpful but is not necessary to guide ongoing management when serial serum sodium levels are available.

The daily fluid maintenance allowance can be calculated with the following algorithm. For each of the first 10 kg of body weight, administer 100 mL/kg; for the next 10 kg (i.e., 10 to 20 kg), add 50 mL/kg; and for each kilogram above 20 kg, add 20 mL/kg. For example, a 28-kg child would require 1000 mL for the first 10 kg, plus 500 mL for the next 10 kg, plus 160 mL for the remaining 8 kg, for a total of 1660 mL over 24 hours. Deficits are added to the maintenance allowance. Clinically apparent dehydration indicated a minimum 5% extracellular fluid deficit. Each percentage of deficit represents 10 mL/kg of normal body weight, so 10% extracellular fluid deficit is 100 mL/kg. In practice, the clinician can use the measured body weight at presentation or the normal weight reported by the parents.

During the initial resuscitation, generally conducted in the emergency department, the therapeutic goal *with respect only to water (the volume deficit)* is to administer 0.9% NaCl (normal saline) solution in increments of 10 mL/kg until the child is hemodynamically stable. Do *not* administer large volumes of fluid to the hemodynamically stable patient, because overly rapid correction of the fluid deficit can exacerbate osmotic shifts in the intracranial, extracellular fluid space, leading to cerebral edema. After stabilization (i.e., cessation of clinical seizure activity), the child should receive a slower infusion of salt to correct the serum sodium level no faster than 2 mM/hr (up to 10 mM over each 24-hour period). The total fluid administered is guided by serial urinary volume assessment. It is appropriate in CSW patients to replace ongoing urinary losses in excess of 3 mL/kg/hr with equal volumes of isotonic saline (0.9% NaCl). This replacement can occur every 2 to 4 hours depending on clinical status. Administration of free water alone (5% dextrose) in the setting of CSW is indicated *only* when overly rapid correction of serum sodium occurs with 0.9% saline. Again, use of the two-bag system (see Figure 16-1) permits exact titration of sodium infusion to match the clinical state. Hypertonic (3%) saline is seldom required.

The use of high-potency mineralocorticoids has been reported in CSW. There is no evidence that this approach is safer or more effective than salt and water replacement as described earlier, and the lack of concomitant glucocorticoid administration is inappropriate if adrenal insufficiency is suspected. Appropriate management of suspected or documented adrenal insufficiency is the administration of hydrocortisone at 50 to 100 mg/m² daily (oral doses should be divided every 8 hours and intravenous doses should be divided every 4 hours). A convenient formula to estimate body surface area (BSA) is:

$$BSA\ (m^2) = \sqrt{\frac{Weight\ (in\ kg) \times Height\ (in\ cm)}{3600}}$$

The most appropriate therapy for SIADH is fluid restriction. Fluid replacement should match sensible losses (stool, urine, emesis, fluid aspirated or drained) and insensible losses (expired water vapor, sweat). In the classic SIADH patient, restriction to two thirds of the maintenance matches ongoing losses.

COMPLICATIONS

Misdiagnosis of SIADH, DI, or CSW and failure to intervene appropriately has proved to be fatal. Overly rapid correction of hyponatremia has been directly linked to central pontine myelinolysis in humans and animal models. Monitoring serum sodium concentration frequently during therapy is the cornerstone to gradual correction of dysnatremia and to anticipate CSW before it results in significant hypovolemia. Acute intracranial injuries, such as trauma, neurosurgery, and subarachnoid hemorrhage, comprise the disorders carrying the highest risk for development of CSW (Box 16-4).

Clinicians, nursing staff, and the patient are inconvenienced by the high urinary flow rates associated with the recommended management of CSW. Nevertheless, the author's experience has shown that this approach safely and effectively manages even the most dynamic and most natriuretic patients. CSW induces ADH unresponsiveness, so administration of exogenous ADH is useless and potentially counterproductive because ADH confounds safe administration of free water. Thiazide diuretics have been administered based on the rationale that they provide competition for sodium excretion. Diuretics are not recommended by the author for the management of CSW, because these agents worsen the hypovolemia, confound the electrolyte management, and unnecessarily complicate management.

Excessive salt administration to SIADH patients worsens their hypervolemic state. However, resuscitation with 3%

saline is indicated to halt acute seizure activity. Left untreated, SIADH can precipitate congestive heart failure or pulmonary edema.

▶ MAJOR POINTS ◀

In the differential diagnosis of hyponatremia, consider cerebral salt wasting, adrenal salt wasting, syndrome of inappropriate antidiuretic hormone, and loss of the renal medullary concentrating gradient.

Suspect cerebral salt wasting in a patient with central diabetes insipidus who becomes unresponsive to desmopressin.

The two-bag system is a universal technique for rapid, cost-effective titrations of intravenous fluids during dynamic electrolyte states.

The safest and most effective therapy for cerebral salt wasting is sodium and water replacement.

SUGGESTED READINGS

Burnett JC Jr, Kao PC, Hu DC, et al: Atrial natriuretic peptide elevation in congestive heart failure in the human, Science 1986;231:1145.

Cogan E, Debieve MF, Philipart I, et al: High plasma levels of atrial natriuretic factor in SIADH, N Engl J Med 1986;314:1258.

Cort JH: Cerebral salt wasting, Lancet 1954;1:752.

Ferry RJ Jr, Kesavulu V, Kelly A, et al: Hyponatremia and polyuria in central diabetes insipidus: challenges in diagnosis and management, J Pediatr 2001;138:744.

Harrigan MR: Cerebral salt wasting syndrome: a review, Neurosurgery 1996;38:152.

Janss AJ, Grimberg A, Ferry R, et al: Neuro-oncology-endocrinology interface: A patient who earned her salt, Med Pediatr Oncol 1999;33:413.

Kappy MS, Ganong CA: Cerebral salt wasting in children: the role of atrial natriuretic hormone, Adv Pediatr 1996;43:271.

Kleinschmidt-DeMasters BK, Norenberg MD: Rapid correction of hyponatremia causes demyelination: relation to central pontine myelinolysis, Science 1981;211:1068.

Laredo S, Yuen K, Sonnenberg B, et al: Coexistence of central diabetes insipidus and salt wasting: the difficulties in diagnosis, changes in natremia, and treatment, J Am Soc Nephrol 1996;7:2527.

Lehrnbecher T, Muller-Scholden J, Danhauser-Leistner I, et al: Perioperative fluid and electrolyte management in children undergoing surgery for craniopharyngioma. A 10-year experience in a single institution, Childs Nerv System 1998;14:276.

Maesaka JK, Gupta S, Fishbane S: Cerebral salt wasting syndrome: does it exist? Nephron 1999;82:100.

Maesaka JK, Venkatesan J, Piccione JM, et al: Plasma natriuretic factor(s) in patients with intracranial disease, renal salt wasting, and hyperuricosuria, Life Sci 1993;52:1875.

Peters JP, Welt LG, Sims EAH, et al: A salt wasting syndrome associated with cerebral disease, Trans Assoc Am Physicians 1950;63:57.

Rodriguez-Soriano J, Vallo A: Salt-losing nephropathy associated with inappropriate secretion of atrial natriuretic peptide: a new clinical syndrome, Pediatr Nephrol 1997;11:565.

Sakarcan A, Bocchini J Jr: The role of fludrocortisone in a child with cerebral salt wasting, Pediatr Nephrol 1998;12:769.

Schwartz WB, Bennett W, Curelop S, et al: A syndrome of renal sodium loss and hyponatremia probably resulting from inappropriate secretion of antidiuretic hormone, Am J Med 1957;529.

Soupart A, Decaux G: Therapeutic recommendations for management of severe hyponatremia: current concepts on pathogenesis and prevention of neurologic complications, Clin Nephrol 1996;46:149.

Verbalis JG: Adaptation to acute and chronic hyponatremia: implications for symptomatology, diagnosis, and therapy, Semin Nephrol 1998;18:3.

Verney EB: The antidiuretic hormone and the factors which determine its release, Proc R Soc B 1947;135:26.

Index

Note: Page numbers followed by f indicate figures; page numbers followed by t indicate tables; and page numbers followed by b refer to boxed material.